Psychocutaneous Disease

Psychocutaneous Disease

Caroline S. Koblenzer, M.D.

Associate Clinical Professor of Dermatology
and of Dermatology in Psychiatry
School of Medicine
University of Pennsylvania
Philadelphia, Pennsylvania

G&S

Grune & Stratton, Inc.

Harcourt Brace Jovanovich, Publishers

Orlando New York San Diego London
San Francisco Tokyo Sydney Toronto

Library of Congress Catologing-in-Publication Data

Psychocutaneous diseases.

Includes index.
1. Skin—Diseases—Psychosomatic aspects. I. Title.
[DNLM: 1. Psychophysiologic Disorders—complications.
2. Skin Diseases—etiology. 3. Skin Manifestations.
WR 140 K748p]
RL701.K63 1987 616.5'08 87-14881
ISBN 0-8089-1865-6

Grune & Stratton, Inc.
Orlando, Florida 32887

Distributed in the United Kingdom by
Grune & Stratton, Ltd.
24/28 Oval Road, London NW 1

Library of Congress Catalog Number 87-14881
International Standard Book Number 0-8089-1865-6
Printed in the United States of America
87 88 89 90 10 9 8 7 6 5 4 3 2 1

Non semper ea sunt quae videntur

Phaedrus c. A.D. 8

(Things are not always what they seem)

For PJK, who knows what it took, and who gave more than should be asked of any man.

Contents

Acknowledgments

Only when the occasion arises to write such an acknowledgment does one become fully aware of the extent of one's reliance on the loyalty and industry of one's colleagues and co-workers, the wisdom and tolerance of one's teachers, and the forbearance of one's family, friends, and perhaps not least, one's patients.

I owe a great debt of gratitude to T.F. McNair Scott, M.D., a wise, humane, and eternally young physician, who, more than 25 years ago stimulated my budding interest in things psychosomatic by the way he handled young patients with atopic dermatitis. A similar debt is owed to Herman Beerman, M.D., himself an early worker in the field, whose support and encouragment have been marvellously reassuring in moments of near-despair, and to Waine Johnson, M.D., my chief at the Graduate Hospital and a long-time and supportive friend. To my partners Melvin Gruber, Booth Durham, and Peter Koblenzer go my thanks for their willingness to support me in this endeavour, and their patience in carrying the extra load when time restraints have been stretched to the limit. To the Institute of the Philadelphia Association for Psychoanalysis, my gratitude for their willingness to take a chance on training a dermatologist.

A work of this type could not come into being without a wide clinical experience. I count myself inordinately privileged to have shared in the lives of so many patients, and to have worked with them to reach an understanding of their physical symptoms in the context of their total life experience. Although often frustrating, this has proved enormously rewarding in the long run, certainly for me, but, I am happy to say, in numerous cases also for my patients.

I am grateful to Fred Urbach, M.D. for generously permitting me to use clinical photographs from the files of the Skin and Cancer Hospital of Philadelphia, and to Gerald Pearlman for his technical skill and infinite patience in providing the prints. Indeed all except Figures 6-4, 6-5, 6-8, 7-1A-E, 7-2, 7-3, 9-2B, 9-6A-E, 9-8C, and 9-10 are from that very rich resource; these latter photographs are from the collection of Peter J. Koblenzer, M.D. and myself, while Dr. Antonio Reginato, M.D. kindly provided those numbered 6-1A-B.

I have benefited greatly from the expertise of two professionals: Anita Schmukler, D.O., psychiatrist, psychoanalyst, and English scholar, has given unstintingly of her time to review the material with regard to content from a psychiatric viewpoint and with regard to style, while my niece, Julia Kagan, a professional editor, has given much needed reassurance and valuable editorial advice.

No one can undertake such a venture without a tolerant and supportive amanuensis, and this I have had in full measure in Virginia Ellis, whose unruffled calm and sharp intelligence have kept me on the straight and narrow throughout.

And finally, my thanks are due to my family and all my loyal friends who, despite my social withdrawal, are still there and ready to pick up where we left off, a year and a half ago.

Preface

The skin is a profoundly important sensory organ. It is the interface between our environment and our soul. As infants the skin functions as a major conduit of sensory stimulation, which is necessary for emotional and physical development. As we mature the sensations transmitted by the skin are a major source of delight and discomfort.

We are perceived by the appearance of our integument. The smooth unblemished skin of a Boticello beauty is aesthetically pleasing and invites our interest, receptivity, and acceptance. By contrast, imagine the same figure covered with the thick red scales of psoriasis or multiple purulent lesions of conglobate acne. Analyze the oberver's response—it is dismay, distress, and repulsion. These perceptions are universal so not only the observer but the individual afflicted with skin disease realizes the impression. No longer is our figure a smiling, optimistic Primavera but she is now a sad, desolate figure of despair. Cutaneous disease profoundly influences our sense of self worth. Witness our obsession with reversing the deleterious effects of actinic radiation on the skin; we want our skin to look younger so we can restore our youthful vigor. The appearance of our skin is a univeral preoccupation of almost all people. The physician who treats patients with skin disease must be continually aware of the psychological ramifications of the patient's dermatoses and the clinician must treat not only the physical ailment but the emotional disability.

The skin is a mirror of our emotional well being. The flare of eczema consequent to marital discord or the self-inflected lesion signalling despair are phenomena that are well known to all dematologists. Frequently, we choose to ignore the underlying psychological etiology and treat the manifestation and then we wonder why our therapy is ineffective.

The 1980s is the era of scientific medicine. Molecular biology, protein chemistry, cellular immunology, and receptor physiology are the bench marks of scientific investigation. Psychiatry has embraced these disciplines with passion and we now witness extraordinary basic science developments in psychoimmunology, psychoneuroendocrinology and psychopharmacology. Unfortunately our captivation with the accomplishments of "scientific medicine" have sometimes resulted in our ignoring the basic psychiatric skills necessary for patient care.

As director of a biologically-based dermatological training program I read Dr. Koblenzer's book with excitement and remorse. I was excited to relearn the structure and strategies of clinical psychiatry made pertinent by my own experiences in patient care. I was remorseful that my psychologial skills may have lost their acuteness because the pressures of professional activities had prevented me from reading in clinical psychiatry. This text is an excellent exposition of the elements of psychiatry pertinent to the therapy of patients with skin disease. It is a welcome, long overdue contribution to both the dermatologic and psychiatric literature, which should be read by all physicians who treat skin disease.

May 1987

Gerald Lazarus, M.D.
Milton B. Hartzell Professor
Chairman, Department of Dermatology
University of Pennsylvania
Philadelphia, Pennsylvania

Introduction

As early as 1925, Joseph Klauder emphasized the necessity of psychotherapy in the practice of dermatology,[3] noting that "the psychological phase of certain skin disease should not be neglected in treatment." Two years later, however, W.T. Sack[11] wrote, "there is scarcely a medical specialty in which modern teaching concerning the neuroses has found so little systematic applications as in dermatology." With the exception of a rather fertile period between the early 1930s and the mid-1950s, this situation continued through the years, and still, I believe, pertains today.

That Rook and Wilkinson consider the management of emotional factors to be of significance in 40 percent of patients attending departments of dermatology,[10] while Medansky and Handler[6] quote a figure of 80 percent, points up the recognition of frequent interactions between psyche and soma in the production and perpetuation of skin disease. Despite this recognition, systematic study of the interaction, application of principles derived from other areas of psychosomatic research, and dialogue between psychiatrists and dermatologists for purposes of mutual enlightenment and residency training are each conspicuous only by their absence. Even those who accord significance to such an interaction do not carry their insight into action; for example, the statement from Rook and Wilkinson quoted above, in a book of over 2000 pages, presages a chapter of only 12 pages. Other texts are equally parsimonious in their allocation of space. For example, Fitzpatrick[2] allocates 10 of a total of almost 2000 pages, while Demis et al.,[5] in their four-volume opus, come up with a winning total—a big 14.

The growth of a discipline, much like that of a child, takes place by virtue of a series of maturational spurts, first in one developmental area and then in another. It is not without awe that we have witnessed over the past two decades exciting advances in the physical sciences. But now it is time for progress in another area; the publication in recent years of Whitlock's monograph, *Psychophysiological Aspects of Skin Disease,*[14] several papers in the American and European dermatologic literature,[7,12,13,15] a section in *Recent Advances in Dermatology*,[1] and most recently, the excellent volume in the *Clinics in Dermatology* series, *Stress and Skin Disease—Psychosomatic Dermatology*, edited by Emiliano Panconesi of Florence, Italy,[8] bear witness to a burgeoning renaissance of interest in the emotional component of physical disease.

And it is those very advances in the physical sciences referred to above that have helped in part to stimulate this renewal of interest, together with the recognition by clinicians that despite all of our exact knowledge, there is always the unexplained factor "X" that influences the course of disease and the results of treatment. Current understanding of chemical mediators, membrane receptors, and hypothalamic function, to name but a few, have made it possible to begin to formulate a theory as to the actual mechanism whereby emotion, ideation, memory, and past experience may be transduced into physical symptom or somatic disease.[9,16] With a goal of this magnitude almost within our grasp, dialogue between workers in all of the related fields becomes exciting and meaningful, and research becomes a compelling challenge.

A second, and perhaps more worldly, imperative that makes important the understanding of the psychosomatic processes is our overwhelming need, as a nation, to curb the spiralling costs of medical care. The cost of the ever more numerous and more sophisticated physical and chemical studies that are developed, as well as the application of new treatment modalities, make it essential that they be used appropriately and in a cost-effective way. If the diagnostic focus, and in its train the therapeutic endeavor, are inaccurate, then inevitably vast sums will be expended in fruitless attempts to unravel the puzzle, while the patient continues to suffer. As an example, over a 5-year period a patient in my practice spent in excess of $12,000 and consulted more than 60 different medical specialists in her search for a physical cause for delusional beliefs that she held about her skin.

In order to tease apart the separate threads of psyche and soma, and approach in logical fashion the diagnosis and managment of the emotional aspects of cutaneous disease, the dermatologist must have a nodding acquaintence with some basic principles of psychiatric diagnosis and managment, which must then be integrated with the physician's dermatologic knowledge. This book is intended as a practical and clinical guide towards that end. Though written primarily with the practicing dermatologist and the dermatologist-in-training in mind, pediatricians, internists, family practioners, psychiatrists, and medical students may also find it useful.

REFERENCES

1. Cotterill JA: Psychiatry & skin disease, in Rook AJ, Mailbach HI (eds): Recent Advances in Dermatology, vol 6. Edinburgh, Churchill Livingstone, 1983, pp 189-212
2. Fitzpatrick TB, Eisen AZ, Freedberg IM, Austen KF: Emotional aspects of cutaneous disease, in Griesemer RD, Nadelson T (eds): Dermatology in General Medicine. 2nd ed. New York, McGraw-Hill, 1979

3. Klauder JV: Emotions and bodily changes, in Dunbar F (ed): Emotions and Bodily Changes: A Survey of Literature on Psychosomatic Interrelationships; 1910-1945. New York, Columbia University Press, 1946, p 375
4. Koblenzer CS: The dysmorphic syndrome. Arch Dermatol 121:780-784, 1985
5. Demis DJ, Dobson RL, Maguire JS (eds): Clinical Dermatology, Vol 4, Section 29-7. Philadelphia, Harper & Row, 1985
6. Medansky RS, Handler RM: Dermatopsychosomatics: Classification, physiology, and therapeutic approaches. J Am Acad Dermatol 5:125-136, 1981
7. Obermeyer ME: Psychocutaneous Medicine. Springfield, IL, Charles C Thomas, 1955
8. Panconesi E (ed): Stress and Skin Diseases: Psychosomatic Dermatology, Clinics in Dermatology 2:4. Philadelphia, JB Lippincott, 1984
9. Reiser MF: Mind, Brain, Body. Toward a Convergence of Psychoanalysis and Neurobiology. New York, Basic Books, Inc. 1984
10. Rook AJ, Wilkinson DS: in Rook AJ, Wilkinson DS, Ebling FJG (eds): Textbook of Dermatology (3rd ed). Boston, Blackwell Scientific Publications, 1979, pp 2023-2035
11. Sack WT: in Dunbar F (ed): Emotions and Bodily Changes: A Survey of Literature on Psychosomatic Interrelationships; 1910-1945. New York, Columbia University Press, 1946 p 372
12. Stokes JH, Beerman H: Psychosomatic correlations in allergic conditions—a review of problems and literature. Psychosom Med 11(4):438-458, 1940
13. Sydenham T: The Works of Thomas Sydenham, Wallis G (ed). London, 1788
14. Whitlock FA: Psychophysiological Aspects of Skin Disease. Philadelphia, WB Saunders, 1976
15. Wilson E: On Diseases of the Skin (4th ed). Philadelphia, Blanchard & Lea, 1857
16. Winson J: Brain and Psyche: The Biology of the Unconscious. Garden City, NY, Anchor Press/Doubleday, 1985, p 34

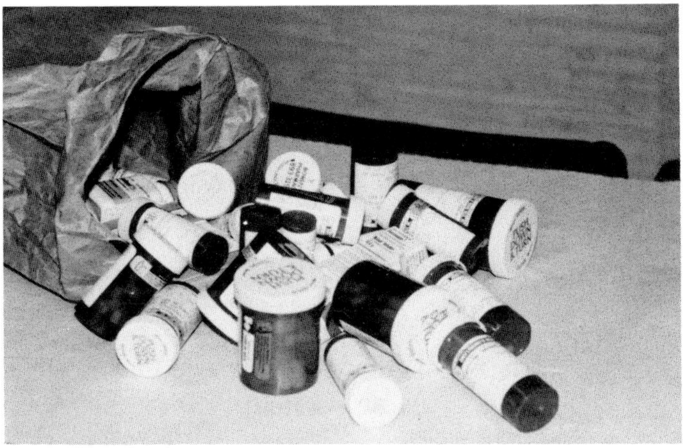

The typical first visit offering from a patient with psychocutaneous disease. The brown bag contains numerous remedies. Many are in duplicate, obtained from several different, recently-visited physicians, but all have been found "useless."

SECTION I

GENERAL PRINCIPLES

Chapter 1

The Skin as an Organ of Perception

Both from work with animals, and from infant observation studies it is clear that the skin of mammals in the early months of life serves, along with the oral cavity, as a paramount organ of perception. The effect of interactions between skin and environment has not only current but also lasting physical and psychological impact on growth and on personality development. Given this fact, it is strange that we dermatologists, whose arena is the skin, with all of its morphologic, physiologic, and pathologic variations, have not turned our attention to a study of skin as a tactile functional unit during this very early developmental phase in order to enhance our understanding of later events.

There is an abundant literature to demonstrate that in a number of mammalian species interruption of normal interaction between mother and infant has a profound effect on the growth and development of those infants.[14] Retardation of skeletal growth and of central nervous system development, and also changes in locomotor activity, heart rate, and learning performance result.[5] Ornithine decarboxylase activity, a sensitive biochemical index of cell growth and differentiation, is reduced in the tissues of the brain, heart, and liver in pre-weanling rat pups if they are separated from the mother, or if all stimuli other than the cutaneous tactile ones are maintained constant by placing the infants with a mother that is anaesthetized.[3,4] This enzyme activity returns to normal levels when normal mother-infant interaction is resumed. The trigger that sets these variations in enzyme activity in motion has been shown to be the active stimulation of the skin that is a normal part of mothering in rats; the process is a neuroendocrine one and is mediated via the secretion of growth hormone.[14] Heavy short strokes with a moist brush to the skin of the head and back of the infant rat substitute for active mothering without adverse sequelae, but light stroking or tail-pinching is not an adequate substitute. Under those circumstances the decrease in enzyme activity will follow. In rat pups there is another vital function that depends also on cutaneous tactile stimulation by the mother: that is the initiation of urination and defecation that follows when she licks her infant's perineum. Rat pups removed from the mother at birth will die because these excretory functions cannot take place.[2] So the perception of tactile stimuli to the skin mediates functions that are involved in life and death processes, and findings analogous to these have been demonstrated in dogs, cats, monkeys, and of course, in humans.

In humans, the syndrome of psychosocial dwarfism is the recognized sequel of maternal deprivation. Once again it is the all-important tactile cutaneous stimulation that is missing, because the syndrome will occur even if nutrition and medical care are adequate. The general slowdown in cerebral maturation that is responsible for suppression of somatic growth, for increase in disease susceptibility, and for the impaired learning ability that characterize this syndrome have as in the case of other mammals been traced to a decrease in the secretion of growth hormone. In conditions of extreme privation even death may occur and indeed up to 90 percent of children in certain foundling homes lost their lives from lack of "mothering" during the last century even though their medical and nutritional needs were adequately met.[14]

The earliest pathways for communication between mother and child are physiologic; inner sensations of hunger inform the neonatal infant of discomfort, the cry is answered with a feed, and the infant is once again comfortable. The appropriate answering of that need comes to be interpreted by the infant as acceptance or love. In analogous fashion the skin forms an equally early channel of communication. Through contact with the mother's skin, by her stroking and touching and by her tender loving care, the infant gradually comes to recognize his or her boundaries—to define the self as an individual and thus separate the self from the mother-child dyad that had existed during pregnancy and in the first few weeks of life. Through skin contact also, mother's attitudes are communicated clearly to the infant, whether they be attitudes of love and acceptance or of rejection. These two facets of the nonverbal "dialogue" between mother and child, the definition of boundaries and the communication of maternal attitudes, are the basis of two important psychological "structures": the psychological body image and self-esteem. Both of these, as we shall see later, are of significance in certain aspects of psychocutaneous disease.

THE DEVELOPMENT OF THE PSYCHOLOGICAL BODY IMAGE

We are indebted to workers in the field of child psychoanalysis for much of the understanding that we have of the development of perception. These clinicians have engaged in the systematic study of childhood by longitudinal infant and child observation from birth. This has by now been ongoing for half a century; the findings have supplemented data available from the psychoanalysis of children, particularly very young children with psychosis, and from reconstruction in the psychoanalytic treatment of adults.[9,16] Additional information gleaned from the experiences of blind-born persons of all ages, who have had to develop visual perception following surgery for congenital cataracts, has lent additional support to these findings.[16]

The psychological body-image is the name given to the internal model that we each carry around with us and that is important for recognition of posture, movement, and localization of sensations.[15] This image is crafted from memory traces that are derived individually as a result of perceived sensory stimuli that impinge on the infant's body in very early life. The stimuli are generated both in the environment and also by the child's own body as the child's hand fortuitously finds his or her mouth or genitals, as the child perceives his or her own odors, and as the inner ear registers shifts in the position of his or her head. So memories of visual, tactile, olfactory, and proprioceptive perceptions all contribute to the total experience of the self that becomes the self-image, of which the inner perception of the body is an integral part. Because it has been shown that the function of memory requires emotional input[6] the perceptual memory traces that come together to form this image are very much influenced by the emotional climate in which it all takes place. For the infant the emotional climate essentially consists of the relationship with mother, or the primary caretaker, in all of its vicissitudes. So at the end of the day, all other factors being equal, it is the quality of mothering, and most particularly one of its important facets, mother's touching and stroking of the skin, that ensures the development of a strong and solid internal representation of the body and its functions.[2,8] When circumstances are less than ideal, the body image may be fragmented, its boundaries may be unclear, so much so, that in some cases self-mutilation is resorted to in order to help define them;[1] alternatively, distorted perceptions of the body-image may arise, as is seen in the dysmorphic syndrome.[10]

THE DEVELOPMENT OF SELF-ESTEEM

As with the body-image, emotional input is also a determinant in the development of self-esteem. It is the quality of the interaction between mother and child that will determine which maternal attitudes the infant will internalize and make his or her own. Warm and accepting mothers who respond to their infants' cries with appropriate gratification—who feed them when hungry, change them when wet, and comfort them when distressed, and who delight in touching their bodies, smiling and talking to them, will make the infants feel loved and appreciated and will allow them in turn to appreciate themselves. By the nature of mothers' responses to their infants, they will learn which behaviors are acceptable, and in their wish to please their mothers, these will be reinforced and new skills will be acquired in which infants and mothers can take pride. And so feelings of self-worth are generated and incorporated as a strong and solid self-esteem.

The quality of the self-esteem in turn is a major determinant in the ability of the individual to handle chronic, disabling, or disfiguring skin disease, unsightly scars, or congenital malformations, as will be discussed later.

THE RELATIONSHIP OF EARLY DEVELOPMENTAL FACTORS TO LATER LIFE EXPERIENCE

In the course of our daily personal and professional lives we tend to take for granted that human life is a continuum, and that one phase inevitably and imperceptibly will merge with the next as it unfolds in its preordained and beautifully organized fashion. As progressive physical stages are traversed, each may leave its mark in the form of scars or "memories" for the future. In the skin, of course, these are there for all to see. The ravages of adolescent acne, the site of an earlier trauma or surgical assault, the actinic elastosis, keratoses and lentigenes that are linked in causal linear fashion to the sun exposures of the past, or the pigmentary changes caused by phenothiazine drugs taken at some earlier time are but a few examples. Intellectual development unfolds in analogous fashion as our capacity for recall makes available to us the information acquired earlier. But what perhaps we sometimes lose site of is that in our emotional life too memory traces persist as an elaborate interconnecting network that reaches right back to infancy;[12] the first evidence we have of the function of memory is usually at about the age of 3 months, when the "social smile" bears witness to recognition of the human face.[15] Because of the complex interconnections between these memory traces, memories from different phases of emotional development may be reactivated by seemingly thematically unrelated events, thoughts, or feelings in the present, and even though these early memories may remain wholly inaccessible to consciousness, inevitably they will make their presence known—if unrecognized—in one form or another. Because of the emotional significance of the skin in very early life that I have described, it will be clear that the memory traces that are the residuum of those early experiences may have important consequences.

Although, like physical development, psychological development is a continuum, there are certain nodal points that have a special significance, both currently and for the future. In order to make clear this concept, I shall return to the discussion of the early months of life, when the skin is of such major developmental significance and when the quality of mothering in relation to the skin influences the child's well-being in ways that I shall describe.

While he was observing institutionalized mothers, with their infants, throughout their first year of life, Spitz noted that a number of quite clearly defined physical syndromes developed in those of the infants for whom the emotional climate, as expressed in the dyadic mother-child relationship, was less than good.[15] He termed these syndromes the psychotoxic diseases of childhood and included among them 3-month colic, rocking, fecal play, and infantile eczema. Spitz found that these disorders were determined by the quality of mothering, whereas infantile depression and marasmus depended rather on the quantity, and occurred when mother was for some reason absent.

In this institutionalized population, 15 percent of the infants had infantile eczema, as compared with 2-3 percent in the population at large. These infants were studied extensively applying many physical and psychological parameters. They received their skin care from the attending physician in the institution, and though clinical records are not available and Spitz was not able to get a consensus from a number of "different dermatological authorities" whom he consulted,[15] yet the clinical description that he gives is consistent with the picture of infantile atopic dermatitis. Further, Rajka feels that atopic dermatitis is the likely diagnosis in most cases of infantile eczema.[11]

As a result of his observations, Spitz postulated that two factors were required for an infant to develop one of the psychotoxic diseases: an inherent predisposition, which of course in eczema we understand as the atopic diathesis, and a quality of mothering that does not meet the emotional needs of the child. In the eczema group, though the deep reflexes did not differ from those of the control group, these infants demonstrated a much greater inherent cutaneous excitability as expressed by the rooting and cremasteric reflexes. The mothers too differed in a rather consistent way from those in the control group; their personality structure was infantile, they masked an unconscious hostility towards their infants behind anxious oversolicitousness, but most importantly, they did not seem to like to touch or care for those infants; they consistently deprived them of cutaneous contact.[15] Interestingly, these same findings are reported by other writers.[13,17] Because of the constant high level of anxiety, derivative of their unconscious hostility, these mothers also gave confusing and inconsistent signals. In this climate, of ungratified wishes for cutaneous contact and stimulation and inconsistent maternal signals, not only did these children, whose inherent need for cutaneous stimulation was greater than normal, develop infantile eczema, but learning was retarded and they were socially less well-adjusted than the control group, showing difficulty in relationships, in controlling impulses, and in handling aggression.

Equally inappropriate is excessive gratification of the need for cutaneous stimulation in the genetically predisposed infant, because a degree of frustration is necessary for growth and development to progress normally.[15] This was well demonstrated by Harlow whose infant rhesus monkeys never developed adult monkey behavior, but persisted in infantile behavior, doing nothing but clinging to each other when kept together in a cage without an adult.[7] I shall refer to this point again in my discussion of infantile eczema.

The type of circumstances here described with these children, an imperfect "fit" between mother and child, leads not only to eczema, but also to the development of a fixation point on the continuum of emotional growth. Frustration of age-appropriate emotional needs at a later stage of development, then, may result in a regression to that fixation point. This regression has both psychological and physical components, for there may be a return to a more infantile behavior as well as an exacerbation of cutaneous symptoms. Other nodal points with analogous significance occur when mouth, ano-rectal area, and external genitalia each, in that sequence, take on for a period special significance as organs of sensual gratification. Each phase merges imperceptibly with the next, with considerable overlap, but roughly speaking the mouth along with the skin holds sway during the first year, the ano-genital region from the end of the first until the third year, and the external genitalia about the fifth or sixth year.[6] A period of latency then follows when attention focuses on intellectual development and the acquisition of motor skills, before the turbulence of adolescence. As with the skin, inappropriate answering of emotional needs in each of these phases may result in a fixation point to which regression may occur at times of stress, not only in childhood, but throughout life, and the regressive features again may be either behavioral or somatic or a combination of the two. The somatic symptoms when present often bear some relationship either real or symbolic to the organ in question, as for example in some cases of persistent pruritus involving the ano-genital region.

REFERENCES

1. Anderson PC, Cross TN: Body cathexis and neurodermatitis. Compr Psychiatry 4:40-46, 1963
2. Brown DG: The relevance of body image to neurosis. Br J Med Psychol 32:249-260, 1959
3. Butler SR, Schanberg SM: Effect of maternal deprivation on polyamine metabolism in preweanling rat brain and heart. Life Sci 21:877-884, 1977
4. Bulter SR, Suskind MR, Schanberg SM: Maternal behavior as a regulator of polyamine biosynthesis in brain and heart of the developing rat pup. Science 199:445-447, 1978
5. Evoniuk GE, Kuhn CM, Schanberg SM: The effect of tactile stimulation on serum growth hormone and tissue ornithine decarboxylase activity during maternal deprivation in rat pups. Comm in Psychopharmacol 3:363-370, 1979
6. Freud S: Three essays on the theory of sexuality. Essay II: Infantile sexuality, in Strachey J (ed): Freud S: Complete Psychological Works (Standard ed). London, Hogarth, 1953, pp 173-206
7. Harlow HF: The nature of love. Am Psychol 13:673-685, 1958
8. Hartmann H, Kris E, Loewenstein RM: Comments on the formation of psychic structure. Psychoanal Study Child 2:11-38, 1946
9. Jackson M: Psychosomatic pathology as developmental failure: a model for research, in Pichot P, Berner P, Wolf R, Thau K (eds): Psychiatry: The State of the Art. Psychotherapy and Psychosomatic Medicine, vol. 4. New York, Plenum, 1985, pp 363-368
10. Koblenzer CS: The dysmorphic syndrome. Arch Dermatol 121:780-784, 1985

11. Rajka G: Atopic Dermatitis. London, Saunders, 1975, p 15
12. Reiser MF: Mind, Brain, Body: Toward a Convergence of Psychoanalysis and Neurobiology. New York, Basic Books, 1984, pp 65-68
13. Rosenthal MJ: Psychosomatic study of infantile eczema. I. The mother-child relationship. Pediatrics 10:581-592, 1952
14. Schanberg SM, Kuhn CM: Maternal deprivation: an animal model of psychosocial dwarfism, in Usdin F, Sourkes TL, Youdim MBH (eds): Enzymes and Neurotransmitters in Mental Disease. New York, Wiley, 1980, pp 374-393
15. Spitz RA: The First Year of Life: A Psychoanalytic Study of Normal and Deviant Development of Object Relations. New York, International Universities Press, 1965
16. Von Senden M: Space and Sight: The Perception of Space and Shape in the Congenitally Blind Before and After Operation. Glencoe, Illinois, Free Press, 1960
17. Williams DH: Management of atopic dermatitis in children: control of the maternal rejection factor. AMA Arch Dermat Syph 63:545-560, 1951

Chapter 2

Psychosomatic Disease as a Concept

Throughout the ages there have been interesting swings back and forth between a unitary and holistic view of disease and its alternative, the "duality" view. The former holds that an interaction between psyche and soma may be involved in the onset and perpetuation of somatic disease, whereas in the latter view the two agencies, psyche and soma, each follows its set course through life, in parallel, but each independent of the other.

In the ancient world, prior to the time of the Greek civilization, the unitary view held sway. Like children who are not given enough information to understand natural phenomena realistically, and who must therefore have recourse to formulating their own theories to answer fundamental questions in ways that they can understand, these peoples believed evil spirits outside of themselves to be the prime force that controlled events and caused disease. Out of whimsy, or out of vengeance, these evil spirits would enter into the body and wreak their havoc on the soma. As increasing sophistication made it possible through the development of tools adequate to the task, a primitive forerunner of psychosurgery evolved, when early man learned to trephine holes in the skull to let out these offending spirits. These primitive beliefs existed from the earliest times through the civilization of Asia Minor and into the world of the Greeks.

Rather than alien spirits residing outside the body, it gradually came to be understood by the Greek philosophers that disease was generated from within. Hippocrates saw the problem as an imbalance in certain body fluids, which imbalance in turn was caused perhaps by imbalance in the external environment, or even by emotional upset. He recognized that emotions could cause physical changes. And as he knew that fear may lead to sweating, or shame to palpitations, he cautioned young physicians to look at patients kindly and not to show impatience, because these negative reactions on the part of the doctor might retard recovery. So already the power of the doctor-patient relationship as a factor in the process of healing was recognized, and was being used to that end. A cult of healer-priests, the Asclepiads, had grown up and presided over temples where patients in isolation might get in touch with their emotions and with their private inner world. Dream interpretation was used in treatment and physical health was regained, these healer-priests believed, through the activation of an inner "life-force." Interestingly, the objectives sought through this ancient belief-system do not sound too different from the goals and modus operandi of a contemporary psychotherapist of the dynamic or psychoanalytic school, whose hope it is to liberate psychic energy for healthy pursuits through the understanding of unconscious conflict and unconscious motivation, using sometimes dream-interpretation as a therapeutic tool. Other facets of medical care also, as practised by the ancient Greeks, suggest treatments extant in the early part of this century in the United States and western Europe, and still in use in Eastern Europe today; I speak of hydrotherapy, for example, prescribed usually in conjunction with rest and special diets. Such seminal thinkers as both Plato and Aristotle supported the holistic view, and expressed the belief that trouble in the mind could bring trouble to the body.

This body of primitive medical knowledge was distilled by Galen during the first century A.D. into a system of medicine that held sway right up until the Middle Ages. It was his understanding that the brain was the center of sensation, motion, reason, and of the rational soul. He at the same time acknowledged the influence of the four humors and understood the importance for health of the interplay between psyche and soma.

A regressive belief in spiritual powers, and in the evil influences of demons and witches, resurfaced during the middle ages, and once again disease became a tool of vengeance for evil spirits. In this climate, the status of doctors sank very low indeed, and the enlightened beliefs of the Greeks were temporarily lost. But with the Renaissance, burgeoning factual knowledge caused the pendulum to swing away from spiritual and emotional issues, and with the capacities for study that new knowledge had brought attention focused once again on the body and its physical attributes as increasingly, anatomical and biological facts became available. The belief that psychic influences could affect the soma was regarded as unscientific, and the holistic posture was totally abandoned as it became a commonplace to focus on the disease, rather than the patient. From autopsy material, Morgagni was able to correlate specific physical symptoms with specific pathological changes, and so demonstrate that more than an imbalance of body fluids was involved in physical disease processes. The detailed microscopic cellular studies of Virchow, and Pasteur's belief that the temple of the future would be the laboratory, made the separation of psyche and soma for the time being complete.

Freud is credited with introducing a new unitarian era, when he demonstrated the importance of the emotions in producing both mental disturbances and somatic disorders, but in fact George Logan of Philadelphia in an address to the Chirurgo Medical Society of Edinburgh, Scotland, in 1777, had already stated that "grief, anxiety, lack of exercise and hard-drinking" were the causes of dyspepsia.[16] Similarly Schweninger (1850-1924), personal physician to Prince von Bismarck, conceiving of man as "the product of his living conditions," suggested that changes in the "product" might require that both the environment and the "inner human being" change[15] while Groddeck (1866-1934), his pupil, found himself "without knowing it, faced with the necessity of evaluating unconscious processes in the treatment of organic disease."[15] Groddeck in fact, working independently, anticipated some of Freud's theoretical postulates when he suggested that a process of "psychic conditioning" could render an organ or system susceptible to the changes of physical disease. Changes that, in turn, served some symbolic or even direct purpose for the individual. But it was through free association, which became the hallmark of the psychoanalytic method,[11] that Freud was able not only to develop a clearer understanding of the relationship between psyche and soma, but to offer an explanation for the development of hysterical conversion symptoms. Through that method also, he brought into focus once again the immense power for healing inherent in the doctor-patient relationship, which he termed "the transference."

Freud's work stimulated a very fertile period in the history of psychosomatic medicine that continued right up into the middle 1950s. Many researchers, trained in the analytic method, notably Dunbar,[7] Alexander,[1] Alexander et al.,[2] and Meninger,[21] attempted to ascribe specific disease entities to specific personality types or specific unconscious conflictual constellations. Their rather simplistic linear approach to causality got a boost in 1959, when Freedman and Rosenman were able to show convincingly with physiologic and personality correlates a relationship between personality type and coronary artery disease.[12] Enthusiasm overrode judgement in many cases, however, and extravagant claims were not always able to be substantiated, so that interest in the application of the psychoanalytic method to the understanding and treatment of physical disease began to flag. Dermatology was a field particularly rich in psychosomatic research and it was not unusual for a psychiatrist to be in attendance during dermatology clinic sessions. Macalpine in London[19] and Seitz,[29] Meninger,[20] and Wittkower[37] in the United States were psychiatrists who wrote on the subject. Among dermatologists, Stokes,[33] Beerman,[31,33] and Ingraham;[34,35] Shaffer;[31] and Obermayer and Becker[26] are names that stand out, while Graham's studies on the urticarial response are classic.[13,14]

Coincident with the disappointing realization that a psychotherapeutic approach was not the answer to all physical ills, during the late 1950s and the 1960s there began a period of advances in the biological sciences of a magnitude never before witnessed. This period has continued to the present time. Just as during the Renaissance, a period of analogous advances in factual knowledge, the pendulum of interest swung away from the psyche, and a separation of psyche from soma was once again accomplished.

Despite, or perhaps because of the incredible scientific advances that we have witnessed in the past two or three decades, and the immense amount of factual knowledge that has accrued, we seem to be experiencing once again a swing back towards the unitarian position of disease etiology. This is, I believe, for two reasons; first, there is still the unknown, the factor "X" that in some cases interferes in the healing process, despite accurate diagnosis and the initiation of appropriate therapy. The second reason provides the greater challenge, the challenge that is sparking excitement in all who work in the field of psychosomatics. I speak, of course, of the possibility that we may one day be able to explain on scientific and biological grounds the emotional and behavioral changes that influence physical disease.

EARLY THEORIES OF SOMATIZATION

As I have discussed in the previous section, changes in the emotional or environmental sphere may result in somatic change. This has been accepted periodically since ancient times. But though we no longer concern ourselves with demons and evil spirits, or with the delicate balance of choleric and phlegmatic humors, yet just how these physical, somatic changes are accomplished, by what particular mechanism they come about, continues to intrigue us.

The Freudian theory of hysterical conversion based on unconscious intrapsychic conflict is still accepted by practitioners of dynamic psychiatry, and of psychoanalysis. This theory holds that the threatened emergence into consciousness of an idea incompatible with the moral position of an individual—should that individual have the inherent ability to somatize—results in the immediate repression of that incompatible idea. A "mysterious leap"[11] occurs from the emotional to the physical sphere, where the appearance of the physical symptom is then allowed. The particular symptom that develops is the result of a compromise between the intrapsychic agencies, and as such serves to satisfy at the same time both the moral position of the patient and the unacceptable unconscious thought or wish that for defensive purposes has had to be repressed. This mechanism is exactly analogous to the development of an obsession or a phobia, and in like fashion it has a symbolic meaning in the life of the patient, who will at the same time derive from it some personal gain.

The following clinical vignette will serve as an example. Some years ago an attractive 13-year-old girl was brought to see me because of pain in the skin. This pain was confined to her legs, and was so severe as to make walking difficult, and strenuous physical activity impossible. She was a talented runner, and anxious to enter junior Olympic competition so it seemed ironic that she should develop such a physical symptom. On examination, no objective abnormality could be detected, despite the fact that she could with consistency delineate for me a sharp circumferential cut-off point that separated pain from normal sensation. This point was one-third of the way up the thigh bilaterally and was quite inconsistent with the anatomic sensory innervation.

This young girl greatly admired her father, a strict, demanding man, and a perfectionist, who worked as an instructor in physical education. In such an emotional climate, physical prowess was quite naturally a loaded issue. The ideas of symbolically "defeating" her father on his own ground by winning in competition, or alternatively of disappointing him by losing, were untenable. So for this patient, competitive running became an area of intrapsychic conflict. The symbolic importance of her legs in the conflict enabled them then to "comply,"[6] by developing a somatic symptom that made competitive running impossible; in other words the nature of the particular physical symptom that she developed enabled the conflict to be avoided altogether. Two other characteristics of the hysterical conversion were exemplified by her symptom: personal gain was provided by a gratifying closeness with her father, now sanctioned by her illness, as she spent with him at his work time that ordinarily would have been devoted to athletic training; a second characteristic, "la belle indifference," was exemplified by her seeming lack of concern about something so incapacitating.

Hysterical conversion symptoms characteristically are mediated via the central nervous system and they form a special group within the spectrum of psychosomatic disease. These patients generally are less psychiatrically impaired than are others who somatize, and one view of the conversion process suggests that the symptom develops in response to a circumstance in which the patient is precluded from bestowing love on an important figure in his or her life, and must instead expend that positive energy on a portion of their own body.[6] Freud was less clear about the mechanism whereby those symptoms mediated by the autonomic nervous system developed.[11] He suggested that under circumstances of tension, recurrent and persistent vegetative changes would result eventually in organic change—a view consistent with the work of Cannon,[4] Selye,[30] and later researchers in the area of stress. Consider, for example, the long-term physical effects of gastric hypersecretion in the ulcer-prone individual, or the effects of palmar or plantar hyperhidrosis in the atopic. This theme will be taken up again in the next chapter, when psychoneuroendocrinology and psychoimmunology are considered.

From the earlier discussion of the relationship of early developmental factors to later life experience, it will be recalled that one understanding of somatization is that it results from developmental failure. This concept has been applied in a number of different ways by workers with differing theoretical bias, and with considerable overlap.

Spitz's view, as I have stated, was that it is an inappropriate fit between the capacity of the mother for emotional giving, and the emotional needs of her infant that result in developmental arrest, or developmental fixation, with the possibility of subsequent regression to that developmental level, under stress at a later date, resulting in somatic symptom formation.[32]

Schur's theory of desomatization and resomatization[28] helps to unify the various developmental views and at the same time incorporate newer concepts. He reminds us that the newborn is capable only of somatic responses to physical or environmental stress. With increasing maturity psychological coping mechanisms gradually develop and through the process of "desomatization," these psychological mechanisms take over from the physical responses and enable the child appropriately to respond to, and control, the stresses of daily life. This is accomplished by binding anxiety through reality-testing, problem-solving thought, and appropriate action. Stress of a magnitude to lead to regression, whether that stress be inherent, maturational, or experiential, will interfere with this mature and effective binding of anxiety, leaving it free to be expressed as somatic symptom through "resomatization." Lipsitt has invoked this process over the entire spectrum of emotionally threatening stimuli, whether that stimulus be the overriding of adaptive ego functions by intensified instinctual demands, an overwhelming loss or separation, or a failure of cognitive skills or of communication.[18] In the alexithymic individual (the name give to persons who for physiologic or psychologic developmental reasons have never developed language to describe feelings, and who apparently have little fantasy life[25]) stress would result from the generation of feelings that are pressing for expression. For others it may be an inability to express only feelings of a particular class. In the area of aggression, certainly there is much evidence to support the concept that atopic patients, at least, are seldom aware of their feelings of anger.[3,22,23] These patients experience improvement in their physical symptoms as they become aware of aggressive fantasies, and as they become able, through psychotherapy, to express hostile feelings. Similarly, physical symptoms have been regarded as a regressive expression of the sexual drive, with scratching and such repetitive movements as trichotillomania being viewed as auto-erotic. In psychoanalytic practice, the uncovering of such unconscious content is not uncommon.[24] Another feeling sometimes expressed in physical symptom rather than in words is depression; burning of lips, tongue, or the soles of the feet are all recognized as being depressive equivalents.[5]

For whatever reason a physical symptom may have developed initially, there is no question that behavioral factors too come into play, and symptoms may be perpetuated as a result of operant conditioning and positive reinforcement.[17] Take for example the case of the atopic child who begins to itch and scratch when frustrated or anxious. Mother may gratify the child's need for attention by soothing the child, thus providing a positive reinforcement of the scratching behavior, or alternatively she may further increase the child's frustration by responding with anger or impatience. Or "illness" behavior may be adopted because through experience and environmental influences the patient's self-image has become that of an "ill" person, and the patient has learned to live his or her life accordingly.[10] As an example, a patient of mine, a 38-year-old single woman with factitial dermatitis, despite consistently normal laboratory values, and benign biopsy findings, had for 15 years carried variously a diagnosis of systemic lupus erythematous and pyoderma gangrenosum. She had been advised as to the seriousness and chronicity of each of these diseases, and recognized the need of appropriate care to avoid exacerbations, particularly since she lived alone and had no one to take care of her. She would stay home from work on the slightest pretext and so great was her fear of a "flare-up" of her disease that she would in panic take as many as 12 tablets of meperidine hydrochloride at a time for a simple headache. Absenteeism put her job at risk, family and peer relationships gradually deteriorated, and alcohol and substance abuse developed as a result of this "illness behavior," although at no time was a systemic disease substantiated.

It now seems clear from the works of Engel[8] and Engel and Schmale[9] that the capacity of a symptom to take on psychic representation, to express symbolic meaning, and to provide secondary gain is of greater importance in the designation of a symptom as hysterical than is the particular mediating pathway. This is well demonstrated in cases of established dermatoses, where the location of lesions may be determined by their symbolic meaning to the patient. For example, a patient of mine with lichen planus experienced a transient, localized episode that was confined to the right hand within 24 hours of shaking hands to say goodbye to a loved and revered teacher who was leaving town. There are many physicians, however, who confine the term "hysterical" to cases that conform to Freud's original formulation (as previously described).

The translation of emotional experience to physiologic change and thence to a physical symptom—known now as "transduction"[36]—has historically been assumed to have a linear causality. But given the nature of memory, with its network of associative links, this assumption is open to question. Are concurrent events necessarily causally related? Is a given reaction a total response to a total experience, or could it be that parallel responses occur concurrently to separately perceived elements of the total experience? For example, could one component acquire psychological meaning, while another results in physiologic change? Animal experiments suggest that this may be so.[9] Can the physical symptoms be traced directly to the emotional experience, or has the experience instead triggered behavior that, in turn, has caused the symptom? An example of this last would be the patient whose guilt surrounding an extramarital affair causes compulsive cleansing, associated with a severe outbreak of atopic eczema. Does reactivation of an old, unconscious conflict by the threat of current stress lead to a state of emotional arousal? Are there, then, autonomic or hormonal responses that heighten brain function, activate ordinarily quiescent neuronal circuits, and ultimately affect other organs? Some of these questions are beginning to be answered, both by animal experiments and by measurements of biogenic amines, hormones, and enzymes, in some of the individuals with psychosomatic disorders.[27]

REFERENCES

1. Alexander F: Psychosomatic Medicine: Its Principles and Applications. London, Allen & Union, 1952, pp 71-75
2. Alexander F, French TM, Pollock GH (eds): Psychosomatic Specificity. Chicago, University of Chicago Press, 1968
3. Bastiaans J: The role of aggression in the genesis of psychosomatic disease. J Psychosom Res 13:307-314, 1969
4. Cannon WB: Bodily Changes in Pain, Hunger, Fear and Rage. New York, Appleton, 1929
5. Coles RB: Glossodynia—a psychosomatic problem. Trans St Johns Hosp Dermatol Soc 52:79-83, 1966
6. Deutsch F: On the Mysterious Leap from the Mind to the Body. New York, International Universities Press, 1959
7. Dunbar F: Psychosomatic Diagnosis. New York, Hoeber, 1943
8. Engel GL: Primary atypical facial neuralgia: an hysterical conversion symptom. Psychosom Med 13:375-396, 1951
9. Engel GL, Schmale AH Jr: Psychoanalytic theory of somatic disorder: conversion, specificity, and the disease onset situation. J Am Psychoanal Assoc 15:344-365, 1967
10. Ford CV: The Somatizing Disorders: Illness as a Way of Life. New York, Elsevier, 1983
11. Freud S: Freud's Psycho-Analytic Procedure, in Strachey J (ed): Freud S: Complete Psychological Works (Standard ed.) Vol VII. London, Hogarth, 1953, pp 249-254
12. Friedman M, Rosenman RH: Association of specific overt behavior pattern with blood and cardiovascular findings: blood cholesterol level, blood clotting time, incidence of arcus senilis, and clinical coronary artery disease. JAMA 169:1286-1296, 1959
13. Graham DT, Goodell H, Wolff HG: Neural mechanisms involved in itch, "itchy skin", and tickle sensations. J Clin Invest 30:37-49, 1957
14. Graham DT, Wolf S: Pathogenesis of urticaria: experimental study of life situations, emotions and cutaneous vascular reactions. JAMA 143:1396-1402, 1950
15. Groddeck A: The Meaning of Illness. New York, International Universities Press, 1977
16. Koblenzer PJ: Edinburgh's influence on medicine in the new world, in Passmore R (ed): Proceedings of the Royal College of Physicians of Edinburgh Tercentenary Congress 1981. Edinburgh, The College, 1982, pp 143-158
17. Lipowski ZJ: Psychosomatic medicine: an overview, in Hill OW (ed):

Modern Trends in Psychosomatic Medicine 3. Boston, Butterworth, 1976, pp 1-20

18. Lipsitt DR: The somatization process and its relation to psychosomatic pathology, in Pinchot P, Berner P, Wolf R, Thau K (eds): Psychiatry: The State of the Art. Psychotherapy and Psychosomatic Medicine, vol. 4. New York, Plenum, 1985, pp 375-380
19. MacKenna RMB, Macalpine I: Application of psychology to dermatology. Lancet 1:65-68, 1951
20. Menninger K: Observations of a psychiatrist in a dermatology clinic. Bull Menninger Clinic ll:141-147, 1947
21. Menninger WC: Functional disorders of the gastro-intestinal tract: the "gastro-intestinal neuroses." Am J Digest Dis Nutrition 4:447-453, 1937
22. Miller H, Baruch DW: A study of hostility in allergic children. Am J Orthopsychiatry 20:506-519, 1950
23. Musaph H: Aggression and sympton formation in dermatology. J Psychosom Res 13:257-264, 1969
24. Musaph H: Itching and Scratching: Psychodynamics in Dermatology. Philadelphia, Davis, 1964, p 3
25. Nemiah JC, Freyberger H, Sifneos PE: Alexithymia: a view of the psychosomatic process, in Hill OW (ed): Modern Trends in Psychosomatic Medicine 3. Boston, Butterworth, 1976, pp 430-439
26. Obermayer ME, Becker SW: Functional studies of patients with neurodermatoses, in Ninth International Congress of Dermatology (Budapest, 1935): Deliberationes, vol. 2. Budapest, Szodoray, 1936, p 495
27. Reiser MF: Changing theoretical concepts in psychosomatic medicine, in Reiser MF (ed): American Handbook of Psychiatry, vol. 4. New York, Basic Books, 1975
28. Schur M: Comments on the metapsychology of somatization. Psychoanal Study Child l0:119-164, 1955
29. Seitz PFD, Shipley RE: An experimental approach to psychocutaneous problems: II. Simultaneous recording of psychotherapeutic interviews and galvanic skin response. J Invest Dermatol 19:49-54, 1952
30. Selye H: Stress. Montreal, Acta Inc. Medical Publ, 1950, pp 12-15
31. Shaffer B, Beerman H: Lichen simplex chronicus and its variants: a discussion of certain psychodynamic mechanisms and clinical histopathologic correlations. AMA Arch Dermat Syph 64:340-351, 1951
32. Spitz R: The First Year of Life. New York, International Universities Press, 1965, pp 224-242
33. Stokes JH, Beerman H: Effect on the skin of emotional and nervous states. V. The rosacea complex: a reappraisal, with special reference to the constitutional background and the rationale of treatment. Arch Dermat Syph 26:478-494, 1932

34. Stokes JH, Beerman H, Ingraham NR: The psychoneurogenous component of cutaneous reaction mechanisms. Am J Med Sci 198:577-588, 1939
35. Stokes JH, Beerman H, Ingraham NR: The psychoneurogenous component of cutaneous reaction mechanisms. Part II. Am J Med Sci 200:560-576, 1940
36. Weiner H: Psychobiology and Human Disease. New York, Elsevier, 1977, pp 630-631
37. Wittkower E, Russell B: Emotional Factors in Skin Disease. New York, Hoeber, 1953

Chapter 3

Current Views of Somatization

Information from a variety of different disciplines has come together to suggest that rather than a specific psychologic or physiologic cause for a specific disease, the "choice" of somatic disease, the time of onset of that disease, and the character of its course are determined by a concatenation of more nonspecific factors that include genetic make-up, past life-experience, and current life circumstance. This has come to be known as the psychosociobiologic view of disease.[43] It is, par excellence, a holistic view.

We shall be looking at early contributions from the fields of experimental physiology, immunology, clinical psychology, and psychosomatic medicine, as well as the more recent and rapidly expanding fields of psychoimmunology and psychoneuroendocrinology, in order to arrive at a consistent and cohesive whole that will satisfy clinical experience and logic.

"Stress" in what follows will be used to designate any one of a variety of different nonspecific events, generated either externally or internally that, by making demands on the organism, set in motion a nonspecific bodily response that leads to a variety of temporary or permanent physiologic, psychologic, or structural changes.[21]

EARLY EXPERIMENTAL OBSERVATIONS

In the late 1940s it was observed that apprehension about impending surgery increased above the previously cited 50 percent level the number of patients who exhibited fibrinolysis immediately prior to, as well as after, surgical procedures.[23] Fifteen years later Ogsten et al. demonstrated that even only quite minor or transient anxiety was necessary in some patients to produce this effect.[34] In the same vein, in 1967 Cash and Allan showed that stress may have a deleterious effect on the production of plasminogen activator in response to physical exercise.[8]

In 1950, Graham and Wolf correlated blood vessel function with changes in life situation, attitude, and feeling state in 30 patients with chronic urticaria. Particularly, they noted a high correlation between situations that generated feelings of resentment in these patients and episodes of urticaria.[14] Arteriolar and capillary dilatation was involved in genesis of the lesions. A similar study undertaken 3 years later in patients with eczema yielded similar findings,[16] and revealed that exacerbations of eczema occurred especially in response to situations in which the patient felt trapped and helpless. Arteriolar and capillary dilatation again was important in pathogenesis, and was accompanied by pruritus. The same group, studying the neural mechanisms involved in itch and tickle sensations, decapitated cartharidin-induced blisters to measure the volume of fluid exudation under various circumstances. This fluid volume was found to decrease when anxious subjects relaxed or were distracted, and after weeping had occurred, but increased if weeping was inhibited.[15,20]

Over a number of years, Black and coworkers studied the effects of hypnosis on allergic reactions in atopic individuals. They were able to suppress the positive immediate response to the intra-dermal injection of known allergens by direct suggestion under hypnosis, despite the persistence of the specific antibody as demonstrated by the Prausnitz-Kustner reaction;[5,29] they were able also to demonstrate a shift in the dose-response curve of the Prausnitz-Kustner reaction by the same means.[7] Hypnotic control of the atopic response was still occupying researchers as recently as 1965, when Dennis and Philippus blocked the Type I allergic reaction by making direct suggestion to the patient that he or she would feel a sensation of coldness at the test site.[10] That the characteristic response to cell-mediated immunity also yields to hypnotic suggestion has been shown by suppression of the tuberculin test response in Tuberculin reactive individuals.[6] Biopsies revealed the expected cellular infiltrate, but erythema and edema were totally absent.[6] Other studies have shown that the vascular response to noxious stimuli, the pain threshold, and the Galvanic skin response also are all responsive to hypnotic suggestion.[9, 44] There are case reports that demonstrate variations in some of these same parameters in correlation with affect change during psychoanalytic interviews.[31,32]

A final note on hypnosis studies; there are intriguing reports of quite remarkable improvement in two cases of genodermatoses using hypnotherapy; in one case of congenital ichthyosis, and another of pachyonychia congenita.[27,28]

In the area of infectious disease, Greenfield found that college students who were emotionally healthy recovered more rapidly from infectious mononucleosis than did those who were less emotionally stable,[18] while Meyer and Hagerty found an increased rate of streptococcal infection in more stressed individuals as compared with those less-stressed.[30] Even in dental disease similar correlations have been made.[25,42] Comparable findings from animal studies have shown that stress impairs host-resistance to the herpes simplex, coxsackie-B, poliomyelitis viruses, and the tubercle bacillus.[13] Studies in patients with autoimmune disease have also yielded interesting results. For example, there is evidence that certain personality traits may predispose towards autoimmune disease and that emotional distress and decompensation of psychological defenses may play a role in its onset and course.[41] These findings are reported in rheumatoid arthritis, ulcerative colitis, Graves disease, systemic lupus erythematous, and multiple sclerosis.

PSYCHOSOCIAL INFLUENCES

Another focus for observation during this same period (1950s to 1970s) has been the relationship of certain life events to the onset or exacerbation of physical illness. For example, Parkes et al., reported an increased mortality rate from cardiovascular disease during the first 6-months post-bereavement. The incidence, not unexpectedly, was highest in bereaved spouses, and the figure had returned to normal within 1 year after the event.[38] Hierarchical tables have been formulated to ascribe to 42 separate life change events a numerical figure. These figures are designated life change units (LCU) and indicate the degree of readjustment in the life of the individual that each of these events would require. Marriage was designated the reference event with an arbitrary score of 50 LCU's. Both pleasant and unpleasant events are included in the schedule, and a number of studies have demonstrated correlations of variable degrees between high scores of LCU's, onset of physical illness, and the severity of that illness. Questionnaires have been completed for specific periods of time, and have been used for both prospective and retrospective studies.[19] But questions as to the usefulness of this modality remain, since it fails to take into consideration the effect of past life experience on present circumstances, or the significance of unconscious meanings of situations, and of experiences to the individual.

The same criticism, failure to take into consideration the effect of past life-experience, or the significance of the unconscious meanings of events, can be levelled also against those studies that rely on personality profile tables, for example the Minnesota Multiphasic Personality Inventory, or scales of anxiety such as the Taylor Manifest Anxiety Scale, as the means of assessing the psyche's contribution to physical illness.

THE GIVING-UP-GIVEN-UP COMPLEX

It is feelings of loss, and of hopelessness brought about by distressing events that seem particularly to be associated with physical deterioration.[28] Engel has written about this as the "giving-up-given-up complex," characterized by feelings of helplessness or hopelessness, self-depreciation, loss of gratification from previously gratifying activities or relationships, a disruption in the sense of continuity between the past, present, and future, and a reactivation of previous and similar feelings of helplessness.[11]

RECENT WORK

It is beyond the scope of this volume to give in detail all of the evidence adduced from more recent work to support many of the earlier observations described, but so crucial is this new information to our understanding of the interaction between psyche and soma that I will summarize a few of the salient findings. The major contributions have come from the work of investigators in two fields, psychoneuroimmunology and psychoneuroendocrinology, in both of which animal and human studies have been undertaken.

Attention has been give to the effects psychosocial factors have on the immune response in a number of different areas in infectious disease, neoplasia, and in autoimmunity. Behavioral factors too have received attention; for example, the possibility of conditioning immunologic responses. It should be stressed that it is not suggested that psychosocial factors can cause disease, but only that they may alter individual susceptibility. The question then is not whether either a pathogenic agent or a psychosocial factor is responsible, but rather to what extent each can be implicated in a given disease episode or course.

PSYCHOIMMUNOLOGY

Recent clinical studies have focused on the relationship between psychosocial factors and measures of host defense. Bartrop found that the mean T-lymphocyte response to phytohemagglutinin and concavalin-A was reduced, 8 weeks after a bereavement, though neither the mechanism whereby this was brought about, other concurrent symptomatology, nor possible late onset somatic effects were considered in this study.[3] Locke found that the ability to cope psychologically with prolonged life change events affected the activity level of natural killer cells and that the level of activity was reduced most significantly in those whose coping skills were least effective.[22] Lymphocyte cytotoxicity has been shown also by Greene[17] to be reduced in those with unsatisfactory psychological coping skills; in similar vein a positive correlation between successful coping mechanisms and level of antibody titer has been reported, 6 months after vaccination against influenza.[40] Finally, impaired neutrophil function has been found to a significantly higher degree in stressed neonatal infants than in those who are healthy.[45]

How can we explain these interesting observations and those from the earlier studies that I have described? By what mechanisms have the various changes been brought about? Recent laboratory studies are beginning to point to some of the answers. Most of these have been animal studies, and though the findings are not uniform in all species, and we cannot assume them to be directly applicable to man, yet I think it fair to assume that comparable events occur that permit psychosocial factors to modify our own immune response.

ANIMAL STUDIES

There can be no question that glucocorticoids are secreted at times of acute stress. In animal studies their effect on the immune response is complex and does not have a consistent effect on the same T-cell subsets, from species to species. For example, in guinea pigs the lymphopenia produced by steroid administration affects circulating T cells to a greater extent than B cells, whilst the reverse is true of mice.[33] Mature medullary antigen-primed effector T cells are spared at the expense of immature uncommitted cortical T cells, in the thymic involution associated with elevated steroid levels.[12] To summarize the work from many different laboratories that demonstrate the effects of glucocorticosteroids on immunomodulation, steroids have been shown at low dose to enhance the inductive phase of lymphocyte reactions, while at high dosage levels they reduce antibody formation, suppress cell-mediated immunity, depress blastogenesis, interfere with phagocytosis and intracellular digestion by the stabilization of lysosomal membranes, prevent lymphokines from activating macrophages, and alter the migration patterns of subsets of lymphocytes.[33]

EXPERIMENTAL STUDIES IN MAN

Palmblad used a 48-hour period of sleep deprivation as the stresser in a number of studies on normal human volunteers. He reported an impaired ability of neutrophils to phagocytose staphylococcal organisms,[35] an increased production of lymphocyte interferon, and a reduction of phytohemaglutinin-induced DNA production; all of these returned to normal within 5 days of the vigil.[36] He also reported an elevation of the erythrocyte sedimentation rate in response to stress and cautioned that psychosocial factors should be included amongst the parameters to be considered when we interpret laboratory values in a clinical setting.[37]

CONDITIONED IMMUNO-PHARMACOLOGIC RESPONSES

The fascinating and reproducible finding that in laboratory rats, the immunosuppression produced by cyclophosphamide can be conditioned to take place on presentation of the neutral stimulus with which cyclophosphamide had been paired at the time of conditioning alone, points to a close association between the central nervous system and the immune system.[1] An association will be considered more extensively below. This concept that conditioning has the capacity to suppress or enhance the immune response, clearly has profound and far-reaching implications for our fundamental understanding of the complex pathogenesis of psychosomatic processes, and of the intimate integration of physical and psychological factors in disease production.

CONTRIBUTIONS FROM PSYCHONEUROENDOCRINOLOGY

Contributions from studies in psychoneuroendocrinology provide the next step in our quest for an understanding of what is by now an apparent, albeit a very complex interaction between the psyche and physical disease.

It was noted in the previous section that a variety of nonspecific psychosocial factors had the ability, apparently, to motivate a number of biological reactions, and that many of these reactions were immunologic in nature. How then is this effected? What governs the "transduction" of neural impulses into chemical secretions—electrical energy into chemical energy?

Central in this complex system is the hypothalamus. Information is received and integrated by the hypothalamus from the prefrontal cortex, the auditory optic and olfactory centers, the brain stem, the reticular formation of the midbrain, and the other components of the limbic system, of which the hypothalamus is a part. The components of the limbic system participate in the regulation of such functions as emotionality and affect, sexual behavior, learning and the imprinting of memory, the vegetative functions of appetite and thirst, and the working of dreams. These various pathways form the afferent limbs of the system as they bring information to the hypothalamus. Most significant among the efferent limbs are the hypophysiotropic hormones, which are secreted into the pituitary portal system by the medial basal hypothalamic nuclei. These hormones act either as releasing or inhibitory factors for the hormones secreted by the anterior pituitary gland. Releasing hormones have been identified for thyroid stimulating hormone (TSH) adrenocorticotrophic hormone (ACTH), somatotropin, or growth hormone (GH), leutinising hormone (LH), follicle-stimulating hormone (FSH), prolactin, β-endorphin, and β-lipotropin while inhibiting factors have been identified only for GH, TSH, and prolactin.[40] Identified also are a growth factor for fibroblasts and a thymocyte stimulating factor. The synthesis and release of all of these is mediated by the biogenic mono-amines norepinephrine, dopamine, and serotonin of which the hypothalamus has a high concentration. So it follows that because, as described, hypothalamic activity is influenced by neural impulses from the visceral brain, by environmental stimuli, and by intrinsic circadian rhythms, and mediated as they are by biogenic amines, any one of the pituitary functions is potentially capable by being influenced by stress, and by the affective state (Fig. 3-1).[26]

A wide variety of other biologically active peptides are also found in the hypothalamus; of these, vasopressin, oxytocin, and neurophysin are transferred for storage and release to the posterior lobe of the pituitary gland, while others, many of which are represented more significantly in the gastrointestinal tract than in the brain, are released from the hypothalamus directly in the circulation.

There are studies to demonstrate alterations in the level of immunologic and inflammatory activity in response to variations in the levels of many of the hor-

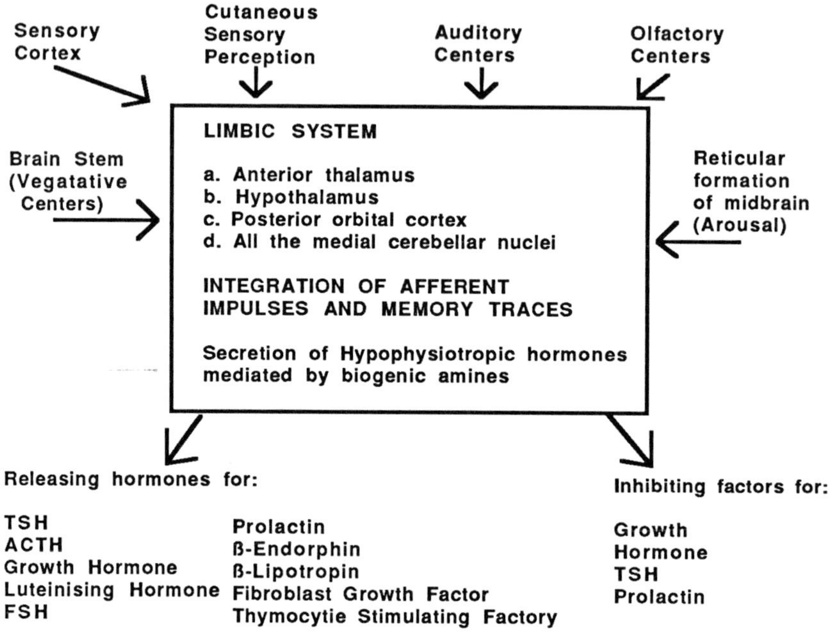

Figure 3-1. The influence of psychological factors on physiologic state.

mones that depend on the pituitary gland for control.[24] It follows then that by means of the hypophysiotrophic hormones, these alterations in activity are in turn mediated by the hypothalamus, in response to the signals that it receives from the wide variety of sources, previously enumerated. These alterations in immunologic and inflammatory activity that occur in response to variations in hormone levels are not consistent from species to species or indeed always in both sexes, or under differing circumstances. These findings do, however, allows us to postulate a control of the body's physiologic defenses that is at least in part exogenous, and closely related to central nervous system activity, rather than the often-held endogenous view that the immune system is entirely responsible for its own modulation. Parallel studies demonstrate that variations in the levels of the biogenic mono-amines serotonin, norepinephrine and dopamine, and acetyl choline, in the central nervous system, in analogous fashion also affect immune function. Indeed, Ahlquist has stated, "I think that I am justified in stating that a denial of the possibility of close links between mental state and immunologic reactions ought to be regarded as scientific suicide."[2]

We are now, I think, in a position to suggest a working hypothesis that will satisfy the requirements of the information that I have outlined, and at the same time give us a unified concept that will go some way towards answering the critical questions—why a disease?—why that particular disease?—and why now?

During the course of early development, each of us adopts a repertoire of psychologic defenses, or coping mechanisms, that become our own. These idiosyncratic responses are called into play whenever we are stressed—stress referring, as mentioned, to any one of the nonspecific events that make demands upon us. From the foregoing discussions, it is clear that stressors may be physical (i.e., a physical injury, a surgical procedure, an illness) psychosocial (i.e., the loss of one's job, failure to pass an examination, perhaps engagement or marriage), or they may be purely internal, the result of intrapsychic processes. The degree to which one can withstand stress will depend on the degree to which a strong, healthy, and mature ego has been permitted by formative forces to develop. I speak of an ego that is flexible and resilient, that has a positive self-esteem, that is capable of forming mature relationships, and that has a secure hold on reality. Physical and emotional health exist when the degree of stress and the defensive response are in equilibrium. Should a stress be so powerful as to overwhelm the defenses, equilibrium can no longer be maintained, and symptoms will develop. Clearly, an outside observer cannot make a judgement about the severity of a particular psychologic stress from its external attributes alone. Ultimately, the effect must depend not only on what is evident—the reality of the situation—but also on the way in which it is perceived by the individual. This perception is the sum effect of the current sensory input, the associational pathways and memory traces that that input triggers, together with the emotions that the processing of all this material generates—material that is both ancient and current—in the limbic system of the brain, of which the hypothalamus is a part. Or put differently, a stress is perceived in terms of its meaning to the individual in the context of the individual's current life; but this current meaning is strongly colored by the stored conscious and unconscious memories that are the residua of past experiences.

With the activation of the hypothalamus then, biogenic amines, hypophysiotropic hormones, and other chemical mediators are generated, which affect their target organs in the ways that I have described earlier, to produce pathophysiologic effects.[4] Reiser has postulated, and has adduced persuasive evidence in support of his theory, that a preprogramming of pathophysiologic circuitry for disease may occur in the brain. This pre-programmed circuitry, then, may be activated by nonspecific stress, to generate a response that is characteristic for the individual. This response has been shaped by three factors: genetic predisposition, personality make-up, and life experience during critical periods of early development. On this basis, the pre-programming circuits, then, will determine whether that patient will develop an affective or cognitive disorder, or a physical disease, and if so, which disease that will be, and by what mechanism it will develop.[39]

REFERENCES

1. Ader R, Cohen N: Conditioned immunopharmacologic responses, in Ader R (ed): Psychoneuroimmunology. New York, Academic Press, 198l, pp 281-319
2. Ahlquist J: Hormonal influences on immunologic and related phenomena, in Ader R (ed): Psychoneuroimmunology. New York, Academic Press, 1981, p 392
3. Bartrop RW, Luckhurst E, Lazarus L, et al.: Depressed lymphocyte function after bereavement. Lancet 1:834-836, 1977
4. Besodovsky HO, Sorkin E: Immunologic-neuroendocrine circuits: physiological approaches, in Ader R (ed): Psychoneuroimmunology. New York, Academic Press, 1981, pp 545-574
5. Black S: Inhibition of immediate type hypersensivity response by direct suggestion under hypnosis. Br Med J 1:925-929, 1963
6. Black S, Humphrey JH, Niven JSF: Inhibition of Mantoux reaction by direct suggestion under hypnosis. Br Med J 1:1649-1652, 1963
7. Black S: Shift in dose-response curve of Prausnitz-Kustner reaction by direct suggestion under hypnosis. Br Med J 1:990-992, 1963
8. Cash JD, Allan AGE: Effect of mental stress on the fibrinolytic reactivity to exercise. Br Med J 2:545-548, 1967
9. Chapman LF, Goodell H, Wolff HG: Augmentation of the inflammatory reaction by activity of the central nervous system. AMA Arch Neurol 1:557-572, 1959
10. Dennis M, Philippus MJ: Hypnotic and non-hypnotic suggestion and skin response in atopic patients. Am J Clin Hypn 7:342-345, 1965
11. Engel GL: A life-setting conducive to illness: the giving-up-given-up complex. Ann Intern Med 69:293-300, 1968
12. Fauci AS: Mechanisms of corticosteriod action on lymphocyte subpopulations. II. Differential effects of in vivo hydrocortisone, prednisone and dexamethasone on in vitro expression of lymphocyte function. Clin Exp Immunol 24:54-62, 1976
13. Friedman SB, Glasgow LA: Psychologic factors and resistance to infectious disease. Pediatr Clin North Am 13:315-335, 1966
14. Graham DT, Wolf S: Pathogenesis of urticaria: experimental study of life situations, emotions and cutaneous vascular reactions. JAMA 143:1396-1402, 1950
15. Graham DT, Goodell H, Wolff H: Neural mechanisms involved in itch, "itchy skin," and tickle sensations. J Clin Invest 30:37-49, 1951
16. Graham DT, Wolf S: The relation of eczema to attitude and to vascular reactions of the human skin. J Lab Clin Med 42:238-254, 1953
17. Greene WA, Betts RF, Ochitill HN, et al.: Psychosocial factors and immunity: preliminary report. Psychosom Med 40:87 (abstr.), 1978

18. Greenfield NS, Roessler R, Crosley AP: Ego strength and length of recovery from infectious mononudeosis. J Nerv Ment Dis128:125-128, 1959
19. Hinkle LE: The effect of exposure to cultural change, social change, and changes in interpersonal relationships on health, in Dohrenwend BS, Dohrenwend BP (eds): Stressful Life Events: Their Nature and Effects. New York, Wiley, 1974, pp 9-44
20. Kepecs JG, Robin M, Brunner MJ: Relationship between certain emotional states and exudation into the skin. Psychosom Med 13:10-17, 1951
21. Lipowski ZJ: Psychosomatic medicine: an overview, in Hill O (ed): Modern Trends in Psychosomatic Medicine 3. London, Butterworths, 1976, pp 4-13
22. Locke SE, Hurst MW, Williams RM, et al.: The influence of psychosocial factors on human cell-mediated immune function. The American Psychosomatic Society, Annual Meeting, Washington, DC, March 31-April 2, 1978
23. Macfarlane RG, Biggs R: Observations on fibrinolysis: spontaneous activity associated with surgical operations, trauma, etc. Lancet 2:862-864, 1946
24. McLean D, Reichlin S: Neuroendocrinology and the immune process, in Ader R (ed): Psychoneuroimmunology. New York, Academic Press, 1981, pp 475-520
25. Manhold JH: Stress, oral disease, and general illness. Psychosomatics 20:83-87, 1979
26. Martin JB, Reichlin S, Brown GM: Clinical Neuroendocrinology. Philadelphia, F.A. Davis, 1977, pp 13-44
27. Mason AA: A case of congenital inchthyosiform erythrodermia of Brocq treated by hypnosis. Br Med J 2:422-423, 1952
28. Mason AA: Letter. Ichthyosis and hypnosis. Br Med J 2:57-58, 1955
29. Mason AA, Black S: Allergic skin responses abolished under treatment of asthma and hayfever by hypnosis. Lancet l:877-879, 1958
30. Meyer RJ, Haggerty R: Streptococcal infections in families: factors altering individual susceptibility. Pediatrics 29:539-549, 1962
31. Mittelmann B, Wolff HG: Affective states and skin temperature: experimental study of subjects with "cold hands" and Raynaud's syndrome. Psychosom Med 1:271-292, 1939
32. Mittelman B, Wolff HG: Emotions and skin temperature: observations on patients during psychotherapeutic (psychoanalytic) interviews. Psychosom Med 5:211-231, 1943
33. Monjan AA: Stress and immunologic competence: studies in animals, in Ader R (ed): Psychoneuroimmunology. New York, Academic Press, 1981, pp 185-228
34. Ogston D, McDonald GA, Fullerton HW: The influence of anxiety in tests of blood coagulability and fibrinolytic activity. Lancet 2:521-523, 1962
35. Palmblad J, Cantell K, Strander H, et al.: Stressor exposure and immunological response in man: interferon-producing capacity and phagocytosis. J Psychosom Res 20:193-199, 1976

36. Palmblad J, Petrini B, Wasserman J, et al.: Lymphocyte and granulocyte reactions during sleep deprivation. Psychosom Med 41:273-278, 1979
37. Palmblad J: Stress and immunologic competence: studies in man, in Ader R (ed): Psychoneuroimmunology. New York, Academic Press, 1981, pp 229-257
38. Parkes CM, Benjamin B, Fitzgerald RG: Broken heart: a statistical study of increased mortality among widowers. Br Med J 1:740-743, 1969
39. Reiser MF: Mind, Brain, Body; Toward a Convergence of Psychoanalysis and Neurobiology. New York, Basic Books, 1984, pp 197-213
40. Roessler R, Cabe TR, Lester JW, et al.: Ego strength, life events, and antibody titers. The American Psychosomatic Society Annual Meeting, Dallas, TX, March 22-25, 1979
41. Solomon FG: Emotional and personality factors in the onset and course of autoimmune disease, particularly rheumatoid arthritis, in Ader R (ed): Psychoneuroimmunology. New York, Academic Press, 1981, pp 159-182
42. Sutton PR: The early onset of acute dental caries in adults following mental stress. New York Dent J 31:450-456, 1965
43. Weiner H: Psychobiology and Human Disease. New York, Elsevier, 1977, pp 630-631
44. West LJ, Niell KC, Hardy JD: Effects of hypnotic suggestion on pain perception and galvanic skin response. AMA Arch Neurol & Psychiat 68:549-560, 1952
45. Wright WC, Ank BJ, Herbert J, et al.: Decreased bacterial activity of leukocytes of stressed newborn infants. Pediatrics 56:579-584, 1975

Chapter 4

Dermatologic Classification of Psychocutaneous Disease and Its Relationship to Psychiatric Diagnosis

From the previous chapters it will be clear that if we adopt the current psychosociobiologic view of disease, then all illness will to a greater or lesser extent represent a disruption of the equilibrium between the stresses of daily living on the one-hand, and the physiologic and psychologic defense mechanisms on the other. In other words, all illness can be viewed in some measure as psychosomatic.

In our daily dealings with patients it is important to keep this in mind, because even in the management of straightforward dermatologic conditions, emotional factors may intrude from time to time and confuse the issue. As an example let me cite the case of a 16-year-old boy whom I treated for severe and intractable cystic acne. It was not until we had struggled aggressively, using every available modality with signal lack of success for 2 years, that I learned that throughout the same period this boy had been under a terrible cloud. He had been present but not personally involved when in the course of high-spirited adolescent horsing around on a country road, two of his friends had contributed to the automobile death of another boy. Distressed by the loss of his friend and by this forcible confrontation with his own mortality, and guilty because he had not somehow magically prevented the disaster, he was also worried about pending litigation in which he was cited by the dead boy's father as one of the perpetrators. Once this information was known to me, I was able to help him to verbalize and master his feelings; but it was not until the case against him was dropped, and he was able to put the whole experience behind him, that we really began to make progress in controlling his acne.

For purposes of evaluation and management, a classification of psychocutaneous disease is helpful. Such a classification must give consideration not only to the dermatologic diagnosis, but also to the level of psychopathology, because rational management will in part depend on the degree of psychiatric impairment.

The classification that I have found most useful is outlined in Table 4-1.

Table 4-1
Classification of Psychocutaneous Disease

I. Conditions with strictly psychological etiology
   A. Dermatitis artefacta
   B. Delusions and hallucinations as they relate to the skin
      1. Delusions of parasitosis
      2. Dysmorphic syndrome
   C. Psychogenic pain syndromes
      1. Glossodynia and glossopyrosis
      2. Atypical facial pain syndrome
      3. Burning of the soles
      4. Some cases of post-herpetic neuralgia
   D. Compulsive habits and obsessional concerns as they relate to the skin
      1. Neurotic excoriations
      2. Trichotillomania
      3. Onychotillomania, onychodystrophy, primary lichen simplex chronicus, factitious cheilitis, etc.
      4. Obsessional concerns about infestation, contagion, bromidrosis, etc.
   E. Psychogenic purpura syndromes
      1. Psychogenic purpura (Gardner-Diamond)
      2. Anti-DNA sensitisation syndrome
      3. Stigmatisation

II. Conditions in which strong psychogenic factors are imputed
   A. The urticarias
      1. Acute urticaria
      2. Chronic urticaria
      3. Dermographism
      4. Cholinergic urticaria
   B. Prurtitus: Generalised and localised
   C. Flushing reactions and rosacea
   D. Psychogenic disorders of sweat glands
      1. Hyperhidrosis
      2. Bromidrosis

III. Conditions probably dependent on genetic or enviornmental factors whose course is often affected by stress
   A. Alopecia areata, telogen effluvium, and hirsutism
   B. Psoriasis
   C. Atopic dermatitis
   D. Acne vulgaris
   E. The remaining spectrum of cutaneous disease

There is some overlap between the three major categories, and although broadly speaking those in the first group are more psychiatrically sick than the other two groups, this is by no means across the board and psychosomatic skin problems can occur over the entire spectrum of psychiatric pathology.

This being the case, and in an attempt to offer a guide to psychiatric diagnosis for dermatologists that is concise and at the same time sufficiently lucid to be useful, I will discuss first the interpretation of signs and symptoms in psychiatric differential diagnosis, and then the individual psychiatric diagnostic categories that we are most likely to encounter in the clinical practice of dermatology.

"SPHERES" OF FUNCTION

Psychiatric symptoms can be viewed in terms of five spheres of mental functioning: the cognitive, affective, perceptual, physiologic, and psychomotor spheres, each one of which is relatively autonomous, though at the same time dependent on the functional integrity of the others.

The Cognitive Sphere

A number of mental functions are subsumed under cognition. These include the level of consciousness as judged by the degree of awareness of self, others, and the environment, the character of the thought process, the capacity to remember recent and distant events, the fund of knowledge, and the use of language.

Consciousness

The level of consciousness will fall somewhere along a continuum that extends from coma at one end, through various levels of sleep and normal wakefulness, to arousal or hyper-alertness at the other. We are interested not only in the level, but also in the quality of consciousness; is it normal, clouded, or expanded? Or are we witness to a dissociative state in which information is split off from the body of conscious knowledge because of its disturbing nature?

Thought

Interest here is in both form and content.

Form of thought. The flow of normal thought is rhythmical. It is goal oriented, comprehensible, and readily followed by the listener, to whom it is specifically directed. Variations from this norm include ideas that are disconnected, circumlocution, flight of ideas, interpenetration of themes, tangentiality, circumstantiality, perseveration, rambling, blocking, and poverty of ideas. Clustering of these various characteristics in certain groupings may suggest certain specific disorders. (See Table 4-2)

Content of thought. Children faced with new situations, if they are not given enough information to understand their observations realistically, will create for themselves an explanation that makes good sense in the context of their infantile world view. They do this in order to relieve the inner tension that ambiguity creates. Disorders of thought content may arise by this same mechanism in adults. They may also arise through the mechanism of neurotic symptom formation wherein thoughts, wishes, or feelings that are unacceptable to conscience must be repressed and kept out of consciousness, whilst attention is displaced onto more innocent thoughts that are linked by association to those that are forbidden. This maneuver provides for the patient a partial solution to intrapsychic conflict, conflict that has arisen between the patient's wishes for gratification on the one hand, and the needs of conscience and reality on the other. It serves at the same time to bind for the patient the neurotic anxiety that is generated. Although to the casual observer, and in the context of the real world, the product of each of these mechanisms may make no sense, yet could we "crack the code," we would find that the ideational content would have symbolic meaning in the context of the patient's early experience and current life circumstances. Understanding of this type is sought and indeed often occurs in the course of psychoanalytic treatment or psychoanalytic psychotherapy. Included in this group would be delusions, obsessions, phobias, and the somatic expression of emotional conflict.

DELUSIONS

A delusion is a false belief that arises without appropriate external stimulus, is not shared by others, and is maintained unshakably in the face of reason. Delusions are pathognomonic of psychosis. It is the intensity of the emotional investment in the false belief that serves to distinguish a true delusion from an obsessional concern or a phobic fear. The spectrum of delusional ideation is broad, varying from a circumscribed and quite discrete belief—such as we see in the patient with delusions of parasitosis, at one end—to complex delusional systems—carefully reasoned and with their own logic, at the other. These latter patients often are flooded with chaotic thoughts and feelings that they cannot understand; much like children, in order to maintain control and to establish order in their chaotic inner world, they develop idiosyncratic theories to explain the puzzling and frightening inner experience. An example would be the 70-year-old woman who consulted me about changes she perceived in her skin. She believed that neighbors had a laser hidden in the adjacent apartment and that the impact of laser energy had caused her to lose scalp hair, develop "bumps" on the cranium, and also a variety of scars on her skin. She spent incalculable time and energy

Table 4-2.

	Paranoia	Mania and Hypomania	Hysterical Conversion	Hyperventilation Syndrome	Organic Brain Syndrome	Schizophrenia	Psychotic Depression	Neurotic Depression (All types Neurosis) Borderline personality disorder	Obsessive Neurosis	Hysterical Neurosis	Neurotic Anxiety (All types Neurosis)	Phobic Neurosis	Personality Disorder	Sociopath
Consciousness														
Hypervigilance	X	X												
Drowsiness					X									
Expanded	X	X												
Dissociated			X	X										
Thought Form														
Poverty of Ideas					X		X							
Circumstantiality					X	X								
Rambling					X	X			X					
Perseveration					X				X					
Disconnected Ideas						X	X							
Blocking						X					X			
Interpenetration of Ideas						X								
Flight of Ideas		X												
Tangentiality		X												
Distractability		X									X			
Pressured Speech		X									X			
Thought Content														
Delusions	X	X			X	X	X							
Somatic Complaints	X		X		X	X	X	X	X	X	X			
Phobias	X					X	X	X	X	X		X	X	
Obsessions	X					X	X	X	X			X		
Memory														
Short Term Loss					X									
Long Term Loss					X									

Table 4-2. (Continued)

	Paranoia	Mania and Hypomania	Hysterical Conversion	Hyperventilation Syndrome	Organic Brain Syndrome	Schizophrenia	Psychotic Depression	Neurotic Depression (All types Neurosis) Borderline personality disorder	Obsessive Neurosis	Hysterical Neurosis	Neurotic Anxiety (All types Neurosis)	Phobic Neurosis	Personality Disorder	Sociopath
Insight Into Illness Present			X	X	X		X	X	X	X	X	X		
Absent	X	X				X							X	X
Abstracting Ability: Absent					X	X								
Joy-Ecstasy	X	X												
Sadness-Despair							X	X	X					
Irritability-Anger	X							X	X					X
Apprehension-Fear	X					X	X			X	X	X		
Perpetual Sphere Pseudohallucinations Hallucinations	X	X			X	X								
Depersonalization										X	X			
Derealization and Deja-vu —Etc								X		X	X			
Physiologic-Sphere Difficulty in Falling Asleep		X				X (Acute)		X			X			
Early Morning Wakening		X			X		X				X			
Hypersomnia								X						
Menstrual Abnormalities		X	X (Pseudocyesis)			X		X			X			
Depressed Appetite							X	X			X			
Increased Appetite		X						X			X			
Sympathetic Nervous System Activation						X (Acute)		X			X			
Sexual Drive Decreased	X				X		X	X	X			X		
Sexual Drive Increased		X												
Psychomotor Sphere, rapid jerky movements		X										X		
Slow, Weight-laden								X	X					

studying in the public library, drawing charts to depict the exact mechanisms of each perceived change, and illustrations of the imagined equipment. She had invested considerable sums in professional photographs and medical consultations in order to bring suit against the offending neighbors. Her arguments had a logic of their own and were quite unshakable.

Though not always so, in some cases of acute psychosis the delusional beliefs may be global; involving as they do every aspect of the patient's life, they are supported by numerous and rapidly changing pieces of evidence. Such a patient is often very anxious, and his or her social functioning is impaired. In contrast, the patient who is more chronically ill, who's delusions are fixed, and more circumscribed, may function quite adequately in other aspects of his life.

OBSESSIONS

Obsessions (and phobias that I shall discuss next) do not have the same implication as do delusions. Though involving thought content, they are not thought disorders in the same sense as are delusions, since the hold on reality remains intact, and though both may occur in psychosis, neither is, like the true thought disorders, pathognomonic of that state.

An obsession is an idea that intrudes unbidden into the mind recurrently and insistently, and that defies all attempts to banish it from consciousness. Although patients may regard it as nonsensical, yet at the same time they recognizes it as their own, rather than an alien thought, even though it must follow to conclusion its own repetitive and stereotyped sequence. Obsessions may occur as isolated thoughts, or as complex ideas, fears, or impulses, and they may be so insistent as to drive the patient to carry out stereotyped actions, which then are known as "compulsions."

PHOBIAS

I have included phobias here, since though like obsessions they are not thought disorders in the accepted sense, as I have suggested thought is involved in the anxiety generated in the patient by the phobic object. As is the case with obsessions, phobias arise by neurotic mechanisms and are symptomatic of unresolved conflict. If an unconscious thought that is inconsistent with the moral position of the patient threatens to come to consciousness, anxiety will be generated. In defense against this anxiety, the forbidden thought is immediately repressed, and attention instead displaced onto an innocent object linked to that thought by historical or ideational association; the innocent object then, comes to serve as a symbolic representation for the patient's forbidden thought. But this mechanism provides only a partial solution, and serves to bind only a portion of the anxiety, so the innocent object in turn will become a source of anxiety, and accordingly must be avoided. As an example, a phobic might try to avoid anxiety concerning infestation, initially by refusing to shake hands. Gradually this action may be extended to avoiding crowded places, public transportation, and public toilets, until finally the poor patient may be confined to the house altogether, to keep safe from all contamination or infestation. Clearly phobic patients come less frequently to the office than do those with obsessions, whose recurring need it is to be reassured that they are not in fact infested.

SOMATIC COMPLAINTS

Somatic complaints for which there is no demonstrable pathologic evidence are frequently seen in association with the psychiatric symptoms of depression, anxiety, or fatigue. There is a spectrum of severity for these somatic complaints, from a simple general concern about health at one end, through over awareness of normal bodily sensations, mild physical symptoms, a strong conviction of physical disease, to frank somatic delusions at the other. Despite a negative medical work-up, one must, of course, always satisfy oneself that in fact there are not subtle signs of occult physical disease present.

Attitudes towards physical symptoms vary tremendously from family to family, and from one cultural group to another, and it is important to recognize that for some patients these symptoms may serve as a culturally acceptable way to communicate conflict, stress, or the need for attention. They may represent a psychiatric or psychosomatic syndrome ipso facto, or alternatively, they may surface as part of a broader psychiatric syndrome, as may be seen, for example, in the various types of depression.

MEMORY

Impairment of short-term memory results from interference in the registration and consolidation of information. It is a nonspecific indicator of a disruption in attention. By contrast, long-term memory suffers impairment when retrieval is disrupted. It too can result from organic or neurotic processes, and it sometimes may serve as a defense against the recollection of painful memories.

INSIGHT INTO ILLNESS

The way in which patients view their illnesses may provide useful diagnostic information. Patients who deny the significance of symptoms, who can find plausible if inaccurate reasons for them (rationalization), or who attribute them to outside agencies rather than to pathology within themselves (projection), have greater psychopathology, and are a more challenging treatment problem, than the patients who find their symptoms alien, and are anxious to be rid of them.

ABSTRACTION

The capacity for abstract rather than concrete thinking is a useful measure both of intelligence and of psychopathology. It can usually be assessed during the normal interaction during history-taking.

The Affective Sphere

It is the emotions that give life meaning, and that serve to endow the stark reality of the present with a richness of color and texture that is in part derived from the past. Because of this coloring of the present by the past, powerful emotions may be generated that may distort current perceptions, and may interfere in effective functioning. In our evaluation of the patient attention must be paid to emotional responsiveness: are the responses appropriate? too frequent? excessive? persistent? or unpredictable? A number of pathologic characteristics of emotional response are described below:

Lability. This refers to rapid shifts from one emotion to another.

Shallowness. The patient with shallow emotional responses cannot experience profound feelings of any sort, and therefore has a somewhat impoverished inner life.

Elevation of mood. Here we refer to joy, ecstasy, and euphoria. These characteristics may be associated with grandiosity or megalomania and with social intrusiveness. They may readily give way to irritability and rage.

Depression of mood. A depressed mood, with feelings of sadness or despair, as with an elevated mood, also may be associated with irritation and anger. Alternatively these negative feelings may be directed inwards, giving rise to feelings of guilt, worthlessness, and poor self-esteem. Apprehension and fear due to depression may be expressed through hypochondriacal concerns about sickness and death, or more globally, as a sense of impending doom.

The Perceptual Sphere

The development, mechanisms, and integration of perceptual experience have been described in previous sections. Perceptions can be regarded as false if they fall outside the normally acceptable biologic, social, or religious context of the individual. They are abnormal if there is a marked disparity between the experience of that individual and the experiences of peers, if the experience interferes with the individual's general functioning, or if there are other signs or symptoms of psychiatric disease, such as distortions of reality based on these false perceptions.

Hallucinations

A hallucination is a false sensory experience. Hallucinations may be auditory, visual, or olfactory. They may be complete and formed, or fragmentary, like odd noises, color flashes, lightening pains, indefinable odors, and the like. Ninty percent of patient's who report a hallucination will also have delusions. Indicating as they do a profound disruption of reality-testing, severe psychopathology is generally implied. While fixed, formed hallucinations are seen in psychosis, fleeting and less well-formed ones may occur in hysterical neurosis; they may be seen in temporal lobe syndromes, intoxication, and in normal individuals under conditions of extreme stress.

Illusions

Illusions arise out of an intense emotional need and are fostered by lack of perceptual clarity. For example, a frightened individual may interpret a shadow in the darkness as an assailant, or a guilty person an overheard conversation as accusation. Clinically, the significance of an illusion will depend on the presence or absence of associated findings.

Depersonalization, Derealization, and Deja Vu

In these states the patient experiences a sense of estrangement; the environment may seem unreal, the patient may feel that he or she is standing outside of the self looking on, or that he or she acts like an automaton, mechanically carrying out tasks. In a related distortion, articles may appear larger or smaller than in reality, or their shapes may be distorted. Deja vu refers to a feeling of familiarity, experienced in a place or situation that is in fact quite strange. Most commonly this is associated with organic, rather than functional disorders.

The Physiologic Sphere

Normal waking consciousness is sustained by the continuous excitation of the cerebral cortex by impulses from the reticular activating system of the brain stem; this excitation is moderated by centers in the thalamus. Sleep occurs when there is a decrease in excitation, while insomnia may result from increased excitation, and may be expressed as an increase in the time taken to fall asleep, lightness of sleep, or early morning wakening.

In addition to sleep, other physiologic functions too may demonstrate aberrations. These include the menstrual cycle, sexual potency, appetite, the autonomic nervous system, and the sensation of pain.

The Psychomotor Sphere

Gait, stance, and the speed and fluidity of movement are of interest to us. Does the patient reveal tics or habit spasms? Are the patient's movements brisk, jerky, and charged with energy? normal? or slow and ponderous? Does the patient complain of weakness, fatigue, or lack of energy?

DIFFERENTIAL DIAGNOSIS

The recent expansion in our knowledge, brought about by the tremendous advances in the area of psychobiology that have taken place in the past two or three decades, has resulted in new approaches to the classification of mental disease. These classifications are by and large based on theoretical bias, and may rely on descriptive characteristics—as is employed, for example, in the Diagnostic and Statistical Manual III—or are determined by whether the precipitant seems to be an apparently spontaneous internal biochemical change, as opposed to a reaction to external events. For our more limited purposes, however, I believe that an older classification based on psychodynamic principles will better suit our needs, since it will provide a guideline as to the appropriate therapeutic approach. Having noted the quality of the various areas of mental functioning that I have described, we are then in a position to evaluate differing clusters of characteristics in terms of the diagnostic possibilities.

The necessary information is summarized in Table 4-2. This is intended as a general guide and is by no means complete. The broad categories that we must consider are psychosis, neurosis, personality disorders, and the organic brain syndrome. In general terms, patients who are psychotic have more profound psychopathology than do those who are neurotic, or who have personality disorders, but this distinction may not be so clear-cut in the clinical presentation; for example, it may be possible in some cases for a patient with psychosis to function better socially than perhaps a patient with a severe hysterical neurosis.

Psychosis

Some patients who become psychotic are thought to have suffered emotional trauma, or privation, in very early life. This early life experience, by interfering with personality development, may result in the formation of a rather fragile ego, unclear about its boundaries, and with poor reality-testing. Such a person is ill-equipped to handle stress effectively, and incapable of forming lasting and mature relationships; instead, such a person relates in an infantile, demanding, and dependent way. Many of these patients do not have the capacity for insight, and therapeutic relationships can be only empathetic and supportive at best. In such a case, one would not recommend insight-oriented psychotherapy, but rather would set up frequent short contacts to provide support, with perhaps psychotropic drugs as the mainstay of therapy. The broad diagnostic categories include schizophrenia, toxic psychosis, bipolar affective disorder (manic-depressive psychosis) and major depression, psychotic reactions occurring in the involutional period, and paranoid states other than those included in the foregoing conditions.

Schizophrenia

CLINICAL PICTURE

Schizophrenia represents the prototype of insanity. Primarily a disease of young adults, the age at onset ranges from the teens to early forties, with a peak incidence in the early twenties; the onset may be slow and insidious, or acute, and the sex distribution is equal.

Particularly when the onset is insidious, the premorbid personality may have had characteristic schizoid features, with loneliness, social withdrawal, a flattening of affect, and vagueness of thinking. Often, there follows a gradual evolution to frank mental illness, with mounting anxiety and fears of dissolution preceding the objective behavioral changes that are characteristic of the disease. The patient experiences confusion, distractibility, inability to maintain a train of thought, and an enhanced sensitivity to extraneous sights and sounds; these subjective experiences are accompanied by a difficulty in maintaining perceptual constancy with regard to the body and the external world.

It is this perception, that the body parts are changing in size or shape, or that the patient has become ugly, that causes the patient to focus obsessionally on his or her physical being, often expressing hypochondriacal concerns. The inconstant nature of their perceptions make them uneasy also in their social contacts, and lead them to create fantasies, and later delusions, in an unconscious attempt to establish constancy and maintain some sort of control. These same physical perceptual changes may cause these patients to engage in perverse sexual behaviors, in a desperate attempt to establish sexual identity, and later in the disease, to a rejection of their bodies expressed through self-mutilation. Confusion about boundaries may become a kind of nihilism that denies that the patient even has a body, or indeed that there is a world. Profound feelings of rejection, and lack of self-respect associated with the changed perceptions that I have described, promote ever increasing defensive avoidance of painful social contact and an increasing indifference, irritability, and unapproachableness.

There follows a progressive dissolution of the personality, with changes in every aspect of mental functioning. Affect is withdrawn from the world of reality, to focus on the inner life, and its expression then may be wholly flat or quite inappropriate to the external circumstances. Feelings of derealization may follow this withdrawal, so that the patient feels like an onlooker, rather than a participant in life.

Because of the displacement of attention inwards, the attention span is poor, associational links become loosened, there may be blocks in communication, and replies to questions seem irrelevant. Symbolism, and condensation of thoughts and words, may make speech incomprehensible. This same symbolism, congruent with inner experience rather than with external reality, is expressed in the delusional ideation that forms the thought disorder characteristic of the schizophrenic. Thoughts often are concerned with sexual issues, or with abstract and often meaningless philosophical or religious ideas, and the delusions express for the patient, in symbolized and condensed form, his or her problems, wishes, and conflicts. They effectively serve for the patient as a solution to his or her problems and a subjective reorganization of the patient's inner life. Perceptual shifts and uncertainties are not confined to the patient, but extend also to those in the patient's environment, so that changing misperceptions of even those closest to the patient, make for suspiciousness, lack of trust, and instability in relationships. Disowned thoughts and feelings, which may often represent parental attitudes, are projected outwards, again in a desperate attempt at restitution, and are experienced as hallucinations.

Just as there are shifts in perceptions of people, so too the patient experiences shifts in goals, objectives, and wishes, and in his or her attitude towards these; it is these shifts that lead the patient to behaviors that appear odd, incomprehensible and impulsive, as both contradictory aspects of conscious and unconscious wishes are expressed in action.

In the motor sphere, lack of activity, apathy, negativism, stereotyped behavior, mannerisms, tics, ritualistic activities, echolalia, and echopraxia are common. With increasing withdrawal, there is a deterioration of social functioning, poor hygiene, and poor grooming; vegetative changes such as insomnia, anxiety, menstrual abnormalities, and absent sex drive may also be seen, but interestingly, despite all of the aberrations enumerated, consciousness, orientation, and memory remain essentially intact.

Historically, a number of variants have been described according to which features of the disease are most prominent, and according to the mode of onset; these include the Hebephrenic, Catatonic, Paranoid, Undifferentiated, and Schizo-affective types, but for our purposes, the broad outline given above will suffice.

ETIOLOGY

Evidence from twin and family studies supports a polygenically determined inherent predisposition to schizophrenia, though genetic studies are hard to interpret since in many, neither associated psychodynamic factors have been considered, nor have schizoid though nonpsychotic persons been included. Associated biological concomitants include a variety of nonspecific findings such as autonomic instability, variation in electroencephalographic sleep patterns, certain urinary metabolites, and in some cases, enlargement of the cerebral ventricles. Attention has been given to the possibility of impaired synaptic transmission due to autoantibodies, and also to abnormalities in various hormones, enzymes, and the intermediate metabolism of cerebral glucose. The most attractive theories currently concern the neurotransmitters, primarily dopamine, which is found to be increased: the question of the specific mechanism involved has generated a number of as yet unproven theories. Important as all of these are to our understanding of schizophrenia, and to improvement in its chemical treatment, they cannot detract from the central importance of developmental and environmental factors in its clinical expression. The nature of the interaction between infant and nurturing figures, as I have pointed out, is crucial to the developing personality, and consistency of nurturing, loving acceptance, an appropriate setting of boundaries, and an appropriate frustration of infantile wishes, are all essential to the development of a healthy and intact ego. Lack of constancy in early parenting may result in ambivalent and unstable relationships, uncertainty as to boundaries and sexual identity, lack of opportunity to learn to master the aggressive and sexual drives, and lack of ability to discriminate fantasy from reality. Often unreasonable expectations are placed on a child, who at the same time does not have the opportunity to develop a healthy self-esteem, and poor parental communication skills expose the child to contradictions between verbal remarks and overt behaviors. All of these contribute to the characteristic inner experience of the patient who is genetically predisposed to develop schizophrenia, should environmental circumstances be such as to permit or promote the clinical expression of the disease.

COURSE AND OUTCOME

The course may be one of progression, or it may be episodic. The younger the age at onset the more acute the presentation; the healthier the premorbid personality, the better the chance for remission, but the risk of personality deterioration increases with each schizophrenic relapse. Some small percentage of patients do experience full and permanent recovery, some will have a full remission but with one or more future relapses, some will have a full social remission, but with personality defects that may or may not render the patient incapable of self-care and self-support, some will go on to stable chronicity, while in a small percentage there will be deterioration to a terminal stage.

TREATMENT

As will by now be clear, schizophrenia remains a complex problem, still only incompletely understood. These patients are extremely sick and in need of informed and specialized treatment in order to control symptoms, prevent exacerbations, and reduce the likelihood of progressive mental deterioration. Treatment is most effective when it combines psychological, environmental, and chemical modalities. Whereas not infrequently the symptomatology includes complaints that may bring the patient to the dermatologist, because of the profound nature of the psychopathology it is unlikely that dermatologic care will help. Given this circumstance, symptomatic and supportive treatment in an accepting environment may enable one eventually to make a meaningful referral.

Toxic Psychosis

The likelihood of a patient with toxic psychosis presenting at the Dermatologist's office is not great, but it is important for us to be aware that chronic abuse of amphetamines, and similarly acting sympathomimetic substances, can lead to a picture not too dissimilar from paranoid schizophrenia, characterized by paranoid delusions, tactile hallucinations, ideas of reference, aggressiveness, hostility, and anxiety. Of greater significance to our interests is the possibility of a distorted perception of the body image, and delusions of parasitosis, which may be accompanied by a sensation of bugs crawling under the skin, known as "formication"; this may lead to extensive and chronic excoriations.

Intoxication from other groups of drugs, such as opiates, cocaine, and the hallucinogens, may also produce psychotic reactions, but their relevance to the practice of dermatology does not warrant their inclusion here.

The Affective Disorders

Under this rubric are included those conditions in which the primary psychopathology is a prevailing mood, either of elation or of depression. This prevailing mood may be expressed in thought and behavior, or alternatively it may be masked by defensive maneuvers, appearing instead as its opposite—for example, elation masking an underlying depression—as paranoid ideas, delusions, or hallucinations, as somatic symptoms, or as neurotic symptoms such as phobias or obsessions. Although depression is a frequent symptom of neurosis, it differs in character and in degree from the psychotic depressions represented in the group currently under discussion. Rather than being the primary pathology in neurosis, the depression represents but one symptom among a whole spectrum that are derivative of the underlying unconscious neurotic conflict.

The affective disorders can be divided into the bipolar type, or manic-depressive psychosis, in which one may encounter either manic episodes alternating with major depressive episodes, or manic episodes alone, and the unipolar type, or major depression, in which one sees only depressive episodes. Genetic, biochemical, and pharmacological research suggests that the bipolar and unipolar variants may represent separate entities, and further, that the unipolar group itself may not in fact be homogeneous. For our purposes, it will be convenient to consider them together.

Fifteen percent of adults between the ages of 18 and 74 may, in any given year, suffer from depression, according to National Institute of Mental Health statistics. Of these, only 5 percent will reach a psychiatrist, and indeed 33 percent of all prescriptions for psychotropic drugs are written by nonpsychiatric physicians. Given these statistics and given the propensity for depressed patients to complain of somatic symptoms, it behooves us to have a basic understanding of these disorders.

BIPOLAR AFFECTIVE DISORDERS (MANIC-DEPRESSIVE PSYCHOSIS)

There is good evidence to suggest that the trait for the bipolar variant is transmitted by X-linked dominant inheritance. The incidence is greatest in those of northern European extraction, and in the higher socioeconomic and professional groups. Women predominate over men in a ratio of 2:1, the median age of onset is 30 years as compared to 45 years for unipolar, or major depression, and the life expectancy for persons with this disorder tends to be shortened. According to some authorities aggressive women with masculine strivings are particularly susceptible, and close observation may reveal symptoms of depression in these patients even as early as childhood.

Symptoms are associated with variations in the level of brain norepinephrine; when these levels are elevated symptoms of elation will develop, while a decrease of this amine in the interneuronal synaptic clefts will have the opposite effect, giving rise to symptoms of depression.

CLINICAL PICTURE OF THE MANIC PHASE Typically, the disorder assumes the form of psychotic episodes, separated by intervals of mental health. These psychotic episodes may be single or numerous, and may present initially either with mania or depression, developing subsequently a tendency towards a swinging back and forth between the two.

The premorbid personality of the patient with manic episodes is usually extroverted, with aggression, self-confidence, wide interests, sociability, and responsiveness. A brief period of mild depression may be superseded by the attack proper. Hypomania refers to a condition of exhilaration, increased assertiveness, buoyant self-confidence, effervescent spirits, and boundless energy; the patient may be demanding, uninhibited, and socially unconventional with childish boasting, tactlessness, intemperate spending, and overindulgence in alcohol. These effervescent good spirits, however, will give way to peevishness, sarcasm, and anger, if the patient is criticized or if his or her wishes are denied, and sudden oscillations of emotion are not uncommon.

The psychotic attack may remain in this attenuated form, or may progress to true mania, wherein the above characteristics become accentuated. Elation gives rise to noisy, boisterous, intrusive behavior, loquaciousness, and grandiose ideas; there is rapid association of ideas, pressure of speech, easy distractibility, and heightened psychomotor activity, leading even to destruction of property and of clothing. Illusions are more common than hallucinations, and wish-fulfilling delusions or delusions of persecution may occur. Sleep requirements are minimal, and symptoms of concurrent physical illness may be ignored. In extreme cases a condition similar to delirium may ensue.

CLINICAL PICTURE—MAJOR DEPRESSION Be it the depressive phase of a bipolar affective disorder, or be it a unipolar depressive episode, the clinical picture of the patient with a major depression is essentially similar.

The premorbid personality may have been timid, friendly, unobtrusive but overdependent, or it may alternatively have been morally rigid, prudish, perfectionistic, and overly sensitive to criticism. The primary emotional need for each of these two groups of patients is to feel loved, respected, and needed. As a result, aggressive feelings are perceived as dangerous and must be defended against, since the direct expression of these might put at risk the primary emotional needs.

A mild depression may not initially be recognized, as it develops insidiously, with exaggeration of feelings that are essentially within the range of normal. If a perceptible mood change is present in a mild depression, it is not usually the presenting symptom; indeed patients will frequently state that they do not "feel depressed." Instead, they are likely to present with one of two clusters of symptoms; either inertia, fatigue, and loss of interest, or alternatively there may be a plethora of somatic symptoms for which no organic cause can be found. Other features include loss of confidence, feelings of inadequacy and lack of personal worth, social withdrawal, lack of interest in their usual pursuits, or difficulty in performing their customary duties. Indecisiveness, and other obsessional features may also be seen, while in some patients the picture may be dominated by anger and hostility.

In more severe cases, the depressive mood is all pervasive, making itself known even in the physical appearance, with slow speech, stooping figure, bowed head, frowning immobile faces, and turned down mouth. Vegetative symptoms are added to those associated with lowering of self-esteem, and include early morning waking, loss of appetite and of weight, constipation, diminished sex drive, impotence, and a decrease in the secretion of sweat. The depressive symptoms are most severe in the morning on waking, improving somewhat as the day goes on; they may be accompanied by a sense of impending doom or by feelings of derealization. In these patients, delusional thinking may occur, concerned with self-deprecation, self-accusation, guilt and remorse, or suspiciousness and paranoid ideation; though there may be pessimistic misperceptions of reality, true hallucinations are not common. A depressive stupor may supervene in the most extreme cases.

A number of variants are described, which include the retarded, in which there is extensive slowing of thought, speech, and psychomotor activity, and the agitated in which increased psychomotor activity is seen as a physical expression of deep intra-psychic anxiety.

PSYCHODYNAMIC INTERPRETATION It is our understanding that depression, like the normal grief reaction, is a psychological response to loss. The loss may be based on reality, such as a bereavement, separation from an important person, loss of job, of prestige, of health, or of a body part, or it may result from an inner experience, an internally perceived or fantasized loss, not immediately understandable to the outside observer. While patients with psychotic depression have more intact personalities than do those with schizophrenia, yet early trauma or deprivation has denied them too, the ability to cope with the frustration of separation and loss. Their helplessness, clinging, and constant need for support represents a psychological regression to an infantile level of mental functioning, while the mania reaction can be interpreted as a massive defensive denial of loss. Loss is experienced by these patients as a rejection and against this, unconscious anger is aroused. Because this anger cannot be tolerated, lest it lead to further rejection, it must be turned against the self, where it is experienced as guilt, depression, and feelings of unworthiness.

The alternating swings between mania and depression in the bipolar illness have been understood also in terms of alternating unconscious identifications with the two parents.

DIFFERENTIAL DIAGNOSIS Because somatic symptoms are not uncommon in patients with depression, it is important for us to be able to differentiate between the various types. Eighty percent of cases of bipolar illness start with an attack of mania, and most will have a manic attack early in the course of the illness. It is important to obtain this history, because the specific treatment for the variant is lithium carbonate, and this treatment should be prescribed and supervised by a psychiatrist.

Mania must be differentiated from schizophrenia, though this is not likely to arise in dermatology practice. Because bipolar patients with mania have less personality disorganization than the schizophrenics, they relate in a more normal, and a closer manner, and one can experience empathy for them. The prepsychotic personality type will be helpful too, in making the differentiation.

Paranoia must be differentiated from those patients with mania, who exhibit anger rather than the characteristic euphoria.

Depression as a symptom of neurosis too must be distinguished. Here the helpless, clinging, and dependent infantile quality of relating will not be prominent, the characteristic vegetative symptoms are less in evidence, and other signs and symptoms of the underlying neurotic conflict will be discernible. The patient will present as an intact individual, able to function though not perhaps to their highest capacity. Alcohol and drug abuse and acting-out behavior may be the expression of depression in the young.

COURSE AND OUTCOME The prognosis for a single episode is good, but recurrences are common. However, 80 percent of patients will recover fully, and only 10 percent will develop chronic illness.

Both early age at onset and a rigid, poorly adjusted pre-psychotic personality slant the prognosis unfavorably. Unlike the schizophrenic, mental deterioration is not a concomitant or a sequel of the affective disorders, and between attacks these patients function quite normally.

TREATMENT As mentioned earlier, the treatment of choice for bipolar illness is lithium carbonate. This drug both controls the manic phase and apparently prevents subsequent depressions. Tricyclic antidepressants may be needed in the depressive attacks.

In unipolar depression, mild cases will respond to analytically-oriented psychotherapy, and even more severe cases will benefit from this treatment in conjunction with either tricyclic antidepressants or mono-amine oxidase inhibitors. Electro-convulsive therapy is reserved for those patients who are resistant to drug therapy.

Psychotic Reactions in the Involutional Period

Involutional psychotic reactions are characterized either by depression or by paranoid ideation.

INVOLUTIONAL DEPRESSION

CLINICAL PICTURE Like neurotic depression, the bipolar and unipolar affective disorders, and the normal grief reaction, patients suffering from involutional depression experience a sense of loss. In this case, however, the loss is related to the physiologic changes of that period of life, and it is their inner meaning, implying as they do impending loss of valued functions through progressive ageing rather than the actual physiologic changes themselves, that have the greatest significance with regard to the onset of depressive symptoms. It is two to three times more common in women, in whom it also appears earlier—in the latter part of the fifth rather than the sixth decade. It is second only to schizophrenia among the functional mental disorders as a cause for hospital admission.

The background history of the patient who develops involutional depression is one of fundamental insecurity compensated for by a compulsive personality configuration, with honesty, frugality, overconscientious perfectionism, rigidity, lack of humor, and a propensity towards guilt and self-punishment; it seems likely that the involutional depression evolves out of a lifelong masked neurosis. The depressive features, however, have a more primitive character than do those in neurotic depression; by their helpless anxiety, repetitive and constant need for support, and clinging behavior, they suggest psychological regression to the level of the dependent infant in a patient who has failed early in life to develop appropriate defenses against loss, due to the early emotional deprivation that I have described.

The frank psychosis may be preceded for weeks to months by irritability, peevishness, loss of interest in usual pursuits, social withdrawal, indecisiveness, and doubt, associated with insomnia and crying spells. Depression, anxiety, agitation, hypochondriacal concerns, and feelings of unworthiness follow, and the patient presents wringing her hands in severe distress, proclaiming her guilt, hopelessness, and total lack of worth.

Misinterpretations and delusions contribute to and are projections of this guilt and shame. This may progress to further impairment of social functioning, sleep disturbance, refusal to eat, loss of weight, and agitation, the patient picking at skin and clothing in a restless agitated fashion.

In severe cases, the treatment of choice is electro-convulsive therapy, which in 50 percent of cases provides rapid improvement. Tricyclic antidepressants are also of benefit, but the prognosis is best in those whose premorbid personality was most healthy, and in whom the regressive deterioration has not reached the most profound levels.

DIFFERENTIAL DIAGNOSIS Involutional depression must be differentiated from the unipolar affective disorder, organic brain syndrome (cerebral arteriosclerosis), and neurotic depression. Age of onset, absence of previous episodes, and an obsessional rather than cyclothymic premorbid personality will distinguish the syndrome from manic-depressives psychosis, while the intense agitation, hypochondriacal and nihilistic ideas, the peevish clinging helplessness, the occasional hallucinations and delusions, stereotypes of speech and behavior, and the vegetative symptoms of insomnia, anorexia, and loss of weight help to rule out neurotic depression. The maintenance of an adequate level of social functioning and interaction, and the occasional characteristic attacks of acute anxiety with their physiologic concomitants of the neurotic are not seen in the involutional patient. Though the patient with organic brain syndrome may exhibit anxiety, hypochondriacal concerns, and unpleasant physical sensations, sustained fear is not present, and other features of organic change will be present.

PARANOID REACTION OF THE INVOLUTIONAL PERIOD

The premorbid personality of the patient with involutional paranoia is characterized by jealousy, suspiciousness, secretiveness, resentment, obstinacy, and a tendency to blame others for the patient's failures. With the onset of the psychosis these traits give way to misinterpretations, and frank but well-organised delusions usually of persecution. Anger, bitterness, hostility, and a propensity to bear grudges are common.

The prognosis in these patients is less good than in those with depression, and electroconvulsive therapy less effective. Antipsychotic drugs may be of some benefit in relieving symptoms.

Paranoid Reactions

There are patients who present with paranoid ideation or delusions, who conform neither to the picture of schizophrenia, nor to that of involutional paranoia. Their psychosis is psychogenic in origin, and develops insidiously as an exaggeration of personality features not uncommon in the population at large. Onset is usually before age 30, it is more common in men than in women, and it tends to be chronic. The family background is usually harshly critical, cruel, and authoritarian, with demanding parents frequently having set unrealistic goals for the patient. This harsh demanding and judgmental parental attitude generates fear and anxiety in the child, who develops a self-image of being "bad," and inadequate. Feelings of hatred, anger, and aggression towards the parents cannot be tolerated in such a repressive milieu, and instead of being expressed must be internalized. It is these internalized negative feelings that provide the driving force for the paranoid ideas and delusions that develop through projection. By this mechanism, internalized negative feelings become externalized again and are experienced by the patient as though directed against the self, cloaked in the structure of the patinet's particular delusional belief system.

As children, these patients are lonely, unhappy, insecure, and unable to relate satisfactorily with their peers. Later, they present with chip-on-shoulder, combative and aggressive as a defense against the perceived hostile environment, critical, intolerant and resentful of discipline. Mild paranoid features gradually evolve into a full-blown fixed paranoid delusional system; unlike the schizophrenic, however, these patients function quite normally in all aspects of their life that do not relate to their specific delusions. Because of the possibility of physical violence in these patients, treatment should ideally be undertaken by psychiatrists.

The Personality Disorders

When we speak of a personality disorder, we refer to a particular constellation of behavioral traits that, though aberrant, are so much a part of the personality structure of the individual that they do not feel alien to that individual. Rather than causing the individual emotional distress, it is those in the patient's environment who suffer on account of his or her idiosyncratic behaviors. Certain of the personality disorders are characterized by behaviors that on the one hand are merely an exaggeration of traits that are to a minor degree common to us all, or on the other hand are those that in patients with neurosis are used as defensive maneuvers to ward off the anxiety triggered in them by the mobilization of unconscious conflict. Included here would be the obsessive-complusive personality, paranoid personality, depressive personality, passive-dependent personality, and hysterical personality. The descriptive names speak for themselves. Though these may be tiresome people to be with, they function well and exhibit no formal disorders of thought. As they are in no conflict with regard to the overt expression of their particular personality traits, they do not develop neurotic symptoms, and are not likely spontaneously to seek treatment. They do, however, sometimes exhibit cutaneous symptoms for which they may come under our care: for example, simple neurotic excoriations are commonly encountered in patients who have an obsessive-compulsive personality configuration.

It will be evident, from the discussion on early development in Chapter 1, that these disordered personality structures result from a combination of factors. These factors include the genetic endowment of the individual, the developmental climate in which he or she grew up, and the specific environmental influences that are operative during critical periods of development. The sum total of these various factors, despite the aberrant features noted, has permitted the patient to develop an intact ego, with sufficient strength and resilience to cope with life in an adequate if not ideal fashion. More seriously flawed are patients with antisocial or psychopathic personalities, narcissistic personalities, and borderline personality disorders. These major disorders do not often exist in pure form, but rather demonstrate a preponderance of the characteristics of one, with an admixture of features from the others.

Antisocial or Sociopathic Personality Disorder

Characteristics suggestive of the antisocial personality disorder often can be detected as early as the early teens. These patients exhibit to a greater or lesser extent a lifelong pattern of social and moral deviancy. They lie, boast, and exaggerate, their affectional ties are shallow, and loyalty is uncommon. Without guilt, they manipulate the environment to serve their own ends, and indulge in a hedonistic abuse of drugs, alcohol, and sex. Impulsivity and poor judgement are prominent, insight into their personal behavior is lacking, and they tend to blame the environment rather than having the ability to take responsibility for their own actions. They do not learn from experience, frustration tolerance is extremely low, and a susceptibility to boredom leads them constantly to seek excitement, often through deviant means.

In addition, these patients are also susceptible to anxiety, insomnia, irritability, phobias, tics, and the development of major psychosis. Multiple somatic symptoms may be present, with secondary gain rather than unconscious guilt as the likely motivation. Under conditions of extreme stress, transient psychotic episodes may supervene.

Narcissistic Personality Disorder

Patients with a narcissistic personality disorder have undergone psychological deprivation very early in life. The deficits that result can be conceptualized as involving two major areas of functioning, the area of interpersonal relationships and the perception that the patient has of her or himself. It is from these two major deficits that the rest of the syndrome follows.

Because the individual has not had the opportunity to experience consistency in important nurturing figures early in life, he or she has failed to learn to integrate the good and bad qualities of others into one "whole" personality. As a result constant positive relationships are uncommon, the patient relating rather with feelings that alternate between idealization and devaluation, a situation known as "splitting." In terms of the doctor-patient relationship this clearly has important implications, but in personal life and in the work place it also has profound ramifications. Stable marriages are uncommon and a poor work history with frequent changes of occupation is the rule.

The other major deficit is a feeling of "entitlement" because of the early deprivation. The patient requires constant admiration and is manipulative and exploitative; insensitive to the needs or feelings of others, the patient sees everything only in terms of her or himself. The patient has a sense of uniqueness, or "specialness," for which he or she expects special favors, and the patient's fantasies are grandiose. However, this grandiosity is brittle and a mask for a sense of profound inadequacy, so that the patient is exquisitely sensitive to criticism, to which he or she is likely to respond with outbursts of rage, or cool indifference that hides shame. Unable to acknowledge failure, the patient resorts to rationalization or outright lying in his or her own defense, and to baseless bragging, in order to impress. Patients with this diagnosis are subject to episodes of depression and under extreme stress, they too may suffer brief psychotic episodes.

Borderline Personality Disorder

More important, in terms of dermatology practice, than either the antisocial or the narcissistic personality disorder, is the borderline disorder, since somatic symptoms in this group are not uncommon.

As is the case with the narcissistic disorder, early emotional deprivation leads to profound deficits in the borderline personality that have ramifications in every aspect of the individual's functioning. In terms of interpersonal relationships, splitting (see narcissistic personality disorder) is common, as is lack of empathy and interpersonal manipulation and exploitiveness. Splitting leads to inconstancy in relationships and in the work place, as described previously.

Two other features of this disorder lead to deviant behavior. These patients have a profound sense of emptiness, boredom, and intolerance of loneliness; this they attempt to relieve by promiscuous and deviant sexual behavior, by a constant search for thrills and excitement, and also by substance abuse. The other feature that I refer to is a deficit in the sense of self and of the self-image. Uncertainty may exist as to gender identity, and as to who they are or what are their long-term goals. Uncertainty about body-image and boundaries may also be a feature, and it is in an attempt to define these boundaries that sometimes these patients will resort to self-mutilation, as will be described later.

Their behavior is characterized by an unpredictability, lack of judgement, and poor impulse control. Gambling, spending, shoplifting, and overeating are common behaviors, as are recurrent accidents, outbursts of rage, and physical fights. As in the other two severe personality disorders that I have discussed, depression and irritability are common and brief psychotic episodes may occur.

The Neuroses

Neurotic syndromes arise as a result of unresolved unconscious conflict between the three intrapsychic agencies. These agencies are exemplified by (1) the needs of conscience; (2) the striving for gratification of the sensual and aggressive drives, in all of their overt, and also their derivative expressions; and (3) the rational requirements of the real world. The cardinal symptom of neurosis is anxiety, which will be aroused whenever unconscious conflict is mobilized, whether it be by external circumstances or by some internal process. The individual neurotic syndromes are each characterized by the particular repertoire of defense mechanisms that they employ to bind anxiety. These mechanisms do not often function perfectly; when this is the case, symptomatic anxiety or guilt or shame may be experienced directly, causing the patient to adopt further defensive measures and perhaps engage in symptomatic behavior to relieve the inner discomfort. Depression, secondary to the neurosis, is also a common symptom, but the majority of neurotic patients are able to function, with varying degrees of impairment, in their personal and social milieu; they experience their symptoms as painful and unwelcome, and their hold on reality is intact. I will review once again the psychodynamic view of neurotic symptoms.

During early child-development, in orderly sequence, certain anatomic sites each, for a period, take on a special sensual significance for the developing child. Experience during each of these phases acquires a coloring characteristic of the phase, while concurrent emotional difficulties will contribute in a characteristic way not only to personality structure, but also to the character of any symptoms that might arise as a result of those difficulties. These characteristic symptoms may also be encountered at a later date, as a result of regression to that level of emotional functioning, under the influence of stress. The mouth and skin hold sway during the first year of life, the ano-rectal area from the end of the first to the third year, and the external genitalia from the third to sixth year. These phases are not sharply separated, but rather, there is an overlapping in either direction, and the emotional flavoring of any one of them can influence behavior at any stage of life as a result of stress-induced regression.

I have previously explained that persons who experience emotional difficulties during the first year, when mouth and skin serve as primary sources of sensual gratification, and before the development of speech, are at risk of being developmentally disadvantaged. Some of these will demonstrate fragile and immature ego development. Not only are they more likely to express their feelings through somatic symptoms—either because they are not emotionally in touch with their feelings or because they have not had the opportunity to acquire language with which to express them—but they are also at greater than normal risk of developing a major personality disorder, or even psychosis. Though we do not believe that neurosis itself derives from the early period, yet some of its behavioral features may color the total symptom-complex of a neurosis, as a result of psychological regression. The features of which I speak would include such things as dependency, a decreased impulse control that might lead to over-eating, excessive smoking, over-medicating, or more severe forms of substance abuse, somatisation, and self-centered behavior that denies the needs of others.

Obsessive-Compulsive Neurosis

Obsessive-compulsive behavior may be seen as a personality configuration, as an obsessional neurosis, or as a part of the picture of a psychosis. It derives from the period during which the growing child is caught in a struggle between the child's wish for omnipotent self-assertion on the one hand and the necessity to conform to parental demands in order to keep their love and acceptance on the other; this coincides with the period of early toilet training when ano-rectal sensuality is prominent during the second and third years of life. Often the mother is rigid, compulsive, and inflexible in her demands for compliance, threatening punishment and withdrawal of love for disobedience. The rage that her demands arouse must be repressed in the child in order not to lose her love. While defiant behavior may gratify the child's wish for the mother's attention, the child must pay for that two-fold, by ultimately giving in to her demands, she being the stronger, and also by undergoing her punishment. Once this behavioral sequence is internalized, during the course of development, it will be activated unconsciously and automatically whenever angry thoughts are aroused. It is this conflict between defiant rage, with the associated guilt and need for punishment on the one hand, and the need to please in order to be loved on the other that accounts for the characteristic ambivalence of the obsessional. In addition to obsessional thoughts and compulsive acts, obsessional defenses include perfectionism, intolerance of mistakes or of being wrong, inability to relax, an over-developed sense of duty, and difficulty in confronting anger directly.

Hysterical Neurosis

Traditionally the genesis of hysterical neurosis has been thought to occur in the period between the third and the sixth years, when sexual identity is becoming firm, and relationships negotiated on that basis. It is during this period that identification with the parent of the same sex, and a loving relationship with that of the opposite sex—with all of its conscious and unconscious implications—sets the pattern for future ways of relating. Some authors suggest a genesis at a much earlier period, but this would seem to cloud the picture by including in the spectrum of neurosis features of the personality disorders. There is a current trend to describe as separate entities the different clinical presentations of hysteria, but because of common psychodynamic mechanisms I shall include here those entities now termed somatization disorder, conversion disorder, psychogenic pain disorder, hypochondriasis, phobic disorder, etc.

Interference during this phase of emotional development then, between the third and sixth years, may result in a failure in the development of adult ways of relating. Most commonly a woman, such a person may retain a childish and dependent attachment to her parents, a flamboyant style of presenting herself, and a wish for early gratification rather than being willing to set for herself long-term goals. Despite a coquettishness, she is frequently confused about sexual issues, and may reject her adult feminine role in a variety of ways. Unconscious conflict may have to do with sexual issues or with aggression or assertiveness, and a plethora of defensive mechanisms are employed against the anxiety that may be aroused when the conflict is mobilized. Foremost among these is repression, by means of which uncomfortable thoughts or feelings are simply lost to consciousness, as though they had never happened. If repression is incomplete, than a number of second-line defenses come into play: there may be displacement onto an innocent, though associationally or symbolically related object, with development of a phobia; there may be a hysterical conversion reaction in which by symbolization and condensation a physical symptom comes to represent both sides of the unconscious conflict; any one of multiple types of somatic symptoms may develop for which no underlying cause can be uncovered; a disassociational state may ensue, in which the patient may engage in activities that she will not later recollect, and during the course of which she has no memory of her usual life situation, as happens most dramatically in patients with multiple personalities; the patient may experience depression; or, it may be that the anxiety will break through, with an outburst of rage, hyperventilation, an anxiety attack, or a full-blown panic attack.

From the foregoing it will be clear that this group of patients is of particular significance in the practice of dermatology because of the multiplicity of physical symptoms that may occur. These may include pruritus, pain in skin, rectum, vagina, or mouth, or concern out of proportion to the physical symptoms of an established dermatosis, among others. Some cases of factitial disease are included here also, either as the result of a dissociative phenomenon or for secondary gain, and these must be distinguished from those occurring in psychosis or in the personality disorders. Unlike patients in these two latter groups, who are intensely involved with the most minute details of their physical complaints, the hysterical patient tends to be rather vague about her symptoms—the well-known "poor historian"—and often dramatic in her presentation. Symptoms of anxiety or depression can often be elicited, and serve as helpful diagnostic features, as does a family history of similar problems, often in the mother, and poor psychosexual adjustment. "Belle indifference" is often noted, and the physical symptoms will be found to provide for the patient a secondary gain in terms of some manipulation of the environment, to satisfy a personal need.

Anxiety Neurosis

This condition, now known as Generalized Anxiety Disorder, may be diagnosed when persistent tension has been present for 1 month or more, and when phobic symptoms or panic attacks do not form part of the picture. Symptoms are those we associate with anxiety, such as palpitations, tachycardia, shortness of breath, sighing, insomnia, urinaria frequency, diarrhoea and vomiting, anorexia, fatigue, shakiness and weakness, etc.

As with hysterical neurosis, this condition is more common in women than in men; it is often attributed to such physical conditions as heart disease, hypoglycemia or thyrotoxicosis, and episodes of secondary depression supervene in as many 40 percent of patients.

Anxiety neurosis is merely a descriptive name for the presenting features in this disorder, and gives no indication of the underlying neurotic conflict, or of a possible psychodynamic formulation. Unstructured psychodynamic interviewing technique is required to uncover this important information, and insight-oriented psychotherapy is indicated in order to spare the patient from a dependence on drugs, or from shopping from doctor to doctor for relief of symptoms. It is possible that stress-management techniques such as are taught by biofeedback and behavior modification programs may be helpful in providing symptomatic relief, but they will of course do nothing to mitigate the underlying neurosis.

REFERENCES

1. Kaplan HJ, Sadock BJ: Comprehensive Textbook of Psychiatry/IV (ed 4). Baltimore, Williams and Wilkins, 1985
2. Kolb LC, Brodie HKH: Modern Clinical Psychiatry (ed 10). Philadelphia, WB Saunders Co, 1982
3. Ludwig AM: Principles of Clinical Psychiatry. New York, The Free Press, 1980

Chapter 5

General Principles of Evaluation and Treatment

This chapter will consider in broad terms the general principles of evaluation and treatment of psychocutaneous disease, based on a logical integration of the physical manifestations, with an understanding of the level of psychopathology as derived from information of the type contained in the previous chapter. I will take up the specific treatment for individual conditions subsequently, in the appropriate sections.

INITIAL OBSERVATIONS

A warm and empathetic approach will enable one to learn much during the first contact in the consulting room. Assume you have a male patient in your waiting room. Is the patient appropriately attired and well-groomed? Does he appear anxious, depressed, or agitated? Has he come alone, or is his spouse along for moral support, or to ensure that he tells his story accurately? This latter observation gives an indication of the way in which the patient views himself, either as a mature and competent individual, or as immature in regard to health matters, denying the significance of symptoms because of anxiety, and so relying on his spouse to take charge and ensure that he is adequately taken care of. If this is the case, then one can anticipate that he will have similar expectations of his physician, and that he will not expect to have to take responsibility himself, for his well-being.

THE INITIAL HISTORY

How is the history given? How sophisticated is the patient with regard to health matters? What is the quality of his thought process? Does he assign to himself a "specialness" with regard to his illness? Does he try to manipulate the circumstances by flattering you, in the unconscious expectation of getting preferential treatment, or of magically ensuring a favorable outcome, or is he belligerent and provocative? Is the history rambling and circumstantial, or is it given in clear and straightforward fashion?

What of the history? Does it make sense in the light of what we know of the anatomy and pathophysiology of the skin, or is there disordered thought, with delusional beliefs or hallucinatory perceptions? Are you but one in a long sequence of unsatisfactory consultants? If this is so, then you must be alert to the likelihood that you will fare no better than your predecessors unless you are willing to address this issue directly. If you can help the patient to look at this, by pointing out to him that he has already consulted Doctors X, Y, and Z unsuccessfully, you can then ask what he hopes you can do that they have not been able to do and in this way you may learn something of his fantasies both about what you can contribute, and about his illness, and the purpose that it serves in his life. Does the patient describe a multiplicity of other symptoms, or is his problem confined to the skin? Has he failed to respond to treatments that on the surface would appear to be appropriate to his condition as you see it? Are there others in the family who have had long or multiple illnesses, or puzzling symptoms with whom he may identify? Has there been a recent illness or death in the family?

What is the history with regard to smoking, alcohol, and medications? Is the use of medication likely to be rational, or is there a possibility of abuse, either of medication, or of recreational or addictive drugs? And what of his relationships—are they able to survive the stresses of daily living, permitting him to maintain a stable marriage and a consistent work-record? Or is he a loner? Is his past strewn with a series of divorces from spouses and from jobs, with intervening periods of loneliness and unemployment?

All of the information in the preceding paragraphs can be gleaned during the initial consultation or in the course of a few succeeding short interviews. The nature of the presenting dermatologic complaint will determine the way that one will view the patient, and the type of history that one will be interested in obtaining. Obviously in the patient with warts, or a simple hand eczema—in most cases straightforward dermatologic problems—one is not likely to take time to concern oneself with a detailed psychological history. On the other hand, the patient with concerns about parasitosis will direct one's interest towards the quality of his mode of relating, and the nature of the thought process, in order to define whether he is psychotic and delusional, or a neurotic, with obsessional concerns. These two examples are fairly straightforward, and the assessment can be made quite quickly. It is the patient whose skin disease falls into the third group in the classification listed in Table 4-1, that falls into the gray area, with issues that are not clear-cut; here one's skills in gathering and applying useful information are most challenged. This question will be taken up in more detail a little later.

THE THERAPEUTIC RELATIONSHIP

The relationship between doctor and patient is a very special one. Both partners bring to it attitudes and expectations that will determine the particulars of its specific nature, but the basic form has its genesis in much earlier relationships, and most particularly in the biologically determined attachment bond of the infant;[22] the quality of this bond colors all future human interactions. Because of this early biological bond, parenting figures commonly provide loving support and acceptance, relieve pain, and alleviate fear; the patient comes into the therapeutic relationship with the expectation that these same needs, occasioned now by illness, will again be met. This positive attitude serves as the first step in the therapeutic process, and the expectation of recovery that it carries is a powerful force for healing. It is important to remember that the therapeutic process is already started when the patient first makes his appointment, and before he even steps into the office.

Apart from the direct physical impairment of function with which as physicians we are all familiar, illness inevitably carries with it profound psychological implications for the patient. For the malingerer this may well be a feeling of superiority and triumph, while for the patient in whom illness is a way of life,[7] who engages habitually in "illness behavior," it will bring gratification in the form of the nurturing and the abdiction of responsibility that he craves. For any patient the meaning may be understood at many levels, the deepest of which can be uncovered only through psychotherapy directed towards the unravelling of unconscious processes. But for most, at a more superficial level, the onset of illness brings with it a feeling of loss of control, through disruption of the familiar, the "taken-for-grantedness" of things, and a split in the unselfconscious harmony between body and self that causes attention to be focussed consciously on the body.[1] This change in experience may give rise to feelings of strangeness and confusion with which patients may need help in coming to terms, while symptoms may also be experienced as a source of weakness, or of shame.

The physician who is empathic, accepting, and nonjudgmental, and who treats the patient with dignity and respect, will by his or her attitude foster the relationship and help it to work for the physician, to the benefit of both. The physician's strength and support will enable the patient to tolerate the anxiety and emotional regression that are generated by illness; frankness and honesty will engender the trust that despite accurate diagnosis, and appropriate medication, is essential for cure to take place.

Just such a positive relationship is the norm, but some patients who, because negative early life experiences have precluded the development of basic trust, bring with them into the therapeutic relationship, as they do into all of their relationships, suspiciousness and hostility, or an angry need to prove the other wrong; in them, profound anxiety may masquerade as truculence, intransigence, depression, tiresome clinging dependence, or noncompliance. These patients constitute the proverbial 10 percent who generate 90 percent of the problems; they have been described in the literature as "the hateful patient."[19]

It is in the management of these patients that to be effective, the physician must be in touch with his or her own feelings. The physician must recognize that his or her own anger is in reaction to feelings of helplessness and defensiveness aroused by the patient's negative behavior, Once this is clear, instead of responding to anger with anger, and so giving the patient justification for negative feelings, and validation for the patient's alienation, or perhaps even driving the patient away, the physician can instead defuse the situation and disarm the patient by addressing directly the anxiety that lies beneath the bombast. As an example, a physician advised a young woman that she should give consideration to having an atypical nevus excised from her earlobe. Some hours later the woman's husband called in extreme anger. "What do you mean she should have this removed? You mean she'll lose half her ear? What do you mean suggesting that? That's a heck of a thing to tell anyone!" To which the physician replied, "I realize that you are angry with me because you are very anxious about your wife and about what may happen to her. It sounds almost as though you feel that it's my fault that she has this lesion." By addressing the underlying anxiety, and so making the patient look at his anger, this physician enabled him to see how inappropriate was his response, and the tension was relieved. He was then able to "hear" what the physician was telling him about the treatment that would be required, and accept it with understanding.*

The physician who does not recognize what is going on in the interaction with a patient may feel threatened, and may find her or himself pressured into making decisions that are not in the long run in the best interest of the patient. The physician may, for example, dismiss the "troublemaker" as quickly as possible to be rid of his or her nemesis, or alternatively, may find her or himself led to over-diagnosing and over-treating for his or her own peace of mind. We must be willing to accept that there are some patients that are simply not open to any kind of treatment, whom we cannot help; these should arouse neither guilt, nor a sense of failure. And we must have the courage to diagnose nondisease, not ordering ever more sophisticated tests, or going to greater excesses of therapeutic endeavor, in our determination to provide a life without discomfort for our patients, or the "cure" that we may implicitly have seemed to promise.

Here, two pertinent examples come to mind. A pediatrician had been called innumerable times by the very anxious and demanding mother of an apparently healthy atopic child, because she could not tolerate his incessant scratching. The physician had patiently tried to reassure the mother but despite his recommen-

*Koblenzer PJ: Personal communication, 1985.

dations for measures to control the itching, and the appropriate medications that he had prescribed, the situation remained unchanged. Finally late on a Saturday, his working day not yet finished and his patience exhausted, another call seemed to be the last straw, making him to feel angry and defensive. In desperation he asked her to bring the child in for an intramuscular injection of triamcinalone. This unhappy sequence of events was followed some weeks later by yet another panic call, when Mother noticed an area of subcutaneous atrophy at the injection site. Had the physician felt less threatened by this mother's anxiety, he might have been free to observe the interaction between her and her child, which by focussing on the itching and scratching served to perpetuate it. He could then have used this knowledge to help the mother interact in a more healthy way with her child, permitting the symptoms to be given up, or at least ameliorated, the child spared much medication, and the couple much misery.

The second example is a young girl of 10 with extensive alopecia areata. This girl's mother was content to pursue an expectant course, and she had herself raised the possibility of psychiatric referral. She believed her daughter to be a perfectionist, and to place demands upon herself that she could not meet—a symptom that is often derivative of unconscious guilt.[9] Instead, the family was referred to a pediatric endocrinologist, who prescribed long-term oral adrenocorticosteroids, adding cushingoid features to her already rather bizarre appearance. While some dermatologists believe long-term oral steroids to be appropriate treatment for alopecia areata,[27] in this case it seemed clear that the treatment choice was largely motivated by the needs of the physician who was made anxious by this bald little girl, rather than the patient, whose need it was to understand why she subjected herself to such unreasonable pressure.

Finally, the physician must be aware of, and have gained mastery over, his or her feelings about diseased skin, lest he or she unconsciously communicate to the patient, by manner or by touch, feelings of revulsion or of lack of acceptance. We must also keep in mind the effect that chronic disfiguring or disabling skin disease will inevitably have on self-esteem and on the body image, and we must be ready to help our patient to come to terms with these, within the context of a supportive and accepting doctor-patient relationship.

CLINICAL MANAGEMENT

Group 1 Patients (see Table 4-1)

These are the patients in whom the skin disease is a secondary manifestation of what is primarily a psychiatric disorder. As has been noted in the literature,[13] when these patients present to a dermatologist, by this act they deny psychopathology and state clearly how they wish to be treated. This wish is based on an unconscious psychological defense, and if we are to be successful, it behooves us to respect it: with very few exceptions, therefore, it is prudent not immediately to confront the patient with our findings, or to suggest a psychiatric referral. Rather, it is more fruitful to hear the patient out, and without judgment empathize with his or her discomfort, and with the restrictions that his or her disease imposes on the patient's life; one can prescribe symptomatic treatment and set up frequent short appointments for its supervision. These frequent contacts, however brief, serve to maintain continuity and permit the best possible relationship to develop, within the context of which symptoms may simply be given up, or a point may be reached where the possiblity of a psychiatric referral can be mooted.

Patients within this group may lie anywhere along the spectrum of psychopathology, from severe psychosis with complete disorganization of the personality and complex and pervasive delusional systems at one end, to the mild neurotic with perhaps acne excoriee at the other. The level of psychopathology will determine the disposition of the patient.

Those who are severely psychotic, who are not functioning in any area of their lives, and who cannot relate in any meaningful way constitute the one exception to the admonition not to confront the patient with the nature of his or her disease. Often these patients have in mind a specific treatment that fits the requirements of their delusional beliefs, and frequently they will reject even recommendations for topical treatment. Better here to acknowledge that you cannot help, and that psychiatric care is indicated; if family members are available, they may perhaps help in ensuring that such help is obtained.

When the personality disorganization is less extreme, however, and if there is some level of personal and social functioning, even though the patient may have little capacity for insight, he or she may respond favorably to an empathic and supportive approach to symptomatic treatment, with the possible addition of psychotropic drugs. The patients included here are those with circumscribed delusions related to the skin, and those who have the borderline personality configuration and an associated skin disease. Their relationships, however, tend to be dependent in nature, and characterized by idealization and unrealistic expectations, but their anger is not far from the surface. While they can continue to anticipate that you will be able to help them, or while things continue to go well in the treatment, these patient will respond positively; should that change, they will feel betrayed, anger will be mobilized, and they will move on to your colleague. The cycle will be repeated over and over again, with doctor after doctor; any attempt at encouraging introspection or at reaching an understanding of the unconscious meaning of the symptom in these patients is likely to be frustrated.

Those patients who are less psychiatrically impaired, for example those with neurosis, will often do well with simple reassurance and appropriate topical measures, and it is only in the persistant and recalcitrant cases that further psychiatric measures might be indicated. Should this be the case, then an estimate of the maturity of the personality will determine the treatment recommended. In patients with greater ego strength, characterized by good impulse control, the ability to distinguish reality from fantasy, willingness to take responsibility for self-motivation and to tolerate frustration, resilience, a capacity for insight, and the ability to develop meaningful relationships, the insight-oriented therapies, and most particularly psychoanalysis would be the treatments that offer greatest hope for real maturational changes within the personality. Patients whose personality development is less mature, on the other hand, and whose mode of relating is more dependent, will do better with supportive psychotherapy. Antidepressants may be indicated in either group. In summary then: patients who present with cutaneous symptoms and who fall into this group are assessed with a view to determining the level of psychopathology (see Table 4-2), based on the information in the previous chapter. Those who are severely disturbed and whose thoughts are grossly disordered should be advised that one cannot help, and although success is by no means assured, an attempt should be made to obtain for them psychiatric treatment. Those whose personality is less severely disordered should not be confronted about their disease or judged, but rather heard empathically, and treated symptomatically; in some cases psychotropic drugs may be added to topical and supportive treatment. This is best accomplished in the course of frequent even quite short office visits. If some level of trust can be achieved, a point may be reached at which the question of referral can safely be mooted, without arousing anger and driving the patient away; unfortunately this is not often successful, and patients seldom follow through. Patients who are neurotic may require only a positive and reassuring attitude together with symptomatic treatment in order to give up their symptoms, even if they do not openly acknowledge any part they themselves may play in the etiology; those with more serious underlying neurotic conflict, however, may require an insight-oriented therapeutic approach. Tricyclic antidepressants may be helpful in controlling symptoms, but there is a less clear place for the use of minor tranquilizers; this, and the use of narcoleptics will be discussed later, in the section on psychotropic drugs.

Group 2 Patients

In each of the conditions included in the second group, there is a physical basis for the pathophysiology, but in each too, psychosocial stress is thought often to be the trigger that sets that pathophysiologic process in motion, once clear-cut physical or environmental factors have been ruled out.

In each case, therefore, the evaluation must include a careful screening to ensure that there is no underlying medical disease, and that the environment is not in some way contributing to the disease process. A trial of symptomatic treatment is then in order, and only should that fail, would there be a need to enquire more deeply into the contribution of the emotions. The time spent in this initial evaluation will have permitted a superficial assessment of the mental and emotional status. Generally speaking one will find that these patients are less impaired psychologically than are those in the first group.

The next step is to explore what is going on currently in the patient's life, in its social, professional, and personal aspects, and to look for patterns in regard to the waxing and waning of symptoms. This information is most successfully obtained by adopting an accepting and nonjudgmental attitude, and a technique of gentle open-ended questioning.[19] Gradually it may be possible to point out the relationships that one has observed, between circumstance and symptom, and so convince the patient that it is his or her emotional life that should be addressed. Not infrequently this information, arrived at in an accepting and supportive environment, will relieve the patient of anxiety, and the symptoms may simply resolve; alternatively the patient may wish to try a more vigorous medical approach, or one of the short-term psychological therapies, for example biofeedback. Another possibility is that the patient may elect to "live" with the symptoms, which are now rendered tolerable by the relief of his or her anxiety. But in a small percentage of patients it will become clear that the somatic complaint is symptomatic of a more pervasive neurosis, that is interfering also in other aspects of the patient's life. In such a case, it may be possible to achieve a successful psychiatric referral by gently reflecting back the information that he or she has given you, and making the connections for the patient between circumstance and symptom.

Group 3 Patients

The patients in the third group are perhaps the most difficult of all to manage, for we are dealing here with the common or "garden" dermatoses, the bread and butter of our practice. What is it then that alerts one to the possibility that this is no ordinary case, and that emotional influences must be given serious consideration? It is in these conditions that the delicate balance between the stresses of daily living—environmental, physical, and emotional—on the one hand, and the sum of the defenses, physiologic and psychologic, on the other, is most tenuous, and most difficult to evaluate because of the multifactorial nature of the possible stresses involved (Fig. 5-1).

Take for example a patient with atopic eczema that suddenly and seemingly out of nowhere undergoes a severe flare; is it because of contact with irritants? Or dermatitis medicamentosa? Has the patient an intercurrent illness, or a pregnancy? Is there a secondary infection with staphylococcus aureus or the herpes simplex virus? Or could it be that the patient has just learned that her husband is romantically involved with his secretary? Any one of these possibilities might apply.

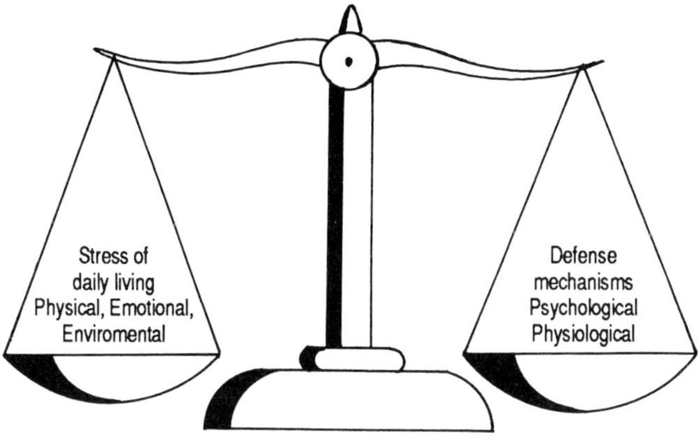

Figure 5-1. It is the balance between the stresses of daily living and the body's defenses that determines health or disease.

In situations where the dermatosis is recalcitrant to treatment despite a careful evaluation of the various possible complicating factors, or alternatively in situations where the symptoms seem to be out of proportion to the manifest disease process, one must be alert to the need to explore the emotional element, proceeding in much the same way as I have described for patients in Group 2.

MAKING A PSYCHIATRIC REFERRAL

It is the rare patient, presenting to a physician with a physical symptom, who will not initially offer resistance to the suggestion of a psychiatric referral. The reasons for this are several. In those patients who are not in touch with their feelings, or who have not developed the capacity for explaining or describing them, resistance may be based on simple disbelief, for lack of supporting experiential evidence. For many patients the concept of psychiatric need carries a negative connotation, with the suggestion of inadequacy or inherent weakness on their part, and the associated painful affects of guilt and shame; these patients, must deny the perceived failure, and avoid the anticipated social stigma. But perhaps the most pervasive underlying reason is an unconscious and irrational fear of what they might find within themselves, and what upsets may be wrought in their lives as a result of psychotherapeutic endeavor; these are risks they are not willing readily to take.

It is usually advisable, therefore, to prepare the patient for referral gradually over several visits. If the referral is to be successful, these visits will be used to obtain information that can be reflected back to the patient in such a way as to make a persuasive case. One can, for example, point out that it has become evident that the cutaneous disease is just one aspect of a more pervasive disorder. Here one can remind the patient of other symptoms you and the patient have uncovered, such as anxiety, depression, insomnia, headaches, difficulties in relationships or on the job, fatigue, and so forth. Remind the patient that the somatic aspects of the disease have been appropriately taken care of. Point out to the patient again the relationship that you two have observed between exacerbations and particular life circumstances. Empathize with the discomfort the patient experiences, and with the ways in which all of the various symptoms interfere in his or her life and ability to function optimally. Empathize with the negative feelings of self-worth that the symptoms arouse, and with the frustration the patient must feel that things have not improved despite all that has been tried. Help the patient also to understand the multifactorial psychosociobiologic view of the etiology of disease. Many patients have an "either/or" view, seeing disease as wholly physical or wholly emotional (and therefore unacceptable and crazy); for them a holistic view is philosophically more palatable, and something that they can gradually come to accept realistically. All of this information one has learned from the patient, and by reflecting it back in a way that appeals to his or her reason and logic, even if the patient cannot accept it at once, often in time he or she will accept a referral.

PSYCHIATRIC TREATMENT MODALITIES

Although most of us as dermatologists have neither time, inclination, or expertise to engage in psychiatric treatment, it is sometimes helpful to know what to expect for one's patients, and to be able to allay some of their anxiety about upcoming consultations; for these reasons I shall describe briefly some of the more usual treatment modalities. Specific indications will be discussed later, in the appropriate sections.

Consultation-Liaison Psychiatry

As with any medical referral, it is helpful to find a specialist in one's practice area with whom one can relate, and who is willing to discuss problems, and work along with you in any given case. Naturally the patient's confidentiality must be respected, but useful information can still be shared, guidance given, and a unified treatment regimen formulated. Sharing of information in this way precludes the patient's unconsciously playing one physician against the other for secondary gain, or getting lost in the cracks between the two disciplines.

The ideal format for integrated care, is the consultation-liaison clinic.[21] Such clinics operate successfully in many centers in Europe, including Florence,[25] Paris, Ghent, Amsterdam, and in Israel; Gould and Gragg have written about their experience at Stanford, in the United States.[13]

The organization and immediate objectives of these clinics vary, but all are oriented towards providing a total care for the patient, by acknowledging the psychosociobiologic multifactorial etiology of disease and addressing all aspects. The ideal would seem to be to set aside space within the confines of the dermatology clinic, designating regular and specific times for the liaison clinic to be in session. Minimal staffing would be a dermatologist and a psychiatrist, jointly to undertake evaluation of patients referred from the regular dermatology clinic. Appointments would be made for 45 or 50 minutes, and the evaluation would include, in addition to a complete dermatology examination, at least one, and perhaps two or three psychiatric interviews in order to make a diagnostic formulation and develop a treatment plan. The ideal, however, is a team approach, including a clinical psychologist to undertake psychological testing where this is indicated, and psychiatric social workers. These ancillary workers can provide valuable help in dealing with reality environmental issues, where the patient's functioning is less than optimal, and also in the evaluation and treatment process, under supervision of the psychiatrist. A Utopian clinic might also include facilities for biofeedback training, and space for various support group activities and the like. Once the evaluation is complete, the patient may either continue in treatment with the dermatologist who will consult occasionally with the psychiatrist, the patient may be referred for biofeedback training, should this be indicated, or for psychotherapy: in this latter case the psychiatrist will consult occasionally with the dermatologist, who will continue the routine dermatologic treatment.

There is great advantage in having the liaison clinic within the confines of the regular dermatology clinic. This permits it to assume a place along with phototherapy, patch-testing, and dermatologic surgery as a part of the normal spectrum of dermatologic practice, rather than some alien, suspect, and terrifying concept.

At Stanford, Gould and Gragg see their objective as primarily educational, affording dermatology residents an opportunity to learn about psychological aspects of the specialty, and to witness at firsthand techniques of interviewing, strategic questioning, and listening.

In Florence, Italy, however, dermatology-liaison is a much more evolved activity;[25] a full staff of psychiatrists and psychologists are exploring the application of sophisticated methods for testing and documentation, in an attempt more clearly to delineate and quantify psychosomatic processes in dermatology. Patients receive integrated but separate dermatologic and psychiatric evaluations that proceed through sequential steps, each determined by the previous findings, and carried out in a multi-disciplinary milieu where jargon is minimized and where any sense of "labeling" or "dumping" is avoided. Work-up in addition to the dermatologic history and physical examination includes an anamnestic psychiatric history and a number of psychodiagnostic tests. Information is stored in a data bank from which graphs and tables are formulated, for use in diagnostic comparison and therapeutic projection. One hopes such facilities as this will, with increasing knowledge and with increasing validation of information, become more widespread and more readily available.

Obviously the harsh economic realities make such cooperation difficult in the private sector. However, exchange of information such as I described earlier, is certainly feasible, and for those dermatologists with a particular interest, it is possible to arrange the work schedule in order to accommodate a small number of extended interviews each week in which to undertake superficial or supportive psychotherapy under supervision of a willing psychiatrist whom you trust.

Insight-Oriented Therapies

The insight-oriented psychotherapies are based on the premise that current attitudes and modes of reaction are governed by past experience, and that phenomena in adult life that are seemingly unintelligible take on meaning when understood in the context of earlier experience. The objectives of treatment are to restructure the personality in such a way as to reorganize maladaptive patterns of behavior, redirect feelings and drives into constructive channels, afford relief from disabling fears and inhibitions, and foster insight sufficient to handle the conflicts and stresses of everyday life. "Free-association" is the medium through which this is achieved, and by means of which unconscious trends are uncovered. Old patterns of relating and old expectations and fantasies are reactivated within the doctor-patient relationship, where they can then be examined, understood, and subjected to change.

Psychoanalysis is the most intensive of these therapies and the one that can produce the most fundamental restructuring of the personality. Not all patients are able or willing to commit the time or money that a psychoanalysis requires, however, and in consequence a variety of short-term and less-intensive therapies have developed that have their roots in psychoanalytic theory. They, too, focus on the "dynamic unconscious," that unconscious component of the mind in which memory traces from the past with all of their attendant emotional baggage live on, influencing current actions, thoughts, and feelings. These brief and less intensive dynamic psychotherapies may be quite formalized, with specific goals set at the outset, and sometimes a time-limit established for the process: studies suggest that the outcome of these therapies will bear a strong relationship to the expectations of the two participants.[8] They may demonstrate a more rapid early improvement than does psychoanalysis, but a plateau is reached between 6 and 12 months, and improvement slow thereafter. In psychoanalysis, improvement will continue through time, and a greater level of general functioning can be achieved.[22]

Other Expressive Therapies

A number of other approaches rely on the therapeutic benefit of insight and emotional expression, but the focus is more superficial, with no attempt at uncovering unconscious material, or understanding the dynamics of unconscious motivation. Problems are addressed at a conscious level, and solutions sought for specific situations. In other cases the therapist may be confronting, or the process may rely on ventilation or abreaction for relief of anxiety.

Hypnosis

Hypnosis has been defined as an induced state of dissociation produced through suggestion.[22] Thirty percent of the population are found to be susceptible to trance induction, and a further 30 percent moderately so.[17] The implication of this type of susceptibility with regard to the expected outcome of other psychotherapeutic treatment modalities is unclear, but the ability to trust, and to give up control both are implicit.

Hypnosis proved to be a valuable tool in the study of psychophysiologic responses in the skin, particularly in the early days of psychosomatic research; some of this work has been discussed in Chapter 3. In psychiatric practice it is a valuable modality for treatment of hysterical conversion reactions, the recovery of lost memories, and in the study of childhood behavior, but memories recovered in this way do not carry the same ring of emotional understanding and emotional truth as do those recovered through the lifting of repression in a psychodynamic therapeutic process; because of this, their use by the patient can only be intellectual at best, and as Freud found, resultant change is by no means assured. Hypnosis has been used also for dental anesthesia,[17] and in obstetrics.[17] Dermatologic applications include among other conditions the treatment of pruritus,[5] warts,[27] and vitiligo,[11] but the reported results are hard to evaluate because of the number of variables, including differing individual susceptibility to suggestion. There are certain drawbacks to hypnotic treatment; while in appropriate subjects it may with dramatic rapidity bring symptomatic relief, the psychodynamic etiologic factors remain unconscious, and the fundamental personality problem remains unchanged. Further, hypnotic suggestions lose their effect over time, so the danger exists that instead of increasing the patient's ability to solve problems independently, the patient may develop a dependence on the hypnotist; this can perhaps be avoided by using insight-oriented treatment in conjunction with hypnosis for long-term change.[22]

Suppressive Treatment

Rather than uncovering unconscious material through free association, treatment here is directed towards strengthening repression and the other psychological defenses. Treatment modalities include persuasion and suggestion as well as supportive psychotherapy. No attempt is made to gain insight into unconscious proccesses, ego strengths are supported by reassurance, and the therapist may assist in decision-making , provide guidance as to action, or intervene to modify the environment so as to relieve the patient of stress. The treatment takes place in one or two sessions per week, and there may be adjunctive use of psychotropic drugs. This treatment is more appropriate to patients who are more severely psychologically impaired, who lack the capacity for insight, who have immature personality structures, or whose capacity for reality testing is incomplete. Included would be patients with severe neurotic depression, psychotic depression, the personality disorders, or psychosis.

Behavior Therapy

Behavior therapy is based on the theory that all behaviors are learned in the process of growing up. Maladaptive behavior represents a breakdown in the learning process, which can be repaired by re-education; emphasis in the treatment is placed on the control of behavior through its consequences. No consideration is given to the inner life, or unconscious motivation, but it has become clear that ongoing and current influences that serve to maintain pathologic behavior must be identified and addressed if the treatment is to be successful.[22] A careful analysis of the various stimulating and perpetuating circumstances must be made, and learning situations designed to bring about change must be individualized; these determinations may be very time-consuming. A variety of techniques are utilized in the re-learning process; these include positive and negative reinforcement, aversive therapy, operant conditioning, and desensitization.

Biofeedback

Biofeedback is a form of behavioral therapy. Through this modality the patient makes a conscious effort to modify his or her physical status, using bioelectric instrumentation to provide immediate visual or auditory feedback in response to physical change. It relies on the learning of relaxation techniques, and although it has been used in stress management, and in a variety of stress-related physical conditions,[28] valid evidence of benefit to date is confined only to the treatment of tension headaches.[26] The feedback of brain-waves has been used in order to achieve the Alpha state of relaxation, a state in which brain-wave activity is at 7.5-13.5 cycles/sec; similar alpha relaxation can be achieved by transcendental meditation.[22]

Some authors claim a 70 percent success rate in the treatment of Raynaud's phenomenon using biofeedback techniques.[23] It has also been used for control of hyperhidrosis,[23] and in its relaxation aspect, for treatment of such conditions as trichotillomania and neurotic excoriations, but anecdotal reports only are available.

Support Groups

Though not strictly speaking a psychotherapeutic modality, groups established for the mutual support of individuals suffering from a particular disease and their families, do operate according to group theory. In dermatology such groups have been established for a number of genetic and nongenetic disabling or disfiguring dermatoses such as ichthyosis, epidermolysis bullosa, psoriasis, and alopecia areata. At a strictly practical and superficial level, these groups permit exchange of information about the day to day handling of different aspects of the disease. At a deeper level, and perhaps more importantly, groups that are cohesive take on the characterisitics of a family, with members unconsciously assuming the roles of parents and siblings;[22] within this context mutual support and comfort are given, and the sense of alienation reduced through the medium of shared problems. Ego strengths and self-esteem are enhanced through identification with other group members and through an increasing awareness and mastery of difficulties associated with the disease that are common to the group.

Psychopharmacology

As with any class of drugs, the plethora of available psychoactive agents can be confusing, and the practitioner will do well to become familiar with one or two only within each class. Unfortunately, not only is the metabolism of these drugs subject to individual variation, but the psychiatric syndromes for which they are used are not homogeneous, so that in practice if one drug does not produce the desired effect, it may be necessary to substitute another.

Tricyclic Antidepressants and Related Drugs

Imipramine hydrochloride was the first in the tricyclic antidepressants group to become available, but as more recent analogues have been developed, their structure has become more diverse, so heterocyclic or "tricyclic-like" are more accurate collective names. Substitution of the basic tricyclic nucleus has not markedly increased the antidepressant action of these drugs, but has in some cases reduced unpleasant side effects and enhanced serendipidous findings.

These drugs are transported bound to protein, metabolized in the liver, and excreted by the kidneys. They have a long serum half-life and accumulate in tissues until a saturation point is reached; side effects frequently precede the onset of the desired pharmacologic effects, which may take 2 to 3 weeks to become manifest. On discontinuing the drug, it is slowly released from the tissues and may appear in the urine for as long as 2 to 3 months after discontinuance. These drugs are less well tolerated in the elderly.

The mode of action of the tricyclic antidepressants is to increase cerebral levels of norepinephrine and serotonin by effecting a reduction in their reuptake in the synaptic clefts, most significantly in the limbic system. Neither euphoriants nor stimulants, these drugs have no effect on the affect of patients who are not depressed.

The side effects are principally those that result from anticholinergic action, which leads then to an atropine-like effect. This is manifest in dryness of the mouth, palpitations, tachycardia, blurred vision, vomiting, constipation, aggravation of glaucoma, and rarely urinary retention or paralytic ileus. Other side effects include sedation, orthostatic hypotension and benign and reversible changes in the EKG; they also block the action of glutethamide hypotensive agents. More severe side effects include defects in cardiac conduction and ventricular arrhythmias, agranulocytosis, which is rare and which appears to be an allergic reaction that may occur in the second to third months of treatment, leukocytosis, leukopenia, and thrombocytopenia. Cholestasis occurs occasionally, increase in appetite and weight gain are not uncommon, and photosensitivity and cutaneous drug eruptions may occur.

The serendipitous side-effect for dermatologists is the ability of these drugs to block histamine receptor sites on cell membrane H_1 and H_2 receptor sites.[2] This capacity gives us an agent with the desirable qualities of a sedative, an antipruritic, and an antidepressant.

The indications for prescribing the tricyclic-like antidepressants then include depression, pruritus, and somatic symptoms that are considered to be depressive equivalents such as glossodynia, glossopyrosis, and some cases of the psychogenic pain syndrome; they are reported to be effective in the treatment of postherpetic neuralgia,[29] which may in some cases in fact be an example of the latter.

The work-up prior to prescribing antidepressants in addition to the routine dermatologic evaluation and your best psychiatric assessment, should include baseline laboratory values, blood pressure, and EKG. The patient should be warned to arise slowly from lying down to sitting because of the possibility of orthostatic hypotension.

Imipramine hydrochloride is less sedating than amitriptyline hydrochloride, but may have less side effects, while doxepin hydrochloride has the greatest antihistamine effect.[14] The same dosage schedule may be used for each of the drugs, but a dose one third to one half of the customary dosage, should be prescribed in the elderly.

Antripruritic dosage is 10 mg at h.s. to 10 mg t.i.d. as mandated by the response. Antidepressant dosage is started at 25 mg to 50 mg at h.s., and increased by increments of 25 mg every 2-3 days to a total of 75-150 mg. This is given as a single dose at h.s. in order to minimize the side effects. Because of the need for tissue saturation with the drug, the full antidepressant effect is not achieved for 2-3 weeks; if after 3 weeks of an adequate dosage there has been no satisfactory relief of symptoms, and provided one is sure that there is patient compliance, an alternative drug, of the same class, should be substituted. Once relief of symptoms has been achieved, the dose may be reduced by 25 percent for maintainance, and after a period of 3-6 months an attempt may be made gradually to withdraw the drug.[22]

Monoamine Oxidase Inhibitors

The application of this class of antidepressant drugs is fraught with more complications than is the tricyclic group, and it does not seem appropriate for the average dermatologist to prescribe them. They are used in the treatment of those cases of severe depression that have failed to respond to an adequate trial of the tricyclic-like drugs, but because of their mode of action and the ubiquitous nature of monoamines, dietary restrictions are required, and hypertensive crisis is a risk.

Lithium Carbonate

Lithium carbonate is the drug of choice for treatment of bipolar depression, and for prevention of relapse in that illness, but as with monoamine oxidase inhibitors, it does not seem appropriate for nonpsychiatric physicians to be prescribing the drug. It is important to remember, however, that lithium carbonate may excaberate both psoriasis and acneiform eruptions,[30] and that there is a competitive inhibition with tetracycline.

Antipsychotic Drugs (Neuroleptics)

Several classes of neuraleptics are in current usage, varying not only in potency but also in the incidence and severity of the extrapyramidal side-effects. Chlorpromazine was the first of the phenothiazine derivatives, and as it is still the most widely prescribed neuroleptic in psychiatric practice, I will use it to exemplify the phenothiazines. The pharmacologic effect is achieved by blocking the uptake of dopamine in the brain, and all of these drugs have therefore Parkinsonian side-effects.[12] Their administration in psychosis results in a decrease in psychotic thinking, and a normalization of psychomotor behavior; hostility, belligerence, restiveness, and uncooperativeness are all reduced, as are suspiciousness and projection. Clearly these are not the patients that we as dermatologists should be treating, and in dermatology the application has been primarily for the relief of pruritus, pain, and delusions related to the skin;[10] dosage schedules are far below the 400-800 mg per day range required often in the treatment of the very disturbed psychotic patients. Because of the lower dosage schedules likely to be employed, usually in the range of 50-150 mg daily, the side effects are likely to be less significant, but I will summarize them briefly.

Chlorpromazine is readily absorbed from the gastro-intestinal tract and widely distributed in the tissues, where it may remain bound for 6 to 12 months after discontinuation. It is metabolized by hydrolysis and glucuronidation in the liver. The adverse side effects are numerous and should preclude the use of the drug on frivolous grounds. Extrapyramidal side effects include acute dystonias, which involve primarily the muscles of face and neck; akathisia, a syndrome in which the patient is unable to keep still; and Parkinsonism. These are treated by lowering the dose of chlorpromazine and adding the antiparkinsonian agent benztropine mesylate (Cogentin Tablets and Injection, Merck Sharpe & Dohme, West Point, PA) in a dose of 1 to 4 mg once or twice daily. Other side effects include orthostatic hypotension, electrocardiographic changes, and a benign pigment deposition in lens, cornea, and retina. There are also anticholinergic side-effects as have been described for the tricyclic-type of antidepressants, and endocrine anomalies that include amenorrhoea and galactorrhea; increased appetite and weight gain occur, and rarely agranulocytosis and disturbances of temperature regulation. Chlorpromazine is also a photosensitizer; drug eruptions, and abnormal cutaneous pigmentation may be seen.

The most significant complication is the development of tardive dyskinesia, an extra-pyramidal syndrome characterized by involuntary dystonic movements that classically involve the tongue and facial muscles and that though painless are extremely distressing and embarrassing. Tardive dyskinesia is usually associated with long-term high-dose therapy; advanced age increases susceptibility. In order to reduce the likelihood of this complication the drug should be used at the lowest effective dose and for the shortest possible time, and the patient should be checked regularly for involuntary movements, since the condition is reversible only in its early stages. The initial work-up prior to prescribing chlorpromazine is the same as is described for antidepressants, but because of the possible opthalmic complications regular eye examination should be recommended.[12]

Two other antipsychotic drugs have recently found favor with dermatologists because of their high potency and therefore low-dosage formula, and their efficacy in the treatment of delusions and hallucinations related to the skin,[3] pruritus, neurotic excoriations,[24] onychotillomania,[15] and post-herpetic neuralgia,[4,6] and other types of intractable pain, with minimal incidence of side effects. The first of these is haloperidol, a butyrophenone, which is a long-acting, non-hypnotic antipsychotic with antiemetic and analgesic properties used in psychiatry for treatment of acute mania, paranoia, and Gilles de la Tourette's Syndrome, in daily dosage schedules of 2-25 mg. In dermatology a dose of 1-4 mg daily generally proves adequate given as a single dose in the morning. Treatment is started with 1 mg daily, and increased by increments of 1 mg at weekly intervals until the desired response is achieved. It may require up to 6 weeks of adequate dosage for delusions to disappear,[16] but if after that period of time the symptoms persist, the drug should be abandoned. After freedom from symptoms of 3 to 6 months, an attempt may be made gradually to withdraw the drug. In many cases, however, it may need to be taken long-term.

Pimozide, a diphenylbutylpiperadine, is the second of the high potency low-dose agents. Approved by the Food and Drug Administration (FDA) for the treatment of Gilles de la Tourette's Syndrome, it has been widely used in Europe and in Canada for the same indications as haloperidol.[20] It is prescribed in similar fashion in a dose range of 1-8 mg daily.

The side-effects and complications of these two drugs are similar to those described for chlorpromazine. It is also important to remember that one must always be alert for noncompliance, particularly in patients who are paranoid, and who may fear that any medication they are given is poisoned.

Carbamazepine

Carbamazepine (e.g., Tegretol Tablets, Geigy Pharmaceuticals, Ardsley, NY) is an anticonvulsant, but it has also been approved by the FDA as a specific analgesic for trigeminal neuralgia. It has more recently been reported to be effective in the treatment of post-herpetic neuralgia.[18] For this reason, I have prescribed it in an number of cases of the psychogenic pain syndrome, but without signal success. Because there are serious hematologic side effects, the physician should be very familiar with all aspects of the drug before prescribing it. The dosage schedule recommended is 100 mg b.i.d. This may be increased by 100 mg every 12 hours as needed for pain, to a total not to exeed 1200 mg daily. Control of pain can usually be maintained on 400 to 800 mg daily, and attempts should be made gradually to withdraw the drug, every 3 months during the treatment period.

Anxiolytics

Essentially all of the anxiolytics or minor tranquilizers currently in use are benzodiazepine derivatives. These drugs reduce the subjective symptoms and the physiologic signs of anxiety and promote an improved level of functioning with greater efficacy and less sedating effect than the barbiturates; they are also effective muscle relaxants. They have a much greater margin of safety than either the barbiturates or meprobamate, and are virtually never lethal unless combined with other drugs; this reduces the risk of accidental or intentional overdose. Since they do not stimulate hepatic microsomal enzymes, tachyphylaxis does not occur with the benzodiazepines, but the potential for habituation does exist and physical dependence can occur when high doses are taken over long periods of time.

The mode of action of the benzodiazepines is not fully understood, but specific receptor sites for diazepam have been identified in the brain and it is postulated that these drugs potentiate the activity of aminobutyric acid, an inhibitory neurotransmitter.

Anxiolytic drugs are indicated when anxiety is sufficiently severe to interfere with the patient's daily functioning, but ideally they should be combined with psychotherapy. They might be considered for the anxiety that is associated with transient inner or environmental stress, or with somatic illness, and they are also used in the treatment of psychosomatic illness; they should be prescribed only if it can be demonstrated that they have a beneficial effect on the specific somatic symptoms. They are not appropriate for the long-term treatment of anxiety associated with the stresses and strains of daily living, or for mild tension or appropriate situational anxiety; under those circumstances the patient would better be taught to improve his or her psychological coping skills.

If anxiety is mixed with depression, and it is not clear which is the primary diagnosis, doxepin, an antidepressant with anxiolytic properties, may be prescribed. Or alternatively, alprazolam, a benzodiazepine with definite antidepressant action.

The dosage range for diazepam must be individualized according to the needs of the patient, but will fall in the range of 2-10 mg 2 to 4 times daily. The usual starting dose for alprazolam is 0.25-0.5 mg 2 to 3 times daily and this can then be titrated according to the individual patient's need to a maximum of 4.0 mg daily.

REFERENCES

1. Baron RJ: An introduction to medical phenomenology: I can't hear you while I'm listening. Ann Intern Med 103:606-611, 1985
2. Bernstein JE, Whitney DH, Soltanik K: Inhibition of histamine-induced pruritus by topical tricyclic antidepressants. J Am Acad Dermatol 5:582-585, 1981
3. Bishop ER Jr: Monsymptomatic hypochondriacal syndromes in dermatology. J Am Acad Dermatol 9:152-158, 1983
4. Cavenar JO Jr, Maltebie AA: Another indication for haloperidol. Psychosomatics 17:128-130, 1974
5. Dennis M, Phillippus MJ: Hypnotic and non-hypnotic suggestion and skin

response in atopic patients. Am J Clin Hypn 7:342-345, 1965
6. Duke EE: Clinical experience with pimozide: Emphasis on its use in postherpetic neuralgia. J Am Acad Dermatol 8:845-850, 1983
7. Ford CV: The Somatizing Disorders: Illness as a Way of Life. New York, Elsevier Biomedical, 1983, pp 7-8
8. Frank JD: The influence of the patient's and therapist's expectations on the outcome of psychotherapy. Br J Med Psychol 41:349- 356, 1968
9. Freud A: The ego and the mechanisms of defense, in The Writings of Anna Freud, vol 2, 1936. New York, International Universities Press, 1974, pp 109-121
10. Frithz A: Delusions of infestation: treatment by depot injections of neuroleptics. Clin Exp Dermatol 4:485-488, 1979
11. Gajwani AK, Sehgal VN: Hypnosis: a new therapeutic approach in vitiligo. Cutis 14:572-573, 1974
12. Gilman AG, Goodman LS, Gilman A (eds): Goodman and Gilman's The Pharmacological Basis of Therapeutics (ed 6). New York, Macmillan, 1980, pp 397-414
13. Gould WM, Gragg TM: Delusions of parasitosis. An approach to the problem. Arch Dermatol 112:1745-1748, 1976
14. Greene SS, Reed CE, Schroeter AL: Double-blind crossover study comparing doxepin with diphenhydramine for the treatment of chronic urticaria. J Am Acad Dermatol 12:669-675, 1985
15. Hamann K: Onychotillomania treated with pimozide (Orap). Acta Derm Venereol (Stoch) 62:364-366, 1982
16. Hamann K, Avnstorp C: Delusions of infestation treated by pimozide: A double-blind crossover clinical study. Acta Derm Venereol (Stockh) 62:55-58, 1982
17. Hilgard ER, Hilgard JR: Hypnosis in the Relief of Pain. Los Altos, CA, Kaufman, 1975, p 6-26
18. Howard JE: Postherpetic pudendal neuralgia (letter). JAMA 253:2196, 1985
19. Koblenzer CS: Psychosomatic concepts in dermatology: a dermatologist-psychoanalyst's viewpoint. Arch Dermatol 119:501-512, 1983
20. Koblenzer CS: The dysmorphic syndrome. Arch Dermatol 121:780-784, 1985
21. Koblenzer CS: Liaison dermatology. Int J Dermatol 25:28-30, 1986
22. Kolb LC, Brodie HKH: Modern Clinical Psychiatry (ed 10). Philadelphia, WB Saunders Co, 1982, pp 66-70
23. Miller Rm: Biofeedback in dermatology, in Richies WH, Sandweiss HJ, Jacob DW, et al. (eds): Biofeedback and Family Practice. New York, Plenum, 1983, p 147
24. O'Regan JB: Treatment of obsessive-compulsive neurosis with haloperidol. Can Med Assoc J 103:167-168, 1970
25. Panconesi E: Psychosomatic dermatology. Clin Dermatol 2:94-179, 1984

26. Shapiro O, Futterman AD, Yamamoto J: Biofeedback in psychiatry, in Pinchot P, Berner P, Wolf R, Thau K (eds): Psychiatry: The State of the Art. Psychotherapy and Psychosomatic Medicine, vol 4. New York, Plenum 1985, pp 275-276
27. Surman OS, Gottlieb SK, Hackett TP, Silverberg EL: Hypnosis in the treatment of warts. Arch Gen Psychiatry 28:439-441, 1973
28. Theirs BH: Cutaneous appendage diseases, in Provost TT, Farmer ER (eds): Current Therapy in Dermatology, 1985-1986. Philadelphia, Decker, 1985, pp 102-104
29. Watson CP, Evans RJ, Reed K, et al.: Amitriptyline versus placebo in postherpetic neuralgia. Neurology 32:671-673, 1982
30. White SW: Palmoplantar pustular psoriasis provoked by lithium therapy. J Am Acad Dermatol 7:660-662, 1982

SECTION II

PSYCHOCUTANEOUS DISEASE —CLINICAL ASPECTS

Part I: Psychiatric Conditions that Manifest in the Skin

Chapter 6

Dermatitis Artefacta

Far from being a specific entity, dermatitis artefacta, or factitious dermatitis, is a facet of a much broader spectrum of factitious disease: this spectrum is broad indeed, for factitious disease has been induced in almost every organ system. Pathomimicry[23] (Fig. 6-1) was the name recently coined by Millard to describe those cases in which a known disease is simulated, rather than a bizarre and inexplicable picture, and reports of self-induced asthma,[7] fever,[2] infection,[26] hemorrhagic diathesis,[18] panniculitis,[1] autoimmune disease,[3] neurologic disorder,[5] psychosis,[34] and diarrhea,[16] etc. abound in the literature, as well as such dramatic presentations as, for example, autoenucleation[12] and autocastration.[17] Fras and Coughlin[10] reported the case of a young woman who lost both kidneys to the surgeon's knife as a result of factitious microscopic hematuria, and Hawkins et al.[13] describe a patient whose simulated thyrotoxicosis led to congestive cardiac failure. Nor is the phenomenon confined to adults, for Meadow[21] tells of 19 young children who underwent needless, prolonged, and often harmful medical investigations and treatments, leading to death in two cases, as a result of the clinical signs that their mothers had fabricated for them, while Stankler[33] reports on a similar situation in a mother and her two small sons.

For purposes of management, self-induced skin lesions are classified into three groups, in each of which the motivation, the psychopathology, and therefore the treatment, are different.

1. Those patients whose lesions result from such conscious and repetitive actions as scratching, rubbing, picking, or pulling. These will be discussed in Chapter 9, under the heading of obsessional habits.
2. Those patients whose lesions are produced consciously and knowingly, but also deceitfully, by the patient for a secondary gain that is other than the adoption or perpetuation of the role of the patient: these are malingerers.
3. Those patients to whom the name dermatitis artefacta most properly belongs. These are patients who produce their lesions with or without their full conscious knowledge, to satisfy a need that is psychological; the secondary gain thus obtained is less obvious, and also less readily under the voluntary control of the patient.

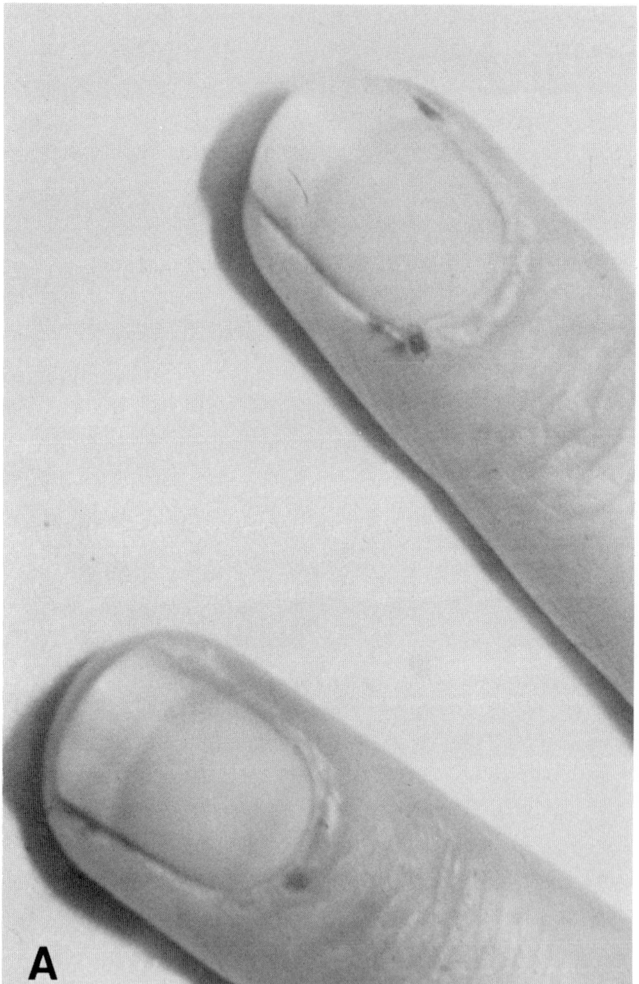
A

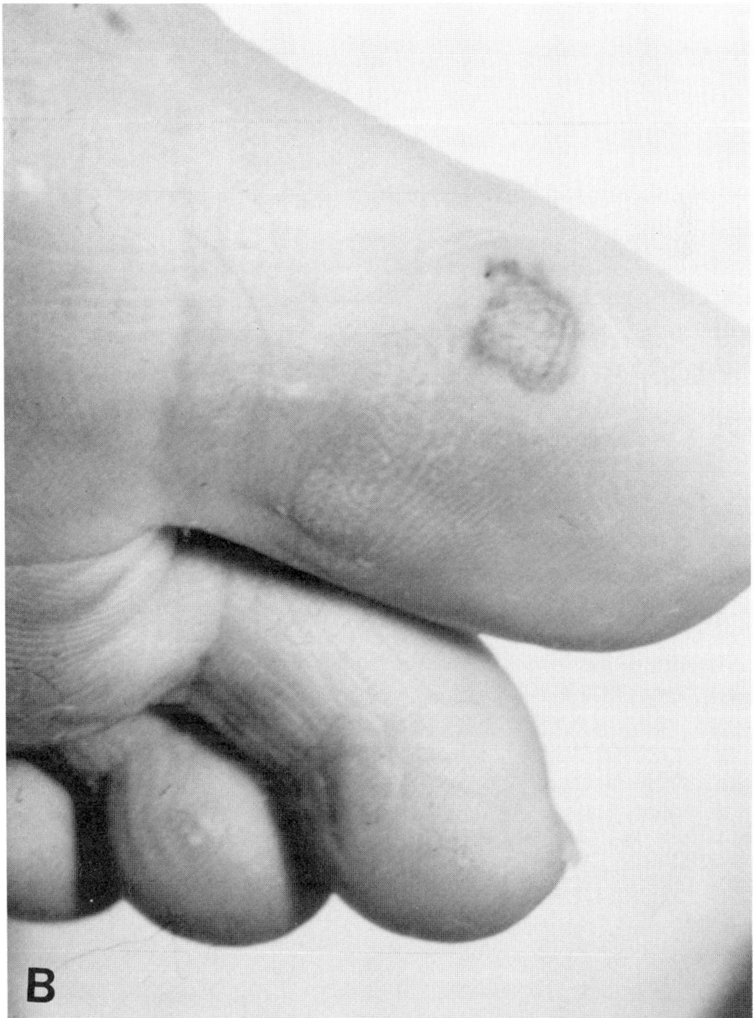

Figure 6-1. (A, B) An example of pathomimicry. A chronic illness of 14 years left this young woman financially destitute. Poor job performance, poor peer and family relationships, and narcotic abuse resulted from the "lupus erythematosus" illustrated here. Laboratory and biopsy findings during seven hospitalizations were within normal limits. Pathomimicry was the final diagnosis and psychotherapy resulted in cure. The pathodynamics of the lesions remains unclear.

MALINGERING

The deliberate and conscious production of artefactual lesions for purposes of a realistic gain, I shall dismiss rapidly. These patients are encountered most commonly amongst those who are incarcerated, in the armed services, in Workers' Compensation clinics, or who are seeking litigation; because their need is to maintain lesions rather than to resolve them, they do not regularly seek our help. Yudofsky[36] has divided malingerers into four categories for purposes of organization.

1. Staged events: an incident is designed in which an injury will occur that can subsequently be embellished.
2. Data tampering: medical data or specimens are deliberately tampered with to simulate a specific disorder.
3. Opportunistic malingering: pre-existing conditions are exploited.
4. Symptom invention: spurious complaints, for example, dysesthesia, are made.

The types of gain that may accrue from such activities include monetary rewards, the avoidance of arduous assignments, receipt of disability pensions, or the long-term prescription of addictive drugs.

In my own experience opportunistic malingering is the form most frequently encountered, and several examples come readily to mind: the recent concern about possible toxic effects from exposure to Agent Orange during combat in Viet Nam has resulted in several patients failing to comply with prescribed treatment for acne vulgaris in the hope of receiving a disability pension on the grounds of having contracted chloracne. A 38-year-old man claimed to have developed contact sensitivity to a paint solvent with which he had been working for 20 years, and sought a pension for life of $1200 per month from the Department of the Navy. Patch tests were all negative and physical examination revealed mild seborrheic dermatitis; this man became quite angry when I suggested he substitute a mild soap for the harsh abrasive industrial cleanser with which he was wont to wash his face. Intermittently patients with perianal condylomata complain of unmitigated pain for weeks or even months post treatment with podophyllin resin and their demands for narcotic drugs may become quite insatiable.

The incidence of malingering is highest in males, from young adulthood through middle age. Usually these are persons of low self-esteem, with poor social and employment adjustment, and an antisocial personality configuration. The malingering is utilized to avoid painful situations or obtain compensation and as such, it tends to be a recurrent phenomenon. As patients, they are often uncooperative and noncompliant, with vague complaints that are hard to substantiate. Often they will become angry if challenged or if a good prognosis is suggested; their symptoms will usually disappear should the goal be achieved, or the stakes become too high.

Most important in the management is for the physician to be aware of the negative feelings that the malingering patient arouses. The physician must be able to tolerate these feelings without acting on them, or overcompensating for them by entering into collusion with the patient to serve the patient's unworthy end. Our role as physician is primarily to rule out serious disease, and we need state only that we could detect no specific disease entity or pathophysiologic process to explain satisfactorily the symptomatology. It is not our job to unmask the malefactor,[17] nor is there much to be gained by psychiatric referral, since these patients lack conscience in this area and are not amenable to psychiatric intervention.

DERMATITIS ARTEFACTA

Clinical Picture

The lesions of dermatitis artefacta, although morphologically of almost infinite variety, do have in common certain characteristics. Single or quite numerous, their distribution is such as to make them readily accessible to the dominant hand; alternatively, they may be bilateral and symmetrical. Characteristically of bizarre configuration, they are frequently angulated or geometric, with surface necrosis often as a prominent feature. When caused by acid or caustic liquids, tell-tale linear streaks may be noted at the margin where they have trickled down. It is hard to obtain a clear history of their evolution; details are vague, and physical examination fails to reveal the usual progression from the earliest beginnings, through intermediate lesions, to the fully developed form—it is as though they had sprung, already fully formed, upon the surface of the skin, and any attempt to elucidate further this "hollow history" [11] is met with anger and obduracy. Lyell has described in detail many of the ingenious and imaginative methods that are used.[20] These include rubbing; scratching; picking; cutting; slashing; gouging; puncturing; application of heat, acids, or caustics; injection of caustics, milk, or other substances; autoinnoculation with infected material, fecal material or blood; sucking; biting; application of suction cups; and strangulation with elastic bands (Figs. 6-2 through 6-6). In some cases an attempt may be made to simulate a known dermatosis, or to perpetuate a pre-existing condition. These patients also tend to be quite suggestible, attempting to simulate lesions that they have seen on someone else, or obligingly producing a lesion at a certain spot, should the physician suggest that that is the expected site next to become involved. Application of an adequate occlusive dressing such as an Unna Boot will almost invariably permit healing of the existing lesions, and prevent extension of the process, although patients are occasionally marvellously ingenious in finding ways to confound us and circumvent even that hurdle by the insertion of knives or knitting needles; as lesions are permitted to heal under the occlusive dressing, new ones will in all probability appear at a secondary uncovered location.

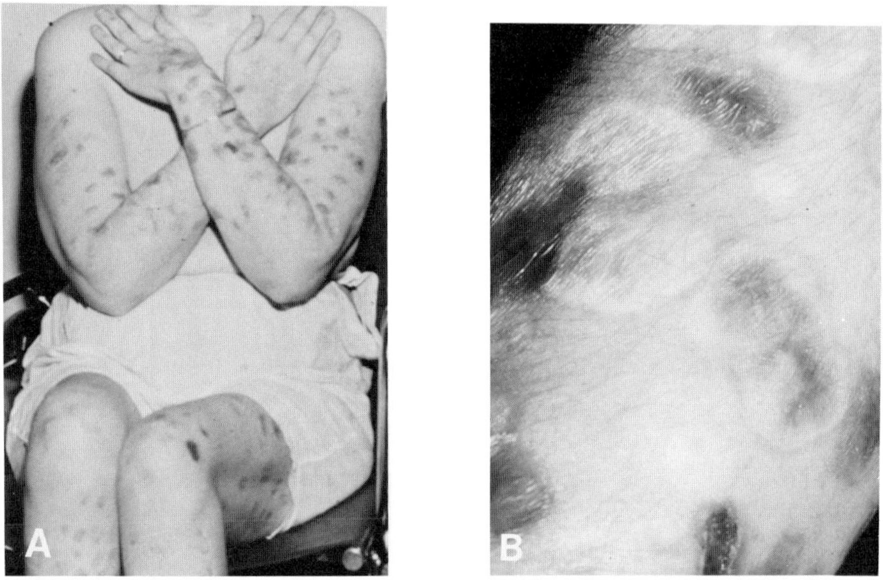

Figure 6-2 . (A, B) An example of dermatitis artefacta; thermal burns. This middle-aged woman induced large bullae by heating with a lighted cigarette a coin applied to the skin. Note the widespread distribution of relatively even-sized ulcerations and atrophic scar in accessible areas; these are more numerous on the left side and are sharply demarcated.

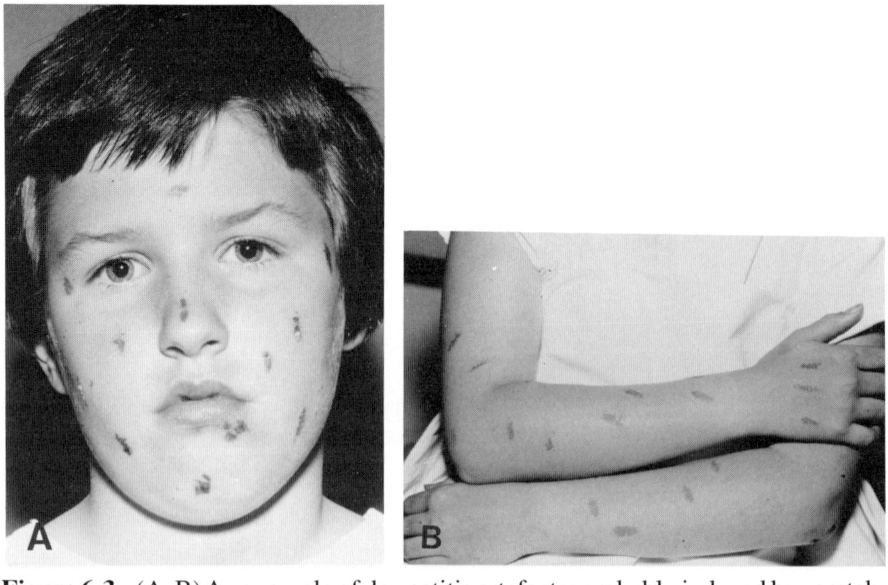

Figure 6-3. (A, B) An example of dermatitis artefacta; probably induced by scratching or rubbing. The superficial, crusted, linear lesions in a beautifully symmetrical but quite "unnatural" distribution leave little doubt as to their true etiology.

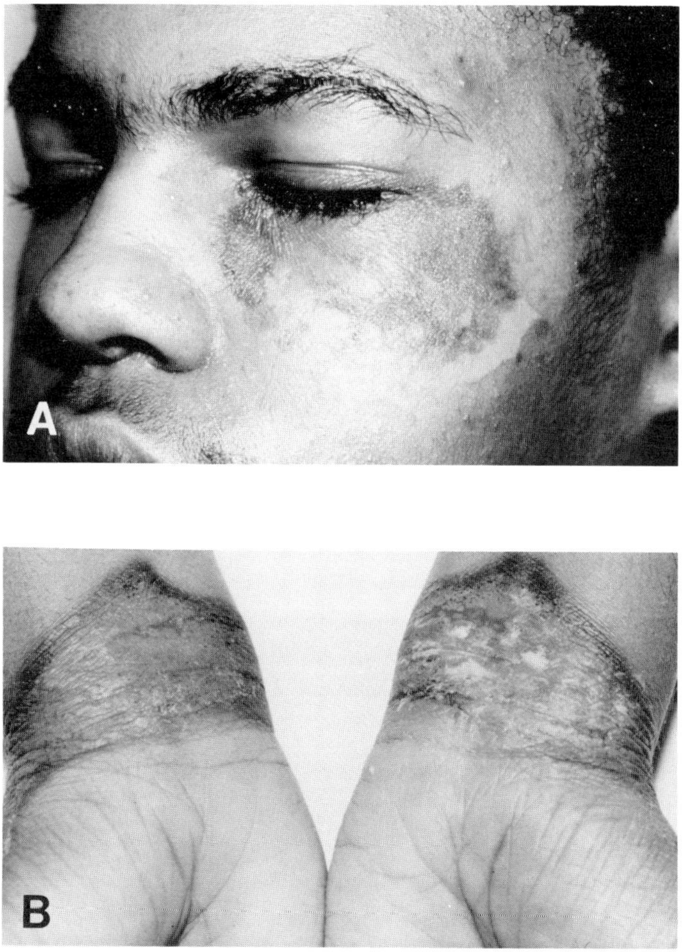

Figure 6-4. *(Continues.)*

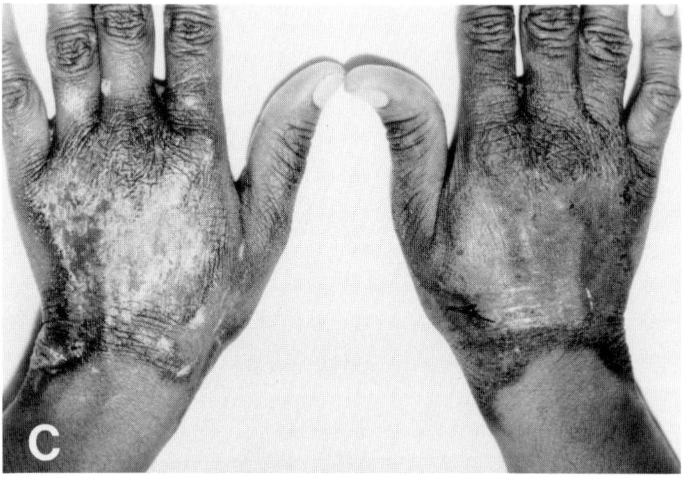

Figure 6-4. *(Continued.)* (A, B, C) An example of dermatitis artefacta; caustic burns. This young man repeatedly induced superficial ulcerations on the dorsal hands, the volar wrists, and the left cheek by application of a caustic. Note the clear-cut demarcation and "glove" distribution. Healing has taken place with hyper- and depigmentation. Permanent scarring may result. Although the bizarre distribution initially suggested an acute contact dermatitis, persistence of the lesions, and extension to the left cheek, suggests dermatitis artefacta. Occupational injuries may be perpetuated in this way.

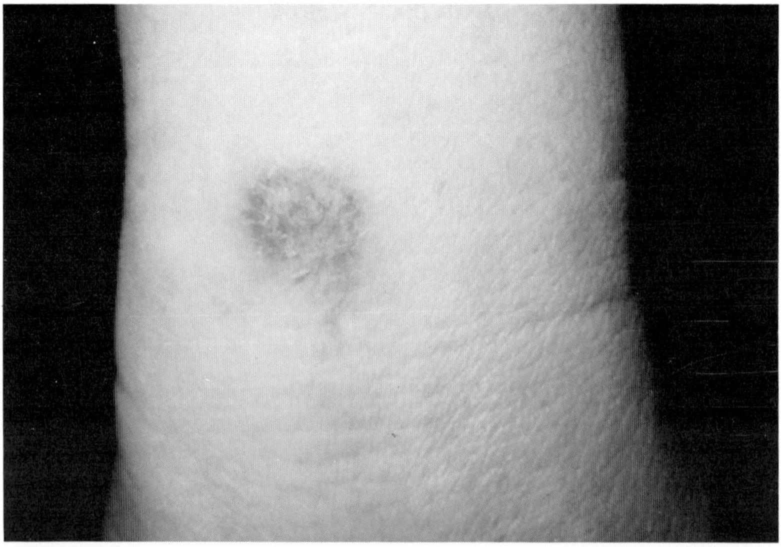

Figure 6-5. An example of dermatitis artefacta. This middle-aged woman presented with several areas of blue discoloration about the wrist following an unsuccessful attempt at suicide by intraveous injection of blue ink.

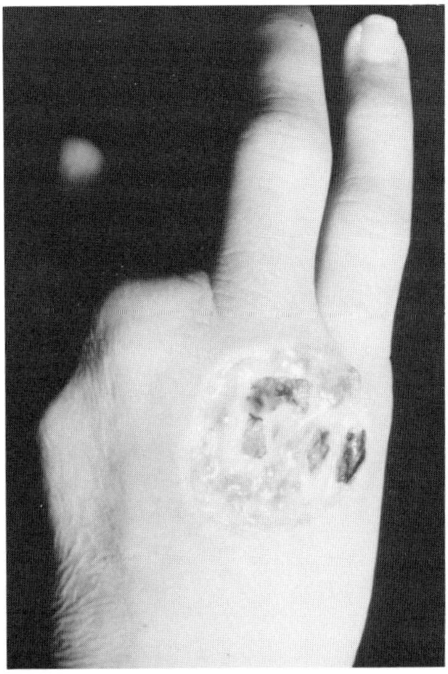

Figure 6-6. An example of dermatitis artefacta; induction and perpetuation of an ulcer by means of a caustic. The purulent and escharotic base of this ulcer suggests the continued application of a caustic agent; the lesion has been slowly progressive for several months despite appropriate therapy.

One of the most striking and perhaps most frustrating of the clinical features of this disorder is the attitude of the (usually female) patient and her family towards the lesions. If challenged, both will deny any possibility of their factitious nature, but whereas the patient will often affect puzzlement and mystification instead of anger, for the family the charge is experienced as a threat that arouses a defensive anger that may be quite extreme, and impatience with a diagnosis they consider inept and insulting; nor is one spared by the primary care physician, who will often join in these same charges.

Whereas the family is clearly anxious about the unexplained symptoms, and solicitous of the patient, she herself may not express appropriate affect; she may accept her lot with extraordinary equanimity, or express excessive discomfort with seemingly inconsequential lesions. Scarring may be quite disfiguring and eminently visible, but it fails to generate in the patient the feelings of shame or embarrassment that one might expect.

Incidence

Unlike malingerers, amongst whom males predominate, the incidence of dermatitis artefacta is higher in women, with female to male ratios quoted variously as anywhere from 3:1-8:1,[8,14,15] Although the condition can be seen at any age, the greatest prevalence is in adolescents and young adults, a disproportionate number of whom have work experience in the health care field or have a close relative employed in that area.[6] A moderate amount of medical knowledge is a not unusual finding, and frequently the dermatitis artefacta is just one incident in a long history of psychosomatic disease.[29]

Psychopathology and Motivation

Cases of dermatitis artefacta can broadly be divided into five categories, according to the level of psychopathology and the unconscious motivation that drives the patient to engage in self-destructive behavior. In each of these except the first, one can uncover two significant elements; first, the early life experiences and personality configuration of the patient that confer on her the susceptibility to factitious disease, and second, a precipitating factor in her current circumstances that determines the onset of the problem. Whereas current stresses that act as precipitants are many and varied, real or symbolic separation from important figures is a not infrequent finding. These five categories are:

1. Patients with metabolic defects or mental retardation.
2. Patients with psychosis.
3. Disturbances in children and adolescents.
4. Patients in whom dermatitis artefacta represents a hysterical conversion or other neurotic reaction.
5. Patients with the borderline personality disorder.

The majority of the patients that we see with factitious lesions fall into category 5, but I will discuss the preceding four categories individually before taking up this group.

Patients with Metabolic Defects or Mental Retardation

Neither patients who engage in self-mutilation because of inherent biochemical anomalies, as for example in the Lesch-Nyhan Syndrome, nor those who are mentally defective can be considered to fit the clinical syndrome of dermatitis artefacta as I have described it, and as the term is most accurately and consistently used in the literature. The subtlety, ingenuity, deviousness, and denial are all absent, and destructive self-induced lesions the only common finding; accordingly these patients will not be considered further.

Patients with Psychosis

Similarly, patients who are psychotic do not fit the clinical syndrome. These patients are not common; they induce lesions in compliance with the requirements of a delusional system and freely acknowledge their participation, along with details of their distorted reasoning; alternatively they may attribute the problem to some external agency, or some higher power, by using the psychological defense mechanism of projection. These patients are usually schizophrenic; it is unusual for patients with psychotic depression to engage in self-mutilation.

An example of psychosis would be a man in middle life who consulted me for treatment of mild facial seborrhoeic dermatitis. In the course of my examination I noted deep ulcerations on the arms and legs for which he sought no treatment. These were entry and exit ports to enable electricity to pass through his body, he explained, and so it was natural that he had no wish for me to try to close such important apertures.

Disorders in Children and Young Adolescents

There are a number of scenarios associated with dermatitis artefacta in childhood; all of these derive from distortion within the parent-child relationship.

In the particular form of child abuse that leads a parent to create lesions on her child's skin, the mother has often herself been a victim of early emotional deprivation, has herself an immature personality, and has a need herself for a continuing close bond with her offspring. Not infrequently she too has a history of similar skin lesions, and may have had multi-system symptoms in the past.[30] The child's lesions serve not only to maintain this close dyadic bond, but also permit a supportive relationship for her with medical personnel, while at the same time allowing moral gratification and increased self-esteem through the praise she receives for her seeming "devoted" parenting. Such parent-child relationships, needless to say, bode ill for the healthy psychological adjustment in the growing child.

A second scenario may occur in homes where there is significant marital or domestic strife. The child learns early that illness, by threatening family stability, causes conflict to be set aside, and a united front formed to care for the invalid. If there is no valid illness to hand when the strife reaches a pitch sufficient to threaten dissolution of the family, then illness must be fabricated, or existing lesions exacerbated by the anxious child, in order to bind the family together;[27] these lesions at the same time serve as punishment for the part the child neurotically fears he or she has played, in stirring up parental conflict. Diagnostically, these children are probably neurotic.

A third scenario occurs in children who have been victims of the worst forms of physical, emotional, and sexual abuse. Factitious lesions may be associated with drug or alcohol abuse and with eating disorders in these isolated and unhappy children, who feel unloved and unloveable, and who find that their deviant activities "make the bad feelings go away."[29] The production of lesions is often planned hours or days in advance, and the severity carefully calculated and controlled. Meninger suggests they may represent a "partial suicide," in order to protect from total oblivion,[22] and it is certainly clear in the literature that successful suicide is not the intent of self-mutilators.[25,28] Other functions that may be served include the expression of negative feelings towards depriving parents, turned against the self; punishment for those negative feelings; and the stimulation, both sexual and physical, that is necessary to prove to the child that he truly exists "somewhere in this world," so overwhelming is the sense of isolation and so unclear the boundaries of the personality, and the sense of self.[28] In some cases it represents even an identification with the punishing parent through which the child expresses "love" towards himself, abuse being the only "love" he has received at the hands of his parents. Diagnostically, these children are generally schizoid or borderline personality disorders.

The fourth scenario, and perhaps the one we most commonly encounter in practice, is a rather more benign situation. A child or young adolescent (usually female) is faced with a task for which she feels inadequate, or a situation where she feels disadvantaged. Anxiety is generated and a solution sought to relieve her discomfort. The parents are perceived as harsh and cold, or judgmental, and the child does not feel free to discuss her concerns. The appearance of skin lesions permits avoidance of the threatening task or situation with which she is faced, while at the same time allowing the child, through adopting the illness role, to regress to a more dependent position. This temporary dependency allows her to regroup her forces and restore her emotional equilibrium, and so move forward to a higher level of maturity. In such a situation then, the factitious illness may be outgrown, although where circumstances do not favor satisfactory personality development, recurrences may occur, or other spurious disorders develop.

Patients in Whom Dermatitis Artefacta Represents a Hysterical Conversion or Other Hysterical Reaction

The reader is referred to the discussion on the neuroses in Chapter 4, and the section in Chapter 2 on hysterical mechanisms, for an explanation of the psychodynamic factors underlying conversion reactions.

Patients whose dermatitis artefacta represents a true hysterical conversion remain quite unconscious of the fact that their lesions are self-induced; the responsible part of the mind is simply split off from that which is available to consciousness; the lesion has always a symbolic meaning in the emotional life of the patient, and a secondary gain will accrue.

As an example, a young woman of 16 consulted me for a curious eruption consisting of grouped erythematous puncta arranged very evenly, each group separated by an equal distance in all directions from the next; this eruption was confined to her right leg (Fig. 6-7). She had planned to apply to nursing school, but her maternal grandmother with whom she had been very close had recently been hospitalized for diabetic gangrene and had died following amputation of her right leg. As I worked with the patient it became clear that she had been profoundly disturbed by her grandmother's illness and death and now wanted no part of nursing. She could not, however, disappoint her parents by giving up thought of her career. The eruption on the right leg symbolically represented both

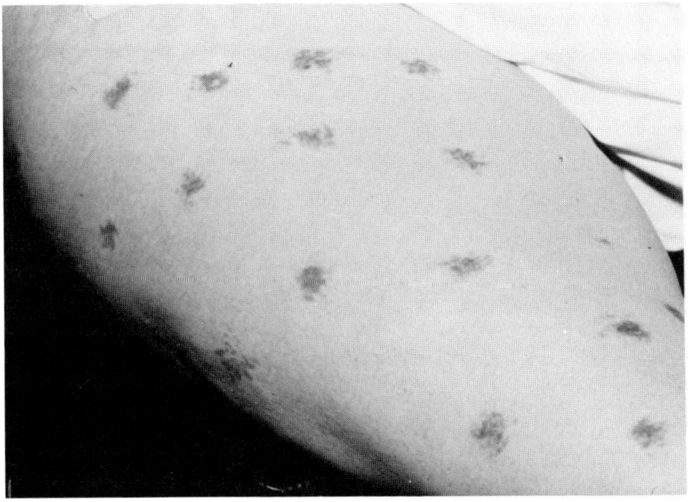

Figure 6-7. An example of dermatitis artefacta; hemorrhagic lesions. These uniform lesions, evenly scattered and readily accessible, were probably induced by pricking.

her grandmother's gangrenous leg, and also the puncta caused by injection of insulin. At the same time because she was sick it allowed her to avoid her conflict about nursing, without losing face. As she worked through these feelings in therapy, the eruption cleared, her anxiety resolved, and she was able to go forward with her chosen career.

Other patients with neurotic conflict and a hysterical personality configuration, may produce lesions that do not have the characteristics of a classical hysterical conversion; even though they may be produced unconsciously or nearly consciously the symbolism maybe less clear, and the gain to the patient understood more as perhaps the expression of forbidden unconscious anger, or a regressive need for nurturing, than as a complete solution for unconscious conflict.

Patients with Borderline Personality

Various authors have discussed descriptively the personality characteristics of patients with dermatitis artefacta, but without giving a specific diagnosis;[9,15,26] these authors recognise the part played by early life circumstances that are characterised by emotional deprivation, in predisposing towards the development of factitious disease, and present, to greater or lesser degree, the clinical picture that has come to be designated the Borderline Personality Disorder. This conclusion is confirmed by Schaffer et al.[28] The reader is referred to Chapter 4 for a description of the features that characterize this disorder.

The creation of factitious lesions helps to relieve the discomfort and tension caused by the different facets of the syndrome: the excitement and stimulation that are generated ease the overwhelming sense of emptiness and isolation; sensations that are aroused in the damaged skin define boundaries and help to establish personal and sexual identity; by adopting an illness role, challenging situations can be avoided, and poor self-esteem not further diminished by failure; the illness role provides a tool for unconscious though self-serving manipulation and exploitation of the environment; an outlet is provided for expression of the characteristic profound unconscious hostility and rage; the discomfort and disfiguration serve as punishment for this rage; and finally through an unconscious identification with hostile early care-takers, early damaging experiences can be reenacted, over and over again, as more lesions are produced.

Differential Diagnosis

Because of the extremely varied morphology, it is virtually impossible to give a complete differential diagnosis. Old disorders are mimicked and new ones created, by every ingenious means. Not only does our training instill in us the fear of missing disease, but the current litiginous climate keeps that fear constantly in mind. Nevertheless we must be prepared to make a positive diagnosis on the basis of physical findings, rather than one by exclusion. First, we must rule out delusions or obsessions concerning parasitic infestation, and compulsive habits such as neurotic excoriations; other considerations to be ruled out include the common and less common bacterial and fungal infections of the skin, septic infarcts, polyarteritis nodosa, pyoderma gangrenosum, panniculitis, spider bites, insect bites, the halodermas, Wegener's granulomatosis, granulomatous vasculitis, and collagen vascular disease.

Management

General Principles

The dermatologic management will not be discussed at length because it will consist of the customary topical measures for the particular type of lesion. Because factitious lesions serve in part as a cry for help, it is essential to create a therapeutic environment that will enable the patient to maintain contact and to keep coming back. Frequent visits ostensibly for supervision of symptomatic treatment provide a satisfactory medium for this, and treatment modalities that require a good deal of patient participation seem to be particularly helpful, focussing attention as they do on constructive rather than destructive activity. Compresses several times daily and antibiotic ointments suffice for most lesions, though deep cavities may be packed with iodoform gauze, necrotic sloughs removed with enzymatic ointments, and granulation tissue stimulated by benzoyl peroxide, granulated sugar, dextranomer beads, etc. Measures for general skin care such as cool baths, neutral soaps and emollients can also be recommended, and appropriate systemic antibiotics prescribed as needed. Bacterial cultures, x-ray and laboratory studies should be undertaken only if indicated, but negative studies should not be repeated, nor should they provide the stimulus to order more and different studies,[4] as in the cascade effect described by Mold and Stein.[24] Whereas occlusive dressings are sometimes helpful in establishing the diagnosis, they are of less benefit in treatment because the patient will be driven by inner need either to breach the occlusion or to start the process at another location.

These frequent visits can be quite short, but should take place not less than once or twice weekly. They will be used to enable the best possible therapeutic relationship to develop, and to permit the physician to get some idea of the level of psychopathology. Only with this information can a rational treatment plan be formulated; the reader is referred back to Chapters 4 and 5 for background information. No matter what the level of psychopathology, it is important to remember that if the patient were in touch with her unconscious conflict, or were she able to verbalize her unconscious needs, she would not have to resort to symbolic communication in the physical language of artefactual lesions. She is driven inexorably to produce these lesions, whether it be consciously or unconsciously, because she needs them. That need is in part internal, but it is also a cry for help to the outside world.

The rest of this section will be concerned with the more difficult aspects of treatment, the psychosocial management.

Earlier dermatologists, regarding self-mutilation as something akin to wickedness, confronted these unfortunates in punitive and judgmental mode. They resorted to hospitalization more, perhaps, for purposes of unmasking the miscreants by stripping and searching their persons and their effects, and of bringing them to their knees in contrition, than for restoring them to health.[19] Lyell suggests,[21] and Sneddon and Sneddon concur,[31] that one must indicate indirectly that one knows of the patient's activities, but that one sympathizes. Van Moffaert[35] takes a similar view. My own approach is to sidestep the issue altogether until I have had the opportunity to evaluate the patient very thoroughly, and until I am comfortable with the quality of relationship that has been established between us. By this means, I hope to avoid mobilizing the psychologic defense mechanisms, and stirring up anger, hostility, disbelief, or such anxiety as to drive the patient away. In an accepting and nonjudgmental environment the symptom is not infrequently given up without any acknowledgment from the patient, and without the actual mechanism ever being disclosed. Similarly it is often difficult to determine whether the patient is actually unaware of her activities, or whether, having obtained the help she needs, she is too embarrassed and ashamed to acknowledge her participation. If and when I bring up the issue of etiology will depend on whether the patient has sufficient stability to tolerate the information, and whether or not the therapeutic relationship is sufficiently strong to enable the information to be accepted without the patient feeling threatened. There are no absolute criteria; these decisions are ones that only the treating physician can make, from knowledge of, and feel for the patient.

The mode of confrontation is critical if one is not to anger or alarm the patient irretrievably. Once one is certain of the diagnosis, and comfortable with the therapeutic relationship, empathy is the watchword. First empathise with the feelings that must motivate the patient to engage in self-destructive activity, before introducing the idea that she is actually doing so. For example, one might say: "I can understand that since your boyfriend left, you must be feeling very angry with him, and very much alone; you must feel that you can't be worth much if you couldn't keep him; you must have felt terrible, and you really needed help with those terrible feelings; I guess that's why you may have injured your skin in that way."

Management of Dermatitis Artefacta in Children and Young Adolescents

Observe the interaction between family members in the office; try to get some feel for the family dynamics: (1) Does mother seem to be overly involved in the child's problems? (2) Is mother warm, affectionate, and at ease with the child? Is she belittling? Is she cold and judgmental? or (3) Is there evident friction between the parents or between the parents and the child?

In the family history: (1) Has mother had many physical illnesses, unexplained symptoms, or curious skin lesions? (2) What is the marital history and work history of the parents? Do they seem able to sustain relationships and hold down a job? (3) Is there a history of poor impulse control, with violent anger, drug abuse, or alcohol abuse in either parent?

In the present history: (1) What was happening in the family situation and in the patient's life when the symptoms began? (2) Are there other evidences of poor emotional adjustment? For example, how are school performance, peer relationships, sleeping and eating habits? Does the patient smoke, or abuse drugs or alcohol? (3) What situations might be currently operative that provide added stress? For example, career choice, relationships, school difficulties, or excessive parental demand for performance?

Information of this kind allows the patient to be fitted into one of the four scenarios previously described. In eliciting the information I find it helpful to see the patient not only with the parents, but also alone; if parents are upset or angered by being separated and as they see it, excluded, I am interested to know why; are they afraid of what the child might disclose about the family? or what the physician might do to the child? Obviously this cannot be asked directly, but one can bring it into focus by expressing puzzlement that such a seemingly innocuous action should cause them such concern.

In the first of the four scenarios previously described, we are dealing with child abuse from a psychologically impaired parent, and the help of the social services must be sought to protect the child and to arrange treatment for the mother. It is likely that the child will require psychotherapy also to avoid impaired psychological development, and poor adjustment later.

In the second scenario counseling should be recommended for the family, whilst the patient is given support and symptomatic treatment. If there is evidence of a more pervasive neurosis, psychotherapy or psychoanalysis is indicated, and appropriate referrals should be made.

The third scenario, like the first, will require all the resources that are available, in order to provide a stable and nurturing background as well as psychiatric treatment for the patient if she is to have any prospect at all of a happy and fulfilling future life.

The fourth scenario is the one in which one is most likely to meet with success, for usually this is essentially a developmental or adjustment problem. A relationship with a warm, supportive, and empathic physician with whom the child can feel free to talk about her concerns, may provide sufficient auxilliary strength for her to be able to regroup her forces, move forward, find ways to handle the at first seemingly overwhelming difficulties, and so permit her lesions to heal. Once a relationship is established, I usually inform the parents of the diagnosis, but not necessarily the child. If within 2 or 3 months there is no evidence of improvement, then the question of psychiatric referral can be considered, with a view to insight-oriented psychotherapy, or psychoanalysis.

Management of Patients with Dermatitis Artefacta and Hysterical Neurosis

1. Try to identify specific precipitating factors.
2. Try to determine to what extent neurotic symptoms are interfering with other aspects of the patient's life.
3. Evaluate the affect; is there significant anxiety or depression?
4. Initiate appropriate topical therapy.

By identifying current stressful circumstances that may have served as precipitating factors, the patient can be helped to recognise her strengths and weaknesses, and improve her coping skills: at the same time, help can be given in manipulating the environment if that is indicated and feasible. If there is significant anxiety or depression, appropriate drugs may be introduced according to the schedules suggested in Chapter 5. Fabisch[8] stresses that these should be prescribed infrequently for short periods only, because dermatitis artefacta tends to be a chronic and recurrent condition.

As a trusting therapeutic relationship develops, the physician will be able to judge to what extent neurotic symptoms are interfering in other aspects of the patient's life. If the physician's supportive and empathic attitude has been sufficient to help her over the current crisis, and point her towards better coping skills and better solutions, she may be enabled to give up her symptoms after a longer or shorter period of time. If, however, dermatitis artefacta is symptomatic of a more pervasive neurosis this will become clear, and the physician will be able to move towards suggesting a psychiatric referral, using the guidelines as suggested in Chapter 5. These patients are psychologically capable of benefitting from a psychodynamic approach, and will do well in psychoanalysis or analytically oriented psychotherapy; they are entitled to be given that option.[32]

An example would be a 34-year-old woman referred to me some years ago with a diagnosis of factitious dermatitis, and a history of recurrent facial acne since adolescence. In 1975 she had developed a large, deep, and intensely painful erosion on the right cheek which had finally healed, after a period of 3 years, leaving a disfiguring scar. The lesion for which I was consulted had started many months previously as a "pimple;" this had enlarged, become indurated, and developed a surface erosion, which progressed to cavitation; as the longer-standing areas healed, the contiguous skin had broken down.

Physical examination revealed a scar on the right cheek, and on the left cheek, a sharply punched-out opening, 1.5 cm in diameter, extending through skin and subcutaneous tissue into a cauldron-shaped cavity that occupied the major portion of the cheek. The base was clean, free of exudate, and composed of muscle tissue; there was no clinical evidence of inflammation, the margins were not indurated, and there was no lymphadenopathy (Fig. 6-8). Extending vertically from the lower margin of the ulceration was a linear scar that reached the mandibular border. Apart from this lesion, the findings were those of acne excoriee. All laboratory tests and x-ray studies had revealed normal findings.

Except for peptic ulcer disease in 1975, the patient had been generally well. From a strongly paternalistic and repressive culture, she had at 18, against parental wishes, travelled abroad to further her education. Whilst overseas she entered into the disastrous marriage that brought her to the U.S. and that gave her three children. Each of the significant facial lesions had coincided with a period of particular marital stress.

After three meetings, my evaluation was that this patient was neither psychotic nor a borderline personality disorder, but rather a patient with severe neurotic conflict. For her, failure of the marriage signified failure as a woman, and all that that implied. Unconscious rage against her husband for his part in the failure was turned against herself, causing symptoms of severe depression. In face of these inner stresses profound psychological regression supervened, and she presented as a pitiful, whining, tearful child, wishing me to put right all the problems that overwhelmed her.

Given the degree of psychological regression, I thought her too fragile to

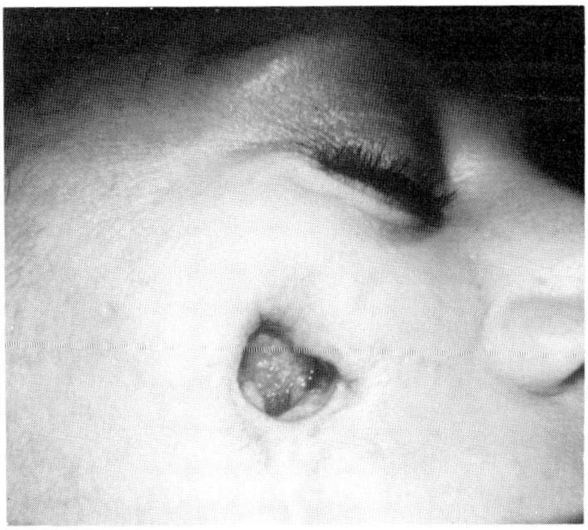

Figure 6-8. An example of dermatitis artefacta. The clean base of this deep ulcer is evidence for factitial etiology. The patient admitted only to "rubbing" the skin with a cotton swab when it itched. The contracted scar at the inferior margin of the ulcer speaks to vigorous attempts at spontaneous healing. A similar disfiguring scar was present also on the opposite cheek.

tolerate my belief that these were factitial lesions. I advised her they came from stress, and arranged to see her on a twice weekly basis.

Work in the therapy was directed first towards supporting her ego strengths in order to restore independence; second, towards helping her to see more realistically the character of her marital relationship, so that she need no longer take full blame for its failure, and third, towards helping her to get in touch with her unconscious anger, and work it through, to liberate psychic energy for constructive use. As her self-esteem improved, and as she worked through her anger, she was able to take charge of her life, fight for the right to custody of her children, and to an equitable financial settlement. She can now see herself as a competent adult, and is currently pursuing her career in this country. There have been no new lesions for 4 years.

Some weeks into the therapy, I suggested gently that she must be very angry, and that she certainly must not like or respect herself very much if she could permit such deforming lesions to develop on her face. She ignored my remark, and spoke as though the facial ulceration was in some way analogous to the peptic ulcer she had had previously. It was not until after healing was complete that she finally acknowledged itchy hive-like lesions that would develop when she was upset or angry; these she "scrubbed" with a cotton swab; so this much of the mechanism at least, we know.

Management of Dermatitis Artefacta in Patients with Borderline Personality Disorder

This constitutes the largest group of patients that we see with factitious lesions, and also quite the most difficult to treat. The same steps are indicated as I have described for patients with hysterical neurosis, but because of the unpredictable, demanding, and impulsive nature of the personality, one must tread very cautiously in order not to arouse anger and hostility, or permit unrealistic expectations to develop. When such expectations are unfulfilled, the patient may experience the physician in the way that she has experienced earlier betrayers in her life, and so vent on the physician the cumulative rage that is derivative of all the situations from early childhood on, in which she has felt unloved, disappointed, and uncared for.

It is helpful to try to identify precipitating factors, support ego strengths, improve coping skills, and intervene to manipulate the environment whenever possible.

Symptomatic topical treatment should be prescribed as suggested, and supervision of this utilized to enable the best possible relationship to develop. Hopefully at some point psychiatric referral may be mooted, if as is usually the case the afore-mentioned measures are not successful; this must be approached very cautiously because these patients are very vulnerable to feelings of rejection, and may respond with ever increased self-destructive activity. Insight is less the goal of therapy than is support, and the quality of the relationship with the psychiatrist is thought by Fras and Coughlin[10] to be a major prognostic factor. Sneddon has found relaxation exercises to be of some benefit.[30] Most authorities feel that the use of psychotropic drugs should be confined to the amelioration of specific symptoms such as, for example, depressive, manic, or psychotic episodes.

Prognosis

Although there are many articles describing the clinical picture, psychodynamics, and treatment of factitious dermatitis and other factitious disease, few authors address the question of prognosis. This facet, as does management, must depend on the psychopathology of the individual patient, and on whether or not this has been appropriately addressed in the treatment. For this reason, statistics drawn from studies in which all categories of patient are included without distinction are not very meaningful in terms of the individual.

Lyell[20] suggests that there may be a single episode, or factitious dermatitis may become a way of life; other authors find that children do better than adults,[9] and that early treatment, by preventing fixation of behavior patterns, is most likely to succeed.[35] Sneddon and Sneddon followed 33 of a group of 43 patients for as long as 22 years; of these 30 percent failed to recover. They found that in those who did, recovery owed more to increased maturity, or improvements in the life situation, than it did to medical intervention.[31]

The following information is based on my personal experience with patients with dermatitis artefacta:

Patients who are psychotic. Only if these patients can be persuaded to accept neuraleptic drugs will delusional thinking improve, permitting cessation of self-mutilating behavior.

Children and young adolescents. (1) Victims of physical or emotional abuse: Unless a nurturing environment can be substituted for the abusive one, and unless psychotherapy can be provided to enable the young person to deal with negative feelings engendered by abuse and by emotional deprivation, the prognosis is not good; these children frequently go on to lives of chronic and recurrent psychogenic disease.[9] Figures are not available for the prognosis under ideal circumstances. (2) Neurotic, or emotionally immature children: These children will do well, if emotional support and appropriate environmental manipulation are undertaken until a more mature ego can take over; this can well be accomplished by the interested dermatologist. Those with more severe and pervasive neuroses will require referral for insight-oriented psychotherapy.

Adult patients with hysterical neurosis. As with (2) above, some of these patients will do well with supportive measures. In the more persistant and recalcitrant cases, or where there is a more pervasive neurosis, insight-oriented psychotherapy or psychoanalytic treatment should in many cases enable the patient to achieve a more favorable adjustment, and give up her symptoms.

Patients with borderline personality disorder. These patients, I believe, are the ones for whom factitious disease becomes a way of life. Even if improvement in the life situation permits a remission, exacerbation can be expected with the next period of stress. Supportive psychotherapy, or modified psychoanalytic technique, can lead to real improvement in some cases, and dermatologists can provide a real service if they can reach a point with the patient where a psychiatric referral can be made. However, one should not be too despondent if one is not successful either in keeping the patient, or in making a satisfactory referral. There are some patients that we are simply unable to help.

REFERENCES

1. Ackerman BA, Mosher DJ, Schwamm HA: Factitial Weber-Christian Syndrome. JAMA 198:731-736, 1966
2. Aduan RP, Fauci AS, Dale DC, et al.: Factitious fever and self-induced infection. Ann Intern Med 90:230-242, 1979
3. Anderson PC, McCaffree MK: Pseudo DNA autosensitivity: A factitial disease. JAMA 196:224-225, 1966

4. Brown HN, Vaillant GE: Hypochondriasis. Arch Intern Med 141:723-726, 1981
5. Carney MWP: Pretending to be unconscious (letter) Lancet 1:358, 1974
6. Coterill AJ: Psychiatry and skin disease, in Rook AJ, Maibach HI (eds): Recent Advances in Dermatology. New York, Churchill Livingstone, 1967, pp 200-201
7. Downing ET, Braman SS, Fox MJ, Corrao WM: Factitious asthma: physiological approach to diagnosis. JAMA 248:2878-2881, 1982
8. Fabisch W: Psychiatric aspects of dermatitis artefacta. Br J Dermatol 102:29-34, 1980
9. Fabisch W: What is dermatitis artefacta? Int J Dermatol 20:427-428, 1981
10. Fras I, Coughlin B: The treatment of factitial disease. Psychosomatics 12:117-122, 1971
11. Gandy DT: The concept and clinical aspects of factitious dermatitis. South Med J 46:551-555, 1953
12. Gorin M: Self-inflicted bilateral enucleation. Arch Ophthalmol 72:225-226, 1964
13. Hawkins JR, Jones KS, Sim M, Tibbetts RW: Deliberate disability. Br Med J 1:361-367, 1956
14. Hollender MH, Abram HS: Dermatitis factitia. South Med J 66:1279-1285, 1973
15. Koblenzer CS: Psychocutaneous disease: neurotic excoriations and other obsessional habits, in Demis DJ, Dobson RL, McGuire J (eds): Clinical Dermatology, vol 4. Philadelphia, Harper and Row, 1985
16. Kramer P, Pope C: Fictitious diarrhea induced by phenolpthalein. Arch Intern Med 114:634-636, 1964
17. Krieger MJ, McAninch JW, Weimar SR: Self-performed bilateral orchiectomy in transsexuals. J Clin Psychiatry 43:292-293, 1982
18. Lababidi Z, Friedman R: Psychosomatic purpura. MO Med 68:386-388, 1971
19. Lyell A: Dermatitis artefacta and self-inflicted disease. Scott Med J 17:187-196, 1972
20. Lyell A: Cutaneous artifactual disease. A review amplified by personal experience. J Am Acad Dermatol 1:391-407, 1979
21. Meadow R: Munchausen syndrome by proxy. Arch Dis Child 57:92-98, 1982
22. Menninger LG: Man Against Himself. New York, Harcourt Brace and Co, 1938, p 88
23. Millard LG: Dermatologic pathomimicry: a form of patient maladjustment. Lancet 2:969-971, 1984
24. Mold JW, Stein HF: The cascade effect in the clinical care of patients. N Engl J Med 314:512-514, 1986
25. Pao P: The syndrome of delicate self-cutting. Br J Med Psychol 42:195-206, 1969

26. Reich P, Gottfried LA: Factitious disorders in a teaching hospital. Ann Intern Med 99:240-247, 1983
27. Richtsmeier AJ Jr, Waters DB: Somatic symptoms as family myth. Am J Dis Child 138:855-857, 1984
28. Schaeffler CB, Carroll J, Abramowitz S: Self-mutilation and the borderline personality. J Nerv Ment Dis 170(8):468-473, 1982
29. Simpson CA, Porter GL: Self-mutilation in children and adolescents. Bull Menninger Clin 45:428-38, 1981
30. Sneddon EB: Simulated disease: Problems in diagnosis and management. J R Coll Physicians Lond 17:199-205, 1983
31. Sneddon I, Sneddon J: Self-inflicted injury: a follow-up study of 43 patients. Br Med J 2:527-530, 1975
32. Sperling M: Psychosis and psychosomatic illness. Int J Psychoanal 36:320-327, 1955
33. Stankler L: Factitious lesions in a mother and two sons. Br J Dermatol 97:217-219, 1977
34. Sussman M, Hyler SE: Factitious disorders, in Kaplan HI, Sadock BJ (eds): Comprehensive Textbook of Psychiatry IV. Baltimore, Williams and Wilkins, 1985, p 1246
35. Van Moffaert M: Factitious affections in dermatology. Arch Belf Dermatol 30:221-224, 1974
36. Yudofsky SC: Conditions not attributable to a mental disorder, in Kaplan HI, Sadock BJ (eds): Comprehensive Textbook of Psychiatry IV. Baltimore, Williams and Wilkins, 1985, pp 1862-1865

Chapter 7

Delusions and Hallucinations as They Relate to the Skin

The reader is referred to Chapter 4 for a conceptual understanding of the disordered thought processes that lead to the clinical expression of delusions and of hallucinations. As has been noted, a delusion is a false belief and a hallucination is a false perception. These both arise without appropriate external stimulation, and are maintained unshakably in the face of reason. While delusions and fixed formed hallucinations are pathognomonic of psychosis, fleeting and less well-formed hallucinations may occur in hysterical neurosis; they may also occur in normal individuals at the moment of falling asleep, during intoxication, or at times of extreme stress.

Because there are different implications with regard to psychopathology, and consequently with regard to appropriate treatment, delusions and hallucinations are to be distinguished from obsessional concerns on the one hand, and phobias on the other. Patients whose concerns are obsessional do not have an unshakeable conviction, but rather a persistant and obtrusive fear about their physical condition. Although this fear may be pervasive and incapacitating, the patient at the same time knows it to be irrational. These patients will be discussed in Chapter 9.

Until recently, there has been confusion in terminology in the dermatology literature, and phobia has been used to designate both true delusions and obsessional concerns:[18] it is a misnomer in either case. The fear of the phobic patient is that he or she may be at risk of contracting a physical disorder. Rather than seeking constant reassurance that he or she is well, as the obsessional does, the patient's defense against this fear is avoidance, and the patient will avoid a progressively expanding plethora of circumstances in which there may be the possibility of exposure to disease.

Traditionally delusions of parasitic infestation have served as the paradigm for delusions as they relate to the skin.[3] More recently it has become clear that the spectrum of delusional ideation concerning skin abnormalities is broad.[37] These delusions are usually circumscribed, and they represent a monsymptomatic disorder more commonly than do they serve as part of a complex delusional system. Authors differ as to whether this syndrome appropriately falls under the rubric of hypochondriasis.[2,4,21,29,42]

DELUSIONS OF PARASITOSIS (EKBOM'S DISEASE)[39]

Clinical Picture

As with dermatitis artefacta, patients with delusions of parasitosis are seen most commonly by dermatologists. They are also seen by gynecologists, and rarely by psychiatrists. Skott,[39] in her very comprehensive monograph, describes acute and chronic phases of the illness. In the chronic phase, the patient having come to terms with the symptoms and learned to live with them, does not seek help, so that our familiarity in dermatology practice is with the acute phase.

This typically female patient is often anxious to the point of agitation. Totally consumed by her symptoms, she is unable to be diverted from descriptive detail. She is often exhausted from lack of sleep and from her unremitting attempts at irradication of the perceived invaders. Prior to the dermatologic consultation she may have seen several other practitioners, and she will have used many pesticides on both her person and her possessions; often she will have repeatedly engaged the services of a commercial pest exterminator, and probably consulted an entomologist or biologist for identification purposes. She may have moved house to escape her nemesis, and fear of contaminating family members, most particularly children and grandchildren, may have led to withdrawal and social isolation. Characteristically the patient appears entirely rational and functions adequately in other areas of her life. She approaches logically the steps she feels necessary for the safety of her family and the irradication of her problem. One patient of mine burned all her clothing including an expensive mink coat, threw out her upholstered furniture and lived in a single room, with only hard wooden furnishings that she thought unreceptive to infestation. She used two sets of clothing only, one of which was kept in a sealed plastic bag after each laundering. She believed herself to have been infested with a cloud of mites from the air conditioner of her car, so she would no longer drive.

The sensations described by patients are more frequently those of "crawling" under the skin, tickling, sharp bites, or stings, than pruritus; Reimer[36a] has proposed the term haptic hallucinosis for this hallucinatory experience on, within, or beneath the skin. The patient has intimate knowledge of her own specific parasites, which are referred to in proprietary and familiar terms. Three possible life-styles commonly are encountered: burrowing into the skin; being trapped under the surface with a need to get out; or descending upon the patient as an overwhelming plague. Such things as lice, scabies, pediculi, beetles, flies, mites, cockroaches, undefined "things," new and as yet undescribed species of bugs, and worms are among the variants described. A patient of mine harbored an organism shaped like a flounder and referred to as "he," whose domicile could be determined only when he emerged from the skin for air; the patient brought slides, microscope, and mounted specimens for my examination (Fig. 7-1). Sometimes there is a complaint of "things" falling out of beard or hair, or jumping on the surface of the skin. Another patient harbored worms around her eyes; these would travel to her mouth when she was eating, to compete for her food. They were apparently finicky eaters, and would move around violently if they did not like what she was eating, so that her diet was governed by the need not to displease them.

But regardless of the exact nature of the infestation described, a consistent feature is the absolute conviction that the patient knows what is going on; also, anger and contempt in face of the perceived incompetence of a physician who cannot irradicate, or indeed even see, the pests that she "knows" to be present.

Cutaneous symptoms may precede the patient's dawning interpretation that she is infested,[43] and in a percentage of cases there is even a valid infestation currently or in the recent or distant past.[25] "Specimens" are frequently brought in, in tins, glass jars, paper tissues, or stuck between two layers of adhesive paper tape. These consist of fragments of skin, hair, fiber, lint, paper, crusts, amorphous debris, or tiny flies or other insects. The history has a persuasive, if idiosyncratic, logic, and the patient may be so convincing that in as many as one third of cases,[39] one or more family members acquire the same symptom in a folie à deux, or folie partagée,—a shared delusion (Fig. 7-1).[10] It is not unusual for a complex life-cycle to be ascribed to the parasite; complicated and detailed diagrams may be provided, with rational explanations as to why conventional methods of treatment and of pest control have not been successful. Common explanations are that the parasites hide under the surface to escape eradication; that they come out only at night; that though adult forms are killed, the eggs escape; or that the species is new, as yet unknown and undescribed, and therefore resistant to current methods of irradication.

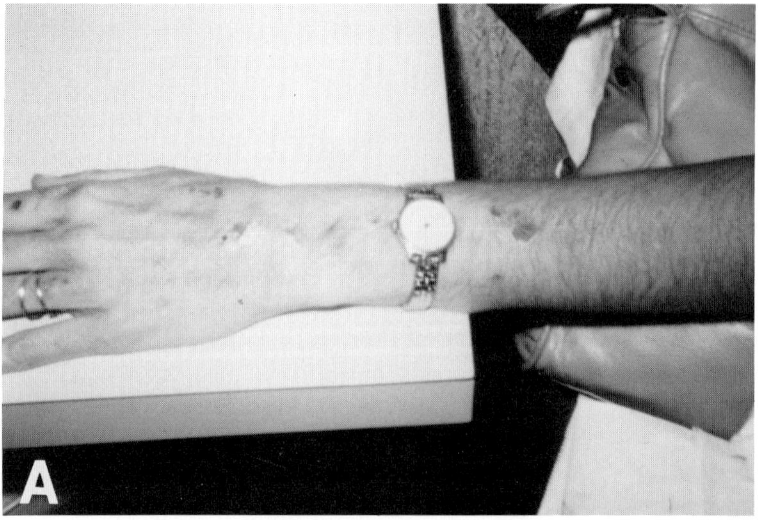

Figure 7-1. *(Continues.)*

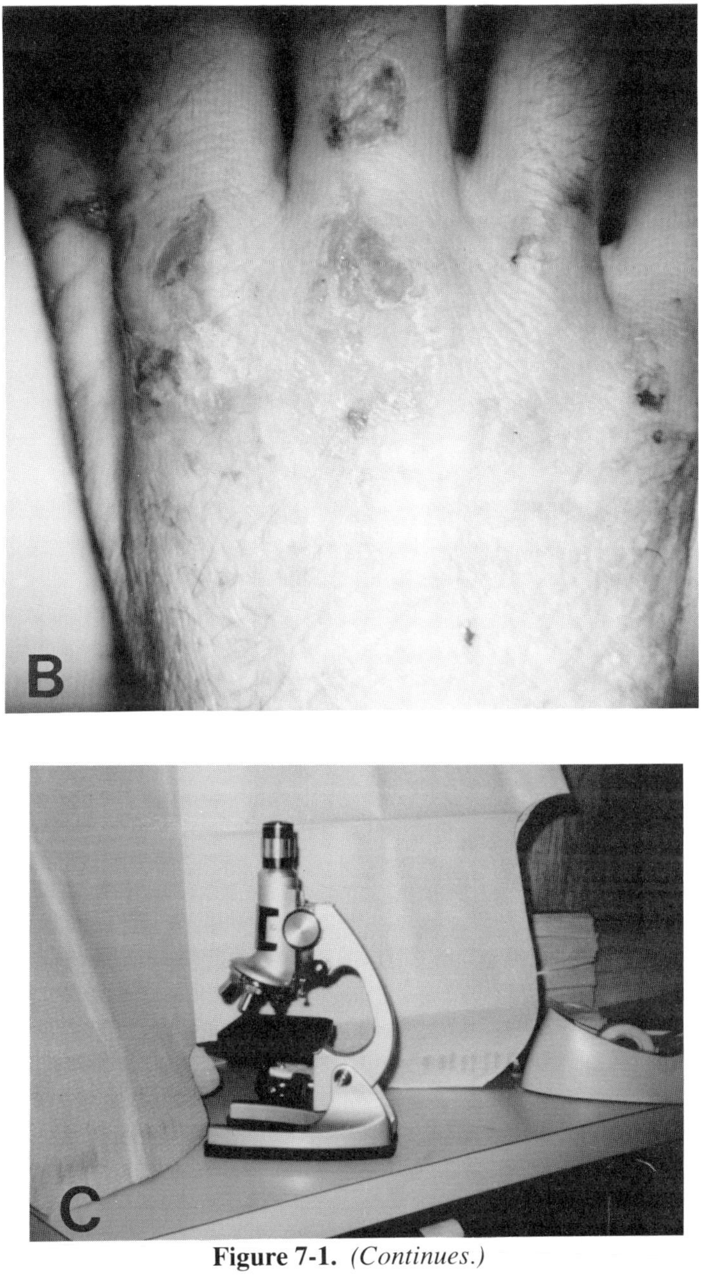

Figure 7-1. *(Continues.)*

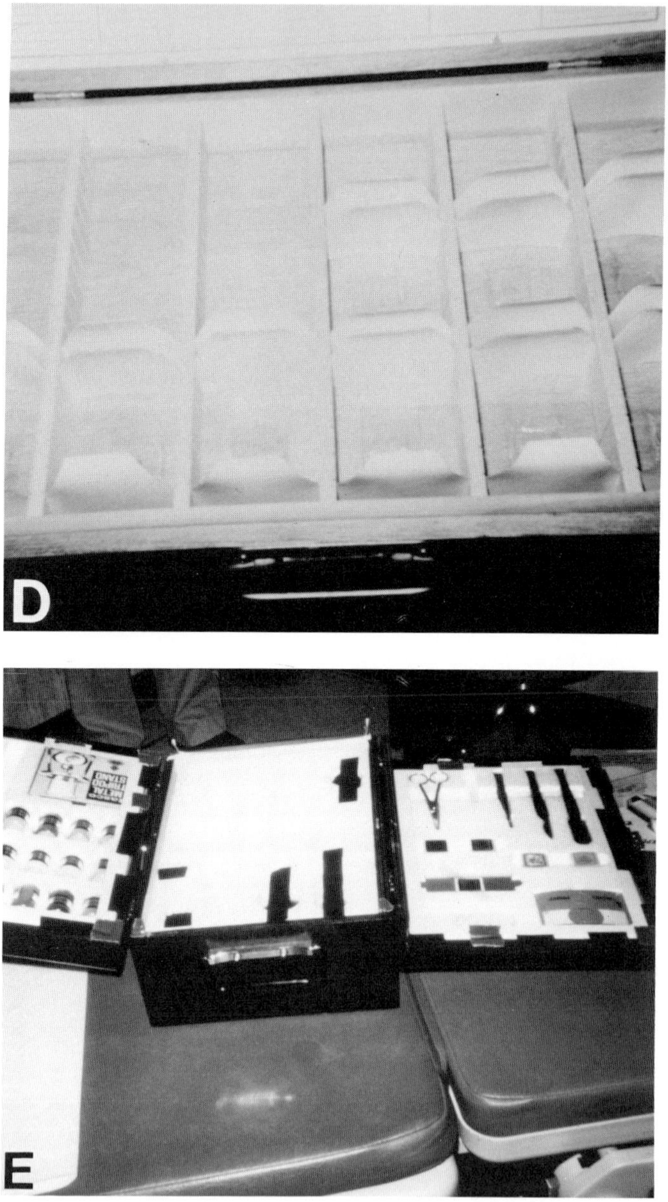

Figure 7-1. *(Continued.)* (A-E) Example of delusions of parasitosis. A and B show the character and distribution of numerous superficial excoriations on this middle-aged lady; the result of her search for elusive parasites. Her son abetted her by providing a dissecting set and microscope. "Specimens" were beautifully mounted on labelled slides in a compartmentalized specimen case. These patients provide a fine example of "folie à deux" (folie partagée), or shared delusion.

Group outbreaks have been reported from a number of occupational facilities; these have been attributed to "phantom biters" and are believed to have a specific though often undetermined cause. Lyell notes that such outbreaks are most common following periods of high temperature and high humidity and may be caused by fragments of carpet fiber or glass fiber.[25] One patient of mine may have been a victim of just such a circumstance; she claimed that she and many other workers were bitten by mites infesting the fiberglass that covered cables in the central telephone exchange where she worked.

Visible cutaneous lesions vary according to the perceived activities of the organisms. In those cases where they "descend like a plague," or "burrow into the skin," there may be no lesions, minor excoriations, or some minor nonspecific dermatosis that is attributed to the infestation. Where they "live under the surface," attempts are made to let them out, and lesions then consist of circular excoriations, deeply gouged pits, or even knife slashes.[25] Not infrequently, in an attempt to demonstrate the creature in the office, the patient will pull out stringy fragments of follicular epithelium with a pair of tweezers, for the edification of the physician. Prominent also may be secondary effects of the frantic and obsessional attempts at cleansing and decontaminating the skin that present as various types of irritant or chemical dermatitis.

Incidence

Delusional parasitosis is a relatively rare condition with a frequency seven times less than that of dermatitis artefacta.[25] The onset may be at any time from the late teens into old age. The highest incidence is from 50-80 years, with a peak in the late sixties.[39] Females predominate overall, with a male to female ratio of 1:1 under 50 years, and 1:3 over 50. Reports vary as to the educational and socioeconomic status of patients,[12,25] but many of them are isolated and lonely. Associated visual or auditory impairment has been noted in a number of patients[39] as well as a variety of concurrent medical disorders that include diabetes mellitus, renal disease, arteriosclerosis, pellagra, Vitamin B12 deficiency, brain tumor, liver disease, lymphoma, and neurosyphilis.[12]

These patients do not form a homogeneous group. Physical status, age, lifestyle, and mental and emotional makeup all contribute to etiology; they contribute also to prognosis and the response to treatment. In many reports no attempt is made to tease apart these separate threads, so that it is not always easy to evaluate the findings. Though the disease carries Ekbom's name, the elderly, abused, institutionalized patients that he describes[9] would seem to be a biased sampling; encompassing a spectrum of very severe cases, they do not conform to the picture of monsymptomatic disease that we commonly see in dermatology practice.

In suceeding sections I will try to tease apart the influence of these factors that I have ennumerated above. My major focus will be on those patients whose condition persists unabated despite correction of other factors of general health. These I will call the "classic" case.

Etiology, Pathophysiology, and Psychopathology

Ambient Conditions in the Skin and Concurrent Medical Disorders

It has been suggested that the condition of the skin, particularly in the aged, because of vascular, sensory, or ambient changes, or concurrent medical conditions, predisposes towards itching, tickling, or crawling sensations that may then be delusionally interpreted by the patient as due to a parasitic infestation.[43] These conditions would include senile xerosis in addition to those listed above. In some cases the delusional state resolves once specific deficiencies or abnormalities are corrected.[1,34,39] In other cases, however, where delusions persist in characteristic fashion despite treatment of concurrent disorders, the condition of the skin can be understood to have served only as an available vehicle for the expression of disordered thinking; had that vehicle not been readily available, then a different delusion might well have been "chosen." It is the persistance of the disordered thinking and its monosymptomatic character that is crucial to the diagnosis, and it does not seem necessary to create a separate classification for those patients with typical delusions, who happen also to have concurrent medical conditions.

Patients with visual or auditory impairment might also be considered here, since we know that sensory deprivation can lead to disordered thought and false perceptions.[40] However, the number of patients with this associated finding is small[39] and it is unlikely to be meaningful in terms of etiology.

Psychopathology

Toxic psychosis. Patients with alcoholic psychosis,[23] cocaine addiction,[15] or amphetamine addiction[23] may complain of parasitic infestation. As in patients with deficiency disease, the delusions do not have the fixed quality that we associate with the classic syndrome, and will resolve on treatment of the underlying condition. Further, the delusion is but one among a multiplicity of symptoms that may well overshadow it in the clinical presentation. It is important to remember that delusions also may occur in steroid psychosis.[23]

Organic brain syndrome. A number of authors have reported delusional parasitosis in association with organic brain disease such as Parkinsonism, dementia, mental deficiency, neurosyphilis, and cerebral arteriosclerosis.[13] These patients also do not fit the classic syndrome because again, the delusional ideation is one of many symptoms, rather than a single symptom in an otherwise apparently healthy person.

The classic case. Because patients with delusions of parasitosis are seen most commonly by nonpsychiatric physicians, a failure to distinguish between obsessions, phobias, neurotic excoriations, and delusions makes many of the early papers in the dermatology literature cognitively misleading, though descriptively rich. Papers in the psychiatric literature are no more enlightening, replete as they are with differing viewpoints as to diagnostic criteria.[12,19,31]

A careful evaluation of these works supports my own clinical experience, which suggests that the majority of these patients fall into one of three diagnostic categories: paranoia, paranoid schizophrenia, or involutional depression in a patient whose premorbid personality was obsessive.[44] Those patients with folie partagée on the other hand, have a delusion that is less firmly fixed—perhaps even an illusion rather than true delusion; they may be immature and suggestible individuals with a hysterical personality configuration.

The psychodynamic underpinnings in each case will be those of the primary psychiatric diagnosis, and so will vary according to whether the delusions are symptomatic of depression, paranoia, or schizophrenia. Skott's very thorough study of 57 patients unfortunately did not address the psychodynamic determinants,[39] but this information has been illucidated by a number of other authors.

Paulson and Petrus[31] studied intensively a series of (unfortunately only) five patients, by psychiatric interview and a complete battery of psychological tests. These tests included those for intellectual as well as for personality functioning. They underlined for us what one might in any case deduce, that only projective tests such as the Rorschach Test, Thematic Apperception Test, Sentence Completion Test, and Draw a Person Test revealed unconscious fantasy themes and areas of unconscious conflict. Tests such as the Minnesota Multiphasic Personality Index, subject as they are to the strictures of the psychological defense mechanisms, reveal only that information that the patient is willing for you to know; they do not contribute to psychodynamic understanding.

Psychodynamic Formulation

Involutional depression. These patients have difficulties in the area of separation and loss. Death of a spouse, the empty nest syndrome, loss of employment, body part, body function, or indeed any event that can be experienced in terms of loss, may serve to precipitate the syndrome. Unconscious guilt because of ambivalent feelings about important figures, often parental figures, contributes to the negative feelings of self-worth; this guilt may be expressed in the fear of contaminating others that so often intensifies the tendency to social withdrawal and isolation. Relief of the sense of abandonment, sadness, and emotional neediness is sought through adoption of the illness role, and through the interactions that constitute the therapeutic relationship.

Paranoia and paranoid schizophrenia. Here difficulties in impulse control, an inability to express aggressive feelings, and unconscious sexual confusion underlie the symptomatology. These patients are suspicious of the external world, harbor intense unconscious hostility, and often also harbor unconscious homoerotic feelings; in this case, it is the sexual conflict, with its attendant guilt, that accounts for the fear of contaminating others. The symptom encapsulates and keeps strongly repressed the primary instinctual drives of aggression and sensuality; this repression serves to prevent disintegration of the ego and further psychotic decompensation.

Differential Diagnosis

In the typical case, it is hard to consider alternative diagnoses. Complete dermatologic and physical examination must be undertaken and appropriate studies ordered if they seem indicated, in order to rule out true infestation, underlying medical disorders, or vitamin deficiency. Dermatitis artefacta is ruled out by the history and by absence of the secrecy and denial typical of that entity. The characteristic total investment in the symptom, the delusional nature of the belief, and the anger and hostility that can be sensed, or that may be openly expressed, serve to rule out obsessional concerns about infestation. Toxic psychosis and the organic brain syndromes are ruled out by the history, and by the monosymptomatic nature of the delusion. A multiplicity of symptoms is the case also in the more florid schizophrenic patient, whose personality disorganization is too extensive to permit inclusion in this syndrome.

Management of the "Classic" Syndrome

The reader is first referred to the section on the general principles of management in Chapter 5, as an introduction to the specific managment of patients with delusions of parasitosis.

Therapeutic Engagement

The work of several authors gives lie to the often stated concept that because somatising patients lack the psychological language for communicating emotional distress, they are not amenable to psychotherapeutic intervention.[5,14,43] Her physical discomfort protects the patient from an even greater emotional discomfort, and at the same time serves as her entree into the medical system. She may feel lonely, isolated, abandoned, and emotionally needy, or alternatively resentful and hostile. She at the same time feels dirty, unacceptable, a source of contamination to others, with her self-esteem at a very low ebb. Finally, she may act in a demanding, provocative, and bizarre way, expressing ideas that answer no logic but their own.

It is important for the physician to bear these points in mind when interacting with the patient, so as not to act unwittingly in ways that may demean the patient further, increase her sense of isolation or hostility, or drive her away. Below is a treatment outline:

1. Do not immediately refer the patient to a psychiatrist; this will be experienced as rejection and will serve to increase the sense of lack of worth of the depressed patient, or the anger and hostility of the paranoid; it may also deprive the patient of some placebo benefit from a treatment that she had anticipated with some optimism.
2. Listen patiently and noncritically to her story, without disputing her idiosyncratic interpretation of reality. This nonjudgemental acceptance will help to reduce her feeling of isolation, and enhance her sense of worth; at the same time it will give the physician an opportunity to try to ascertain what current situation may have precipitated her illness.
3. Let the patient know that you believe her symptoms to be real, but do not enter into collusion with her as to etiology; this latter course can only serve to reinforce the delusion. Give her the courtesy of examining her specimens—they may indeed be parasites!—but also she will know that you take her problem seriously. I am usually frank about the nature of the specimens. If the issue of etiology cannot be sidestepped, a number of different approaches can be taken, depending on the particular circumstances.
   a. "I have successfully treated patients with this problem before; they give a history very similar to your own and though we don't exactly know why the problem arises, the medication that I am going to prescribe is usually helpful in eradicating the symptom."
   b. "You may very well have had an infestation initially that was adequately treated, and the only sign now is the residual sensation you feel in your skin. Given the experience you have had, I can understand how you feel that parasites are still there. This is a situation that I have seen before, and the medication that I am going to prescribe is usually very helpful in getting rid of this last remaining discomfort."
   c. "You have been in a situation where it would certainly have been possible for parasites to infest your skin, and I can quite understand that when you developed sensations such as you described to me, you might interpret those sensations in that light. But that isn't quite how I understand it. I think that

given the information available to you, you arrived at the only explanation that made sense. You added two and two together, but came up with five. Sometimes we do see this, and the medication that I am going to prescribe is usually helpful."

4. Prescribe whatever topical measures and symptomatic treatment you feel indicated by an objective evaluation. Do not get drawn into ordering unnecessary or repeated tests, or repeated treatments with parasitocides; again, this only serves to reinforce the symptoms. Set up return visits at intervals preferably of one week, and no greater than two, for supervision of treatment, to establish rapport, and for support.

Treatment as outlined up to this point is within the competence of any practising dermatologist, and is something that the physician must be willing to undertake if the patient is not to be deprived of help.[5,14] Those with special interest, however, may be willing to essay the next step.

5. Try to help the patient to reverse the displacement of focus from the somatic to the emotional sphere. Instead of talking about discomfort in somatic terms, help her to learn to talk about it in the emotional terms more appropriate to it.
   a. Frequent appointments should be continued. Once or twice weekly is optimal; extended visits of 30-45 minutes are of course ideal, but much can be accomplished in even quite short visits.
   b. Speak of her discomfort in generic terms, not in specific terms related to the delusion; this opens up the way for a broader consideration of her life's circumstances, and its discomforts.
   c. Try to ascertain how the disease affects her life and ask how she experiences the restrictions that it imposes. This will enable you to find areas for empathy. For example, say, "It must be awful for you to thus and so," or "I don't know how you have tolerated x, y, and z" and so turn up the "volume" of her discomfort[5] rather than making light of it by saying, for example, "I hope you feel better." This empathic understanding will ensure that she does not have to act out the emotional pain, by intensifying the physical symptoms.
   d. Recognize that it is because you accept her emotional pain at a somatic level and do not challenge her that the patient is able to keep coming back. Your acceptance permits her to extend the expression of her feelings to the emotional sphere, and so gradually be freed to give up their somatic expression.
6. Although some authors feel that insight should not be the goal of therapy, I find it useful to help patients to try to understand their disease in the context of their current life circumstances and their past experience.

As an example of point 6 above, a young woman of 27 consulted me about "bugs" in her hair. She had been selling door-to-door to make a little extra money and during a sales visit had heard a customer talk at length about having to treat head lice and pet fleas. Shortly thereafter, the patient saw a "bug" crawl out of her infant son's hair. She became very worried, and her own head began to itch. The symptoms became progressively worse; she found many "bugs" in her son's hair, and her own; when anyone scratched, she felt guilty—certain that she was spreading contagion through the family; she cut down social contacts and devoted her entire time to cleansing and disinfecting her self, her son, and her home. She was very anxious about the child because many doctors had told her not to treat him, as the medication was "toxic." She had been told the "bugs" were grass seeds. She complained of insomnia, anxiety, and epigastric distress.

The patient had lost two children prior to the birth of her son, and his had been a difficult pregnancy with a threatened abortion, emesis, and toxemia. She wanted a larger family but was afraid to try again because of obstetric difficulties.

Her father had had an accident that prevented his working just before the onset of her symptoms, and his business was now failing; she was partially dependent on him financially and his reverses caused her considerable financial distress. She had always been close to him, and had depended on him in many ways. In fact the "bug" was noted in her son's hair during her father's birthday party at her house.

It was helpful to this patient to begin to look at her feelings about herself as a mother, in light of her previous poor obstetrical history, and her close and dependent relationship with her father. These two factors made her feel inadequate as a mother and this inadequacy together with ambivalence about a baby who had given her so much trouble physically and who added to her financial difficulties aroused fears that she might injure the child in some way. These fears were expressed in her delusion that she had infested him, and in her guilt, in the exaggerated efforts to eradicate the infestation. Guilt about her ambivalence towards her father because of his financial and physical weakness was expressed through her own infestation and her constant concern about contaminating others.

She readily acknowledged her fear of injuring her baby when this was suggested to her in context, and this enabled her to look more realistically at the "infestation" and its consequences. The precipitating event was her father's accident, which threatened her security.

Drug and Other Treatment Modalities

Many agents have been used in the drug treatment of delusional parasitic infestation. Early authors refer to the use of opium[30] and of tranquilizers for relief of anxiety,[29] and tricyclic-like agents for the secondary depression that so often accompanies the syndrome, but they state that the delusion itself remains unchanged.[30] Various of the neuroleptics have also been reported, prescribed both by the oral route and by injection of depot preparations, and there are many reports documenting the seemingly specific efficacy of one of those neuroleptics, pimozide.[16,27,29,36]

Although not a homogeneous group diagnostically, a unitary approach to treatment has been the rule, and most would agree that pimozide is the drug of choice at this time. Certainly this is so in patients whose symptoms result from paranoia, but in my experience patients with involutional depression, whose delusional symptoms are of relatively short duration, a 6-8 week trial with a tricyclic-like antidepressant is worth considering, before resorting to pimozide. Roberts and Roberts report success with monoamine oxidase inhibitors[38] but as noted previously, these drugs are better prescribed by those who are thoroughly versed in psychopharmacology.

When possible, drugs should be prescribed in conjunction with a psychotherapeutic approach such as is outlined in the previous section; it is recognized that patients on psychotropic drugs prescribed in conjunction with psychotherapy do better than do those who receive drugs alone.[23]

Tullet finds electroconvulsive therapy to be ineffective,[44] but there are reports of modest success with psychosurgery; this rather radical modality, however, is unlikely to be resorted to at this time.

Course and Prognosis

Untreated, the prognosis for spontaneous remission is very poor indeed, if not hopeless.[45] The acute phase, with its characteristic high level of anxiety, its frenetic search for cure, that takes the patient from doctor to doctor and from entomologist to exterminator, and its frantic efforts at cleansing and sterilizing, gives way gradually to a chronic phase in which the patient renounces her quest for help and resigns herself to living with her symptoms.[39,43] The symptoms indeed may span many years, but as the patient is no longer seeking help, she is usually lost to follow-up.

With treatment, the prognosis will vary according to the underlying psychiatric disorder. Up to 80 percent of those patients who are paranoid will gradually improve over a period of up to 6 weeks once pimozide is prescribed, and the drug may need to be continued lifelong.[29] In a small percentage of cases pimozide can be discontinued, but may need to be reinstituted at a later date should symptoms recur. In patients who cannot take pimozide, haloperidol has been reported effective.[22]

In my experience, patients with involutional depression may achieve remission or even cure with treatment either with a tricyclic-like antidepressant or with pimozide, particularly if it is augmented with psychotherapy as outlined in the previous section.

OTHER DELUSIONS AND HALLUCINATIONS

Frequently reported under the rubric mono-symptomatic hypochondriasis, hypchondriacal psychosis,[32] dysmorphophobia,[8] dysmorphic syndrome,[22] or dermatologic nondisease,[7] a number of clinical syndromes are described that consist either of a monosymptomatic delusional belief about the structure or function of the skin, and/or its underlying supports, or a hallucinatory perception of abnormal feeling, color, or odor.

Dysmorphophobia, a term coined by Morselli[26] to describe a distortion of the "psychological" body image (the inner representation or perception of the somatic self in all its aspects) is nosologically no more accurate than is parasitophobia, as has already been discussed at length. While all the symptoms to be taken up in this section could with accuracy be perceived as distortions of the psychological body image, or subsumed under the title monosymptomatic hypochondriasis, I have proposed rather the term *dysmorphic syndrome*[22]; this is at the same time nosologically more accurate and also, one hopes, a diagnosis that a patient with an unconscious need to deny psychopathology might be able to accept; it avoids the negative connotation of such words as hypochondriasis and psychosis.

Clinical Picture

Like the patient with delusional parasitosis, these unfortunate patients are totally consumed by their physical symptoms, which occupy their every waking thought and fill all conversation. Their distress is all-pervasive, anxiety is at a high level, and depression lies over them like a pall. Though overwhelmed by the somatic symptom, with all of its ramifications, their functioning in other areas is relatively unimpaired and their personality intact (Fig. 7-2).

The onset is often insidious. Though in 30 percent of the cases a precipitating event can be identified,[29] at presentation symptoms have existed for an average of 5 years.[29] These symptoms include such dysesthesias as burning, itching, coldness, dull aching, or intense throbbing pain; altered structure such as a change in body contour, degeneration or dissolution of the skin, the rapid appearance of unexplained lines or wrinkles, and ugliness or offensiveness of appearance, most particularly of the nose; increase in facial hair, increase or decrease in scalp hair, matting or weaving of the hair on or under the scalp; or altered functioning such as bromidrosis or olfactory reference syndrome, in which an odor, offensive to others, is believed to emanate from skin or body orifice. As Cotterill has noted, these symptoms most commonly affect face, scalp, or anogenital region.[7] In every case the findings are entirely normal to objective examination.

The history is given in exquisite detail. The patient in all probability has already consulted specialists in every field even marginally related to the problem,

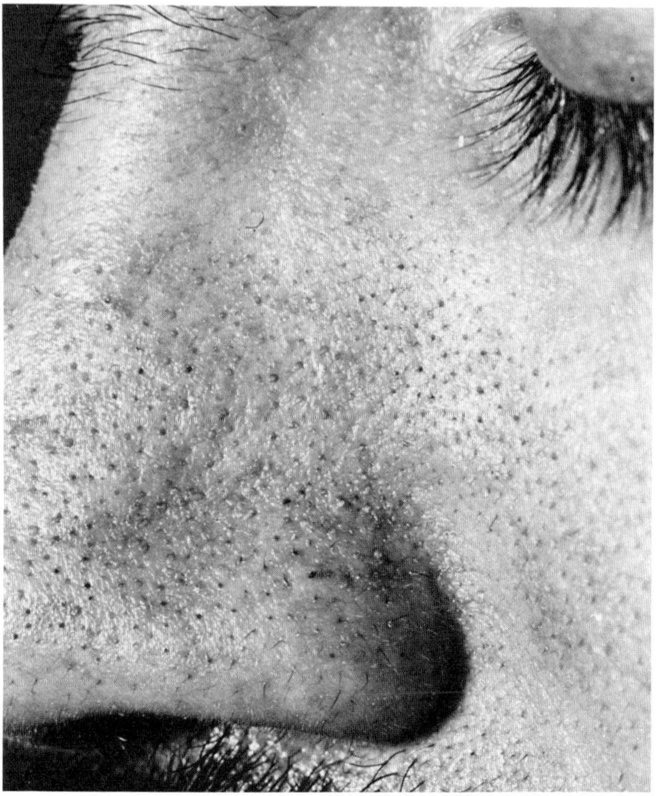

Figure 7-2. An example of cutaneous delusion. This 30-year-old university professor had a firm and unshakeable belief that his skin would dissolve into holes were it to contact water. He refused all medication for the same reason. After 2 years without washing, apart from an oily cast and light brown surface debris, the skin appeared perfectly normal.

every conceivable relevant and less relevant study has been undertaken, with invariably negative findings, and vast resources, both financial and medical, conventional and alternative, have been expended before the dermatologist is ever consulted. A patient of mine in a 5 year period saw 60 specialists in almost as many disciplines, at a cost of more than $12,000, and visited multiple centers in this and other countries in her relentless pilgrimage to seek relief from unremitting facial pain and perceived facial deformity (Fig. 7-3).[22] The unsuccessful outcome of such a course inevitably leads to anger, disappointment, and resentment towards doctors, who are often seen as uncaring if not incompetent; it leads also to intense hostility towards those who suggest that symptoms are not real, or that the perceived physical abnormality or change is not apparent.

The relentless quality of the quest for relief and the driven and accelerated

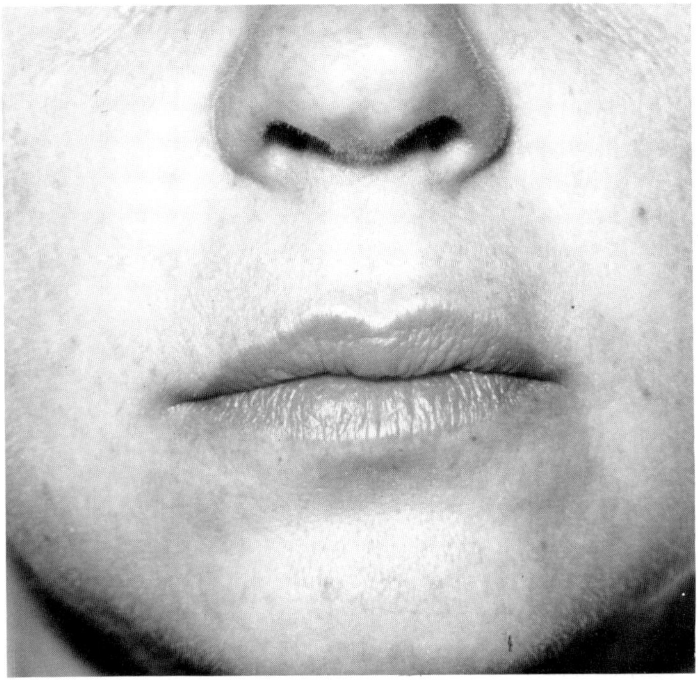

Figure 7-3. An example of dysmorphic delusions. This 50-year-old woman believed her skin to be decomposing and her facial contours so distorted that she had become grotesque and unrecognizable. All of her time and financial resources were expended in an unsuccessful search for relief from unbearable pain and progressive "deformity."

quality of the search for positive laboratory findings[28] are characteristic; they deplete personal and family resources, impair relationships, and may ultimately erode the level of functioning in various areas, albeit the personality remains intact.

Incidence

Reports in the literature vary as to the age and sex incidence. Hay[17] reports a male:female ratio of 2:1 and an age span of 15-55 years; the sex ratio in Connolly and Gipson's series was almost 1:1, with a mean age incidence of 27 years;[6] Cotterill's series of 28 patients ranged in age from 16-76 years, with a mean of 46, and a male:female ratio of 3:4.7[7]; whilst in my own series of 18 cases,[22] the age span was 19-79, of whom 66 percent were 45 years or older, and the male:female ratio was approximately 1:2. Two percent of women seeking cosmetic surgery in one series had this syndrome. Munro and Chimara[29] in a study of 50 patients quote an age incidence anywhere from adolescence onwards, with equal representation in both sexes and in all races and cultures. They found that those of lower socioeconomic status are more frequently affected, as are those males who are unmarried, separated, or divorced, and who have few or no children. In light of the above findings it seems that there is probably a slight preponderance of females, who tend to be affected at an older age than do males, but the onset of the disease in either sex, and from any race or socioeconomic group, may be from the mid-teens into old age.

Psychopathology

There is a tendency in the literature to treat as homogeneous this heterogeneous group of patients, making meaningful interpretation of the data difficult. Cotterill recognises the need to distinguish between obsessional concern and true delusion,[7] while Thomas suggests that dysmorphophobia be applied to obsessional concerns, ("overvalued ideas") and monosymptomatic hypochondriasis to true delusions.[41] But this would seem to be arbitrary, as the distinction between these two is not always clear-cut; an idée fixe may, over time, acquire the qualities of a true delusion.[18]

In the interests of clarity, and to avoid confusion about the level of psychopathology, only those cases whose disordered thinking leads to a true delusion, or hallucination, will be considered here; "over-valued ideas" will be taken up in Chapter 9.

Patients with schizophrenia may as part of the syndrome experience dysmorphic symptoms, and indeed such symptoms may represent a prodrome of that disorder.[17] The vast majority of those seen in dermatology practice, however, have a monosymptomatic picture that represents a sub-type of paranoia in a person whose pre-morbid personality was obsessive.[28] Depression is frequently part of the clinical picture and while some authors regard this as secondary, there is a question as to whether the dysmorphic symptom in these cases may not, in fact, have represented a masked depression at the outset.[11] Hay reports 5 schizophrenics in his series of 17 cases, and Korkina[24] 35 of 41, while Connolly and Gipson quote an incidence of 7 percent.[6] In Cotterill's series, depression was prominent,[7] while in my own series of 18 cases,[22] I classified 7 as involutional depression and 8 as paranoia; the three whom I termed personality disorder, in retrospect would, I believe, fit the sub-group of paranoia as described by Munro.[29]

Psychodynamic Formulations

Many authors speak of repressed hostility and covert self-reproach.[3,29] Negative feelings in response to bereavement, loneliness, or unacceptable aggressive impulses are initially directed against the self, as self-reproach; in defense against this reproach physical symptoms develop, which are more acceptable to the patient as cause for complaint; now, rather than a direct charge to important figures that have caused hurt, the patient instead tells them endlessly about his or her genuinely felt, but displaced, physical hurt. By this maneuver the patient is relieved of the intolerable discomfort of self-reproach, and also of the direct expression of aggression, while at the same time he or she punishes with his or her illness those perceived to have caused the hurt, or their symbolic substitutes. The relief of unconscious guilt implicit in this manoever is in line with Pryse-Phillips' concept of the patient "primed" for signs of "personal badness."[35] Negative feelings of self-worth because of unconscious conflict in areas both of aggression and sexuality are evident in such symptoms as perceived ugliness, tissue destruction, physical deformity, or body odors, while dependency needs are satisfied by the constant demands for care-taking and medical attention. In contrast, Bebbington understands the syndrome in behavioral terms, as learned behavior, suggesting that patients through stimulus augmentation have come to seek care-taking by deviant means.

Differential Diagnosis

As with delusions of parasitosis, diagnosis is not difficult in the classical case. The level of anxiety, the concomitant depression, the global involvement of emotional energy, the inability to divert attention to any topic other than the somatic symptom, the violence with which the beliefs are held, in face, often, of conflicting objective evidence, the stack of studies, sophisticated and mundane, often many times repeated and invariably unrevealing, and the multiplicity of physicians previously consulted, all speak for themselves.

If it is early in the course, and if this has not already been done, appropriate and reasonable tests must be undertaken to rule out whatever physical condition may be suggested, but the dysmorphic syndrome should be a positive diagnosis, and not one only by exclusion,[22] so tests should not be repeated, or more abstruse ones sought, with the physician entering into desperate collusion with the patient to identify a physical cause.

Although virtually any change in morphology or in function, and at any site, might form the substance of a delusion, that face, scalp and ano-genital area are the most common is a diagnostic pointer. Schizophrenia will be ruled out by the multiplicity of symptoms that characterize that syndrome, and obsessional concerns in the neurotic, by the quality and lack of delusional intensity with which they are held.

Management

Managment is essentially on the same lines as that for delusional parasitosis, and the reader is referred to that section, and to the section on general principles of management, in Chapter 5, for a fuller discussion.

Therapeutic Engagement

1. Do not refer the patient immediately to a psychiatrist.
2. Listen patiently and noncritically to the patient's story. Empathize with the patient's distress, and with his or her unsuccessful attempts at obtaining relief.
3. Let the patient know that you believe his or her symptoms to be real, but do not enter into collusion with the patient as to etiology. If that issue cannot be sidestepped, then one of several approaches can be taken.
   a. "There's a lot we don't know about the nerves in the skin, but I've seen a number of patients with problems like yours, and the medicine I am going to give you has been very helpful."
   b. "We believe that this change that you notice in your skin is due to some shift in the balance of certain chemicals in the brain. We don't know exactly what sets it off, but the medicine that I am going to give you will help to restore the balance. It may be that (the precipitating event, if you have been able to uncover one) in some way triggered the shift."
   c. If tricyclics are to be used, then reference can be made to their antihistaminic and analgesic effects, for symptomatic relief.
4. Prescribe appropriate topical and symptomatic treatment, if indicated. Set up return visits as previously outlined.

Treatment as outlined up to this point is within the competence of any practising dermatologist, and is something that the physician must be willing to undertake if the patient is not to be deprived of help altogether. Those with special interest however, may be willing to essay the next steps:

5. Try to help the patient to reverse the displacement from the somatic to the emotional sphere, as outlined in the previous section.
6. Try to help the patient see the current situation and its precipitant, in the context of his or her current circumstances and past experience; this is also outlined in the previous section.

As an example of these last steps, a woman of 69 developed intense pain in the skin of her right arm within days of an automobile accident in which her car was disabled. She called her daughter to take her first to the hospital, and then home, but she felt guilty because she interrupted her daughter's work. Her injuries were minor, but the localised pain persisted despite competent dermatologic care for many months. It kept her up at night, caused her to withdraw socially and to become indecisive; she was clearly overtly depressed. Her husband of 30 years had died 2-½ years prior to the accident. He had been an invalid for the last 15 years of his life and had demanded her attention day and night. She had married him because she had felt sorry for him; she had always "been there" for everybody, behavior that had its roots in childhood. Now that she was alone, and her son and daughter busy with their own lives, the accident made her realize that no one would take care of her, and she would reap no reward for her years of devotion; she felt lonely, abandoned, and helpless; what would happen if she really became ill?

This woman felt better when she could see the sequence of recent events against the back-drop of her life; she was then able to acknowledge both ambivalent feelings about the 15 years of her husband's illness, and strong resentment that her children were involved in their own lives when she needed help; she had deep longings to be taken care of, yet could not ask without feeling guilty.

Drug and Other Treatment Modalities

Patients whose dysmorphic symptoms derive from depressive illness, especially when these are of short duration, may improve with tricyclic-like antidepressants, especially when prescribed in conjunction with psychotherapy.[22]

Monoamine oxidase inhibitors, electroconvulsive therapy, and leukotomy have all been found effective, and there are also several reports of the successful application of behavioral techniques.[3,20] Of the various neuroleptics that have been used, haloperidol seems to be the most effective; it has been shown particularly helpful in the treatment of paranoid symptoms and halucinations. Pimozide is the specific neuroleptic for treatment of delusional parasitosis, but the reports of its efficacy in the dysmorphic syndrome are conflicting; it has been suggested that this may be because it functions primarily as an antipruritic, by binding opiate receptor sites.[21] This is certainly not the whole story, however, because it has proved effective in many cases of dysmorphism and also in the treatment of pathological jealousy,[32] among other conditions.

Course and Prognosis

The dysmorphic syndrome has been termed a morbid syndrome, and indeed it is, for untreated the symptoms will continue unabated, indefinitely. A percentage of these unfortunate patients will eventuate in florid schizophrenia, and there will be a number of suicides and attempted suicides, particularly in women with facial symptoms.[7]

Patients may be reluctant to take medication out of a paranoid fear of poisoning, or because it does not fit their delusional concept of the disease. Often, also, the drug will be discontinued because the patient lacks the insight to recognize causality when symptoms clear, and therefore claims the drug to be ineffective, when as is almost inevitable, they relapse.

Cotterill found neither tricyclic-like antidepressants nor pimozide helpful in his series of 28 patients, while Munro states that 80 percent of patients improve with pimozide, and of these, 75 percent will be able to resume a normal life. In my own series of 18 patients, all who received haloperidol responded; 5 of these had been antidepressant failures; all relapsed when the drug was discontinued, though apparently a small number of patients may remain symptom free if the drug is gradually withdrawn. A further three patients responded to antidepressants and psychotherapy, and have been able to be weaned off their drugs after a period of between 6 and 12 months.

REFERENCES

1. Aleshire I: Delusions of parasitosis: Report of successful care with antipellagrous treatment. JAMA 155:15-17, 1954
2. Bishop ER Jr: Monosymptomatic hypochondriasis. Psychosomatics 21:731-747, 1980
3. Bishop ER Jr: Monosymptomatic hypochondriacal syndromes in dermatology. J Am Acad Dermatol 9:152-158, 1983
4. Brotman AW, Jenike MA: Drs. Brotman and Jenike reply. Am J Psychiatry 142:1121, 1985
5. Brown HN, Vaillant GE: Hypochondriasis. Arch Intern Med 141:723-726, 1981
6. Connolly FH, Gipson M: Dysmorphophobia—a long-term study. Br J Psychiarty 132:568-570, 1978
7. Cotterill JA: Dermatological non-disease: A common and potentially fatal disturbance of cutaneous body image. Br J Dermatol 104:611, 1981
8. Crisp AH: Dysmorphophobia and the search for cosmetic surgery. Br Med J 282:1099-1100, 1981
9. Ekbom KA: Der prasenile dermatozoenwahn. Aus Derm Krankenhause Beckomberga, Angby (Stockholm) Vorstrand: Chefarzt Dr. F. Wiesel, pp 227-259
10. Evans P, Merskey H: Shared beliefs of dermal parasitosis: folie partagee. Br J Med Psychol 45:19-26, 1972
11. Feinmann C, Harris M, Cawley R: Psychogenic facial pain: Presentation and treatment. Br Med J 288:436-438, 1984

12. Freinhar JP: Delusions of parasitosis. Psychosomatics 25:47-53, 1984
13. Goltz RW, Derbes V: Delusions of parasitosis, in Orkin M, Maibach HI, Parish LC, Schwartzman RM (eds): Scabies and Pediculosis. Philadelphia, JB Lippincott, 1977
14. Gould WM, Gragg TM: Delusions of parasitosis: An approach to the problem. Arch Dermatol 112:1745-1748, 1976
15. Grinspoon L, Bakalar JB: Drug dependence: Non-narcotic agents, in Kaplan HI, Sadock BJ (eds): Comprehensive Textbook of Psychiatry IV. Baltimore, Williams and Wilkens, 1985
16. Hamann K, Avnstorp C: Delusions of infestation treated by pimozide: A double-blind crossover clinical study. Acta Derm Venereol (Stoch) 62:55-58, 1982
17. Hay GG: Dysmorphophobia. Br J Psychiatry 116:399-406, 1970
18. Hopkinson G: Delusions of infestation. Acta Psychiatr Scand 46:111-119, 1970
19. Hopkinson G: The psychiatric syndrome of infestation. Psychiatr Clin 6:330-345, 1973
20. Jenike MA: A case report of successful treatment of dysmorphophobia with tranylcypromine. Am J Psychiatry 141:1463-1464, 1984
21. Johnson GC, Anton RF: Pimozide in delusions of parasitosis (letter). J Clin Psychiatry 44:233, 1983
22. Koblenzer CS: The dysmorphic syndrome. Arch Dermatol 121:780-784, 1985
23. Kolb LC, Brodie HKH: Modern Clinical Psychiatry (ed 10). Philadelphia, WB Saunders Co, 1982, pp 328-329
24. Korkina MV: On the clinical significance of dysmorphophobic syndrome. I. On the phenomenological characteristics of dysmorphobic sundrome. Zh Nevropat Psikhiat Korsakov 59:994-1000, 1959
25. Lyell A: Delusions of parasitosis. Br J Dermatol 108:485-499, 1983
26. Morselli E: Sulla dismorfofobia el sulla tafefobia. Boll Accad Sci Med Genova 6:110, 1866
27. Munro A: Delusions of parasitosis (letter). Br Med J 1:1219, 1977
28. Munro A: Hypochondriasis revisted: From “Le Malade Imaginaire” to alexithymia. Ann R CRSC 18:405-409, 1985
29. Munro A, Chimara J: Monosymptomatic hypochondriacal psychosis: A diagnosis checklist based on 50 cases of the disorder. Can J Psychiatry 27:374-376, 1982
30. Obermayer ME: Psychocutaneous Medicine. Springfield, IL, Charles C. Thomas, 1955, pp148-163
31. Paulson MJ, Petrus EP: Delusions of parasitoiss: A psychological study. Psychosomatics 10:111-120, 1969
32. Pollock BG: Diagnosis and management of hypochondriacal psychosis. Can Med Assoc J 123:722, 1980

33. Pollock BG: Successful treatment of pathological jealousy with pimozide. Can J Psychiatry 27:86-87, 1982
34. Pope FM: Parasitophobia as the presenting symptom of Vitamin B12 deficiency. Practitioner 204:421-422, 1970
35. Pryse-Phillips W: An olfactory reference syndrome. Acta Psychiatr Scand 47:484-509, 1971
36. Reilly TM, Jopling WH, Beard AW: Successful treatment with pimozide of delusional parasitosis. Br J Dermatol 98:457-459, 1978
36a. Reimer F: Das syndrom der optischen haluzinose. Stuttgart, Thime, 1970
37. Riding J, Munro A: Pimozide in the treatment of monosymptomatic hypochondriacal psychosis. Acta Psychiatr Scand 52:23-30, 1975
38. Roberts J, Roberts R: Delusions of parasitosis (letter). Br Med J 1:1219, 1977
39. Skott A: Delusions of infestation: Dermatozoenwahn-Ekbom's syndrome. Goteborg, Sweden, Departments of Psychology II, St. Jorgen Hospital, and Clinical Neurophysiology, Sahlgren Hospital, University of Goteborg, 1978
40. Solomon P, Kleeman ST: Sensory deprivation, in Kaplan HI, Sadock BJ (eds): Comprehensive Textbook of Psychiatry IV. Baltimore, Williams and Wilkins, 1985
41. Thomas CS: Dysmorphophobia: A question of definition. Br J Psychiatry 144:513-516, 1984
42. Thomas CS: Dysmorphophobia and monosymptomatic hypochondriasis. Am J Psychiatry 142:1121, 1985
43. Torch EM, Bishop ER, Jr: Delusions of parasitosis: Psychotherapeutic engagement. Am J Psychother 35:101-106, 1981
44. Tullett GL: Delusions of parasitosis. Br J Dermatol 77:448-455, 1965
45. Wilson JW, Miller HE: Delusions of parasitosis (acarophobia). Arch Dermatol Syph 54:39-56, 1946

Chapter 8

Psychogenic Pain Syndromes

There are a number of other pain syndromes of psychogenic origin in which the patient is not quite so intensely involved with his or her symptom as are those who have the dysmorphic syndrome. The differentiation between these two groups is by no means clear-cut, and some over-lap is inevitable, but in general the pain experienced by patients in this group, though intrusive and uncomfortable, does not become the focal point of their entire lives. Unlike those in whom dysesthesia is an expression of the dysmorphic syndrome, these patients can continue to function relatively normally, can be deflected to some degree from discussion of their symptoms, and are not driven with quite the same inexorable relentlessness to squander their resources in the quest for ever more obscure, diverse, and even deviant tests and treatments. The delusional quality of the thought process is absent and the level of understanding of the causality of symptoms more closely approximate to reality.

Pain is one the most frequent complaints that patients make, yet because of the myriad possible etiologies, and the enormous variations in individual response, it is perhaps one of the most difficult of symptoms to treat.

Engel has suggested that while we know that sensations of sight and sound can be experienced without peripheral stimulation, as in hallucinations or in dreams, it is sometimes hard for us to accept that the same can be so for pain; that we have stored memories of pain, and of body parts affected by pain, with all of the emotional baggage of those memories, and that these, like other memories, can be reactivated centrally without stimulation of the peripheral end-organ, and so without organic cause. Pain is never neutral; there is always an affective tone, whether it be of unpleasure or of relative pleasure. This affective tone gives pain its central psychic significance and its special meaning to the individual. The special meaning is developmentally derived. Some of these developmental paths in persons who seem unconsciously to seek out pain, the "pain-prone" individual,[5] are listed below; all of these mechanisms operate unconsciously:

1. Pain is important in the earliest of human relationships. For example, the cry of the infant brings the mother, who gives comfort and relieves "pain"; this association of pain with comfort and mother for some permits suffering to be-

come a pathway through which closeness with important figures is achieved; anticipation of this closeness makes it worthwhile to endure the pain.

2. Pain becomes associated with punishment, and so with guilt; thus pain may become a signal for guilt. If one is in pain, one must have been "bad"; it serves also as a means of expiating that guilt. Pain may be welcomed if it brings with it the anticipation of forgiveness, and therefore reconciliation with an important figure.
3. Pain becomes associated with aggression. If overt expression of the aggressive impulse is not tolerated by the individual, it may be expressed instead against the self in the form of pain. Because in this displacement of aggression to the self, the pleasure of expressing the impulse is retained, pain may be sought out.
4. As a corollary to the above, pain becomes associated with ideas about the loss of an important nurturing figure, whether the loss be fantasied, threatened, or real. It may serve to expiate guilt for negative wishes or feelings towards that figure; it may also provide a substitute for that figure, encapsulated in a painful part of the subject's own body, that can be loved instead. The site "chosen" for the pain may be the same as the site of pain suffered by the lost figure, allowing it through identification to keep that person "alive" for the patient, and so alleviate the patient's feelings of loss.
5. Pain may come to be involved in sexual feelings, in those sexual relationships that are sadomasochistic in character.
6. Pain may be used in exhibitionistic and demonstrative fashion both in order to satisfy a wish to be looked at and to satisfy a need for sympathy.

Contrary to common belief, one cannot differentiate between functional and organic pain on the basis of a differing response to placebo. Indeed 30 percent of normal persons, and of persons whose pain is organic in nature, derive some benefit from placebo. Furthermore, it is possible to raise the pain threshold by as much as 40 percent through a number of psychological maneuvres that include biofeedback, the creation of a positive emotional state, relaxation exercises, physical therapy or other physical activity, meditation, guided imagery, suggestion and hypnosis, as well as by placebo or analgesics.

Just as these techniques, which are designed to reduce stress, may raise the pain threshold, factors that increase stress will lower it. Among such factors are the anticipation of pain to come. The element of suspense, the conscious and unconscious fantasies of what is to be endured, increase the level of tension and lower the pain threshold. This fact argues persuasively for the adequate education and reassurance of patients who are scheduled for potentially painful procedures; most particularly is this so in children.

Psychogenic pain may, as explained, be entirely central in origin, while central determinants, including of course memory, are known to influence the experience of peripherally induced pain. For example, the extent of peripheral tissue damage due to injury need not necessarily correlate with the perceived pain; psychological and sociocultural aspects of the meaning of injury to the individual play a part in the degree of pain that is perceived; soldiers in battle may experience less pain and require less narcotics than do civilians with equivalent injuries.[13] Central determinants are involved also in post-traumatic pain, when chronic and intractable pain at the site of an injury may persist long after the pathophysiologic effects of that injury are resolved.

Engel found that aggression, pain, and suffering were prominent in the early relationships of "pain-prone" patients.[5] A number of family scenarios were observed:

1. Parents who were verbally and physically abusive to each other and/or to the child.
2. One submissive and one brutal parent, often an alcoholic father.
3. A parent who punished frequently, but overcompensated for guilt and remorse by shows of affection; this caused the child to come to believe that there would only be love and affection if there was first suffering.
4. Cold and distant parents who expressed love and affection only if the child was sick or suffering.
5. Important figures who suffered pain or illness, for which the child somehow came to feel responsible; fantasies of this type arise from guilt over aggressive feelings towards the important figure.
6. A child who had initially been overtly aggressive and hostile until some event caused abandonment of the behavior through guilt, and a turning of the aggression onto the self.
7. A child who manifested guilt by deflecting parental aggression away from the other parent or a sibling, onto him or herself.

The pain-prone person is at risk on two counts; first, the physician who has been unable to relieve the patient's distress may experience frustration and unconscious anger. This anger may lead the physician to make a hasty psychiatric referral without adequate somatic evaluation, to "dump" the patient, or alternatively, the anger may drive the physician to undertake some medical or surgical procedure not, perhaps, entirely warranted by an objective evaluation of the physical findings. Second, it must be kept in mind that the presence of a psychiatric diagnosis does not preclude a concomitant physical illness. For this reason, a change in the nature or the intensity of pain always demands further evaluation; 10 percent of patients with chronic pain who have been appropriately evaluated are ultimately found to have an occult malignancy or other medical condition that gradually becomes manifest.[13]

There is a consistency to the patterns of pain of peripheral organic origin; the character, location, and periodicity, for example, allow one to identify with reasonable confidence the pain of renal colic, duodenal ulcer, or myocardial infarction, on the basis of the history. The purpose of these pains is to alert their host that something is amiss, and that physical damage may ensue; if there is no super-added psychological component, the description will be terse, economical, and to the point; it will also be consistent with our understanding of anatomy and physiology.

In contrast, as Engel has observed, the more complex the ideation and the imagery, the more are psychic processes likely to be involved in the pain experience.[5] Descriptions are vague as to specific details of timing or duration, yet replete with colorful metaphor; rather than terms like sharp, dull, or throbbing, we hear of gnawing, crawling, burrowing, or feelings of being on fire or caught in a vise. The location of the pain is also vague, and consistent rather with some idiosyncratic view of anatomy and body function than with structure and function as we know it. Should such a patient have a peripheral organic lesion, the pain sensations arising from it are likely to be subjected to such psychic distortion and elaboration that its typical organic qualities are at risk of being obscured.

While a number of psychiatric disorders cause chronic pain syndromes, chronic pain itself constitutes a stress for the individual. This may result in a degree of personality disorganization, and such symptoms as irritability, anxiety, depression, fatigue, insomnia, and interpersonal difficulties in the family and on the job. Such symptoms as anxiety, hypochondriacal concerns, and depression all may be decreased if chronic pain is treated adequately.

ETIOLOGY

It is of crucial importance to recognize that depression may be manifest entirely through "physical equivalents," without there being any overt evidence of affective change. That the patient does not "feel" depressed, and claims to have "nothing to be depressed about," is in no way a bar to this diagnosis, and it should be assumed that masked depression is present until an adequate trial of antidepressants has failed.[13] In other cases, the cause is hysterical neurosis, hypochondriasis, or schizophrenia as discussed in Chapter 7.

INCIDENCE

Patients suffering from psychogenic pain tend to be of middle age or older; they come from larger families with more numerous siblings, and often from the lower socioeconomic groups. They tend also to have more relatives with painful illnesses, more relatives receiving disability compensation, and themselves to have had more painful illnesses and injuries than do controls.

TREATMENT

The reader is referred to the section on general principles of treatment in Chapter 5, to provide a background. Specific modalities for the treatment of psychogenic pain include: (1) Antidepressants, rather than analgesics, nerve-blocks, or neurodestructive procedures.[11] (2) Be encouraging and supportive lest a pejorative or threatening attitude require the patient unconsciously to "make a point" by intensifying the symptom. (3) Avoid hospitalization if possible, in order to prevent further regression into the passive, dependent, invalid role. (4) Psychiatric referral according to the guidelines previously outlined, if this is indicated, with a view to: (a) Insight-oriented psychotherapy or psychoanalysis where applicable; (b) Behavior modification techniques, with a focus on rewarding healthy, "well" behavior, rather than passive, dependent "sick" behavior; or (c) Hypnosis.[18]

SPECIFIC SYNDROMES

A number of specific presentations of psychogenic pain crop up with some regularity in dermatologic practice; these will be discussed below.

Glossodynia and Glossopyrosis

Burning pain or other dysesthesias may involve the tongue, palate, or buccal mucosa; dryness of the mouth, and a persistent metallic taste are other occasional complaints. In a percentage of cases this syndrome is caused by such conditions as ill-fitting dentures, moniliasis, Vitamin B12 or iron deficiency, geographic tongue, diabetes mellitus, Type II allergic reactions to inhalants or ingestants, heavy metal poisoning, and xerostomia secondary to Sjogren's syndrome or drugs.[1] But there is abundant evidence in the literature, most particularly in that of oral medicine and dentistry, to suggest that masked depression is the most frequent cause of these conditions.[2,7] Zegarelli, in a very thorough analysis of 57 patients,[19] found psychogenic influences responsible in 37 percent, and a factor in a further 11 percent; moniliasis was responsible in 21 percent, geographic tongue in 26 percent, multiple etiologies in 12 percent, while only 2 percent each were accounted for by trauma and pernicious anemia; in no case was diabetes mellitus the cause. The psychogenic group was comprised primarily of post-menopausal women; the tongue and palate were the sites most frequently involved. Grushka[9] and Coles[3] also found post-menopausal women to predominate in the psychogenic group; in explanation of this fact, it has been suggested that atrophic changes induced by the menopause may create a special vulnerability to dysesthesia in the mucosae of these women; biopsy material reveals no significant difference, however, from that of age-matched controls who are free of symptoms. There is some dispute as to the beneficial effects of replacement estrogen therapy and this approach remains to be evaluated definitively. The onset in the majority of Grushka's cases followed by a few weeks relatively extensive dental procedures; these procedures may have served to focus anxiety on this particular anatomical location. Haneke[10] and Coles[3] both confirm a psychosomatic etiology, while a number of authors write about the need for the dentist to be able to recognise and manage the depressed patient.[7,17]

Psychogenic Facial Pain

In addition to the dysesthesias of tongue, palate, and buccal mucosa described above, other types of atypical facial pain are reported that also appear to represent depressive equivalents, and that respond to treatment with tricyclic-like antidepressant drugs.[8] Among these are facial arthromyalgia (tempero-mandibular joint dysfunction syndrome) and a variety of other types of deep throbbing pains experienced in teeth or bones, or referred to other areas of the head.[14] Facial arthromyalgia has been attributed to bruxism and to malocclusion, but the incidence of malocclusion in these patients is no higher than in the population at large, and occlusal adjustment is reported not to afford relief.[6]

The response of all these variants to tricyclic-like antidepressant drugs is good, with 81 percent of 84 patients in one series becoming pain-free in 12 months.[6]

Burning of the Soles

Burning of the soles of the feet also is a recognized entity, and in absence of a clear-cut physical cause (such as tarsal tunnel entrapment of the tibial nerve or peripheral neuropathy) is believed to represent a depressive equivalent.[15]

Post-Herpetic Neuralgia

The etiologic position of post-herpetic neuralgia is not clear, but the 33 percent incidence in the age group over 60 years[12] (that group most subject to depressive disorders), together with the good response in many cases to tricyclic-like antidepressant drugs[16] and neuroleptic drugs,[4] raises the question as to whether or not this entity too, in some cases, may represent a depressive equivalent.

REFERENCES

1. Basker RM, Sturdee DW, Davenport JC: Patients with burning mouths. Brit Dent J 145:9-16, 1978
2. Beck FM, Kaul TJ, Weaver JM II: Recognition and management of the depressed dental patient. J Am Dent Assoc 99:967-971, 1979

3. Coles RB: Glossodynia—a psychosomatic problem. Trans St. John Hosp Derm Soc 52:79-83, 1966
4. Duke EE: Clinical experience with pimozide: Emphasis on its use in postherpetic neuralgia. J Am Acad Dermatol 8:845-850, 1983
5. Engel GL: "Psychogenic" pain. Med Clin North Am 42:1481-1496, 1958
6. Fenimann C, Harris M, Crawley R: Psychogenic facial pain: Presentation and treatment. Br Med J 288:436-438, 1984
7. Gobetti JP: The psychological aspects of dental therapy: A diagnostic problem. J Am Dent Assoc 102:662-663, 1981
8. Goldie L: Psychiatric aspects of otolaryngology. Practioner 221:701-706, 1978
9. Grushka M: Burning mouth: A review and update. Ont Dent 60: 56-61, 1983
10. Haneke E: Glossodynie. HNO 30:208-212, 1982
11. Kolb LC, Brodie HKH: Modern Clinical Psychiatry. Philadelphia, WB Saunders Co,1982, p 826
12. Oxman MN: Varicella and herpes zoster, in Fitzpatrick TB, Eisen AZ, Wolff K, et al. (eds): Dermatology in General Medicine. New York, McGraw Hill, 1987
13. Thompson TL: Chronic pain, in Kaplan HI, Sadock BJ (eds): Comprehensive Textbook of Psychiatry IV. Baltimore, Williams & Wilkins, 1985
14. Thomson H: Mandibular dysfunction syndrome. Br Dent J 130:187-93, 1971
15. Tuchman JH: Painful burning feet (letter). JAMA 251:657, 1984
16. Watson PC, Evans RJ, Reed K, et al.: Amitriptyline versus placebo in postherpetic neuralgia. Neurology (NY) 32:671-673, 1982
17. Webb HE, Lascelles RG: Treatment of facial and Head pain associated with depression. Lancet 1:355-356,1962
18. Wilkenson JB: Hypnotherapy in the psychosomatic approach to illness: A review. J R Soc Med 74:525-530, 1981
19. Zigarelli DJ: Burning mouth: An analysis of 57 patients. Oral Med Oral Pathol 58:34-38, 1984

Chapter 9

Compulsive Habits and Obsessional Concerns as They Relate to the Skin

Patients who have either compulsive habits or obsessional complaints related to the skin, come to us with symptoms that on the surface may sound very like those of the patients described in previous chapters, who have dermatitis artefacta or delusions. Those with obsessional concerns may complain of parasitic infestation, of emitting an odor, excessive hair loss, herpes, AIDS, or cancer, while the patient with a compulsive habit engages in such self-destructive activities as creating deep excoriations, licking their lips, pulling out hair or eye-brows, or picking at their nails.

These patients are in general less profoundly disturbed than are the first group. They do not as a rule suffer from psychosis or a personality disorder, but rather from unconscious neurotic conflict. Some are concerned lest they may really have the condition of which they complain, though they at the same time know that they do not, while others know full well that it is they who are creating lesions, driven by the demands of an uncontrollable inner force; usually they freely acknowledge this and do not engage in elaborate secrecy or deceit.

The reader is referred back to Chapter 4 for a discussion of our theoretical understanding of neurosis.

COMPULSIVE HABITS

The conditions to be discussed here include neurotic excoriations, traumatic chelitis, trichotillomania, onychotillomania, some cases of lichen simplex chronicus, and prurigo nodularis. These conditions have many features in common, but there are also significant differences, so each will be considered individually.

Neurotic Excoriations

Clinical Manifestations

One of three common mechanisms usually serves to initiate neurotic excoriations. An interruption in the smooth continuity of the skin surface may be perceived by the patient as an imperfection that cannot be tolerated and that must therefore be removed; such mundane lesions as insect bites, acne papules, or inconspicuous keratin plugs may serve in this way. Alternatively, an intolerable itching sensation may develop on apparently normal skin, which on scratching forms an urticaria-like papule that must be erased. The third method is for the patient to rub the skin very firmly with the fingertip until the surface is abraded; this rubbing may or may not be preceded by an itching sensation.[1,22,28,34,37]

Once initiated, the course is rather consistent. Whenever the patient becomes aware of the lesions either by the restless wandering of the hands over the surface of the skin, by a momentary sensation, or by a chance catching sight of them, a ritualistic picking of all lesions one by one, sometimes even in a particular order, gets underway. For some patients this must be done in a particular location or at a particular time of day, often at bed-time.[31] While for some the whole process is accomplished with full conscious awareness, there are others who fall into a trance-like state during the picking ritual;[29] often no pain is experienced until the ritual is over.

To complete the ritualized picking may take anywhere from a few minutes to several hours, and while fingers and fingernails are most commonly used, some patients resort to the pointed tips of knives or other accessory tools.[37] Regardless of how the manoeuvre is carried out, in common with other compulsive rituals, a consistent feature is the mounting inner tension that cannot be relieved until the requirements of the compulsion are satisfied.[50] With each successive repetition of the cycle, lesions become larger, more prominent, and more intrusively "imperfect," and therefore more pressingly in need of being "removed"; thus, the condition is inevitably progressive. As the patient is caught in the struggle between the need to pick and the wish to give up the habit, repeated failures contribute often to a profound secondary depression.

Characteristically, lesions vary in size from a few millimeters to 1 or 2 cm (Fig. 9-1). They are symmetrically distributed, within easy reach of the hands, and most commonly on the extensor aspect of arms, fore-arms, legs, thighs, face, and upper back, although any accessible site may be involved. Round, oval, or with a linear configuration, they may have a hemorrhagic crust, or alternatively a clean base in which follicular structures can be identified as minimally elevated puncta. Healing, when permitted, takes place centripetally from the margins, which in older lesions are hypertrophic, violaceous, and surround the central ulceration like a Celtic barrow.[37] Superfical lesions may heal with minimal atrophy and a halo of hyperpigmentation, while older and deeper lesions heal first as a hypertrophic nodule, followed by a leukodermic scar, with variable degrees of atrophy.[34] In the full-blown case, multiple lesions in all stages of development are the rule, but one may occasionally see a patient with only one or two lesions. These arise and heal in the same manner as described, but seem to be on a continuum with lichen simplex chronicus or prurigo nodularis, rather than typical neurotic excoriations (Fig. 9-2); these latter conditions will be discussed in a later section.

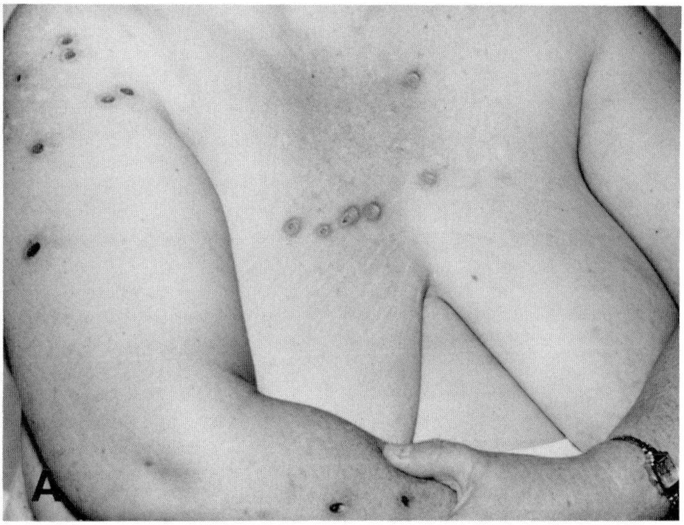
A

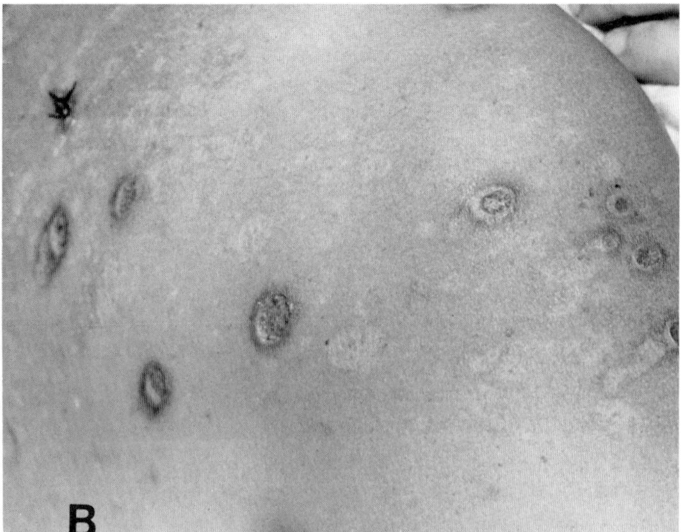
B

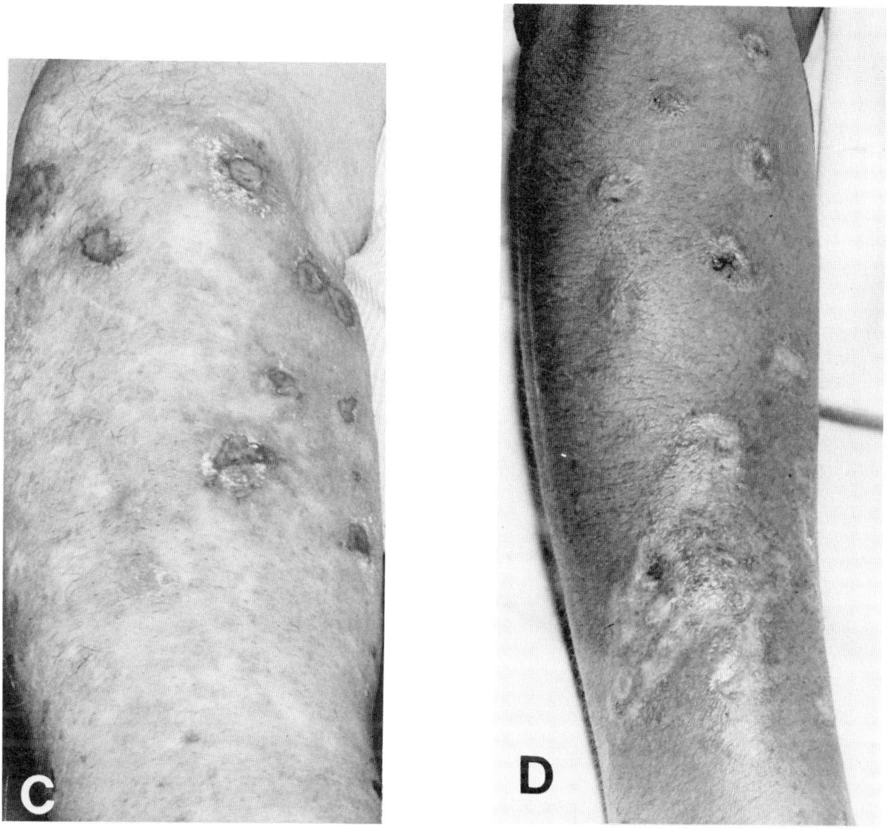

Figure 9-1. Neurotic excoriations; ulcer type. The most characteristic of these lesions are approximately 10 mm, shallow, scooped-out ulcers—often with a clean base—some scabbed over and with a regular outline (A, B). Irregular and bizarre-shaped lesions are sometimes seen (C, D). Pathodynamically, they are created by constent or episodic excoriation with finger-nails, knife, or other implement. Some lesions are allowed to heal and many scars may be seen in the same general area (B, C). The condition is chronic and may continue for years, even decades.

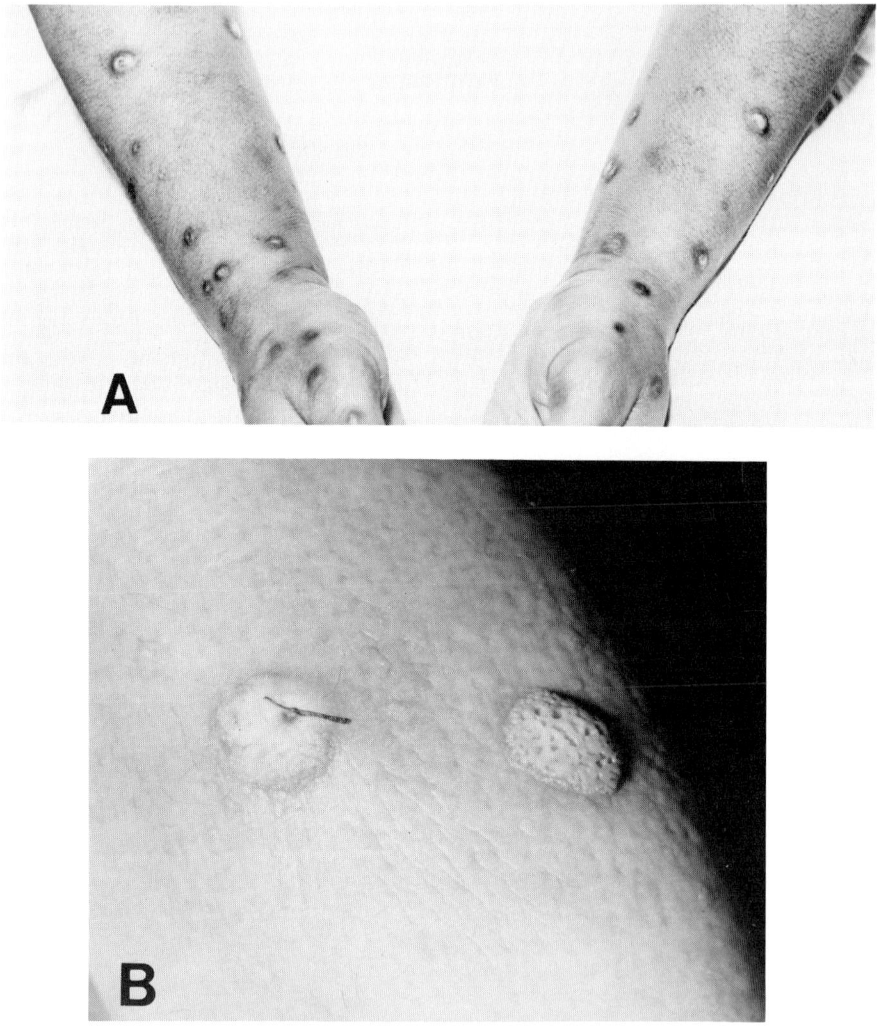

Figure 9-2. (A, B) Neurotic excoriations; hypertrophic type (nodular prurigo). Lesions may be single or multiple; single exophytic lesions may resemble warts, or neoplasms of epidermal or dermal origin.

Incidence

Michelson[31] described two distinct types of patient with neurotic excoriations. The first group were primarily young women in the second and third decade of life, who excoriated lesions of some preexisting dermatosis such as acne, in the typical ritualized fashion described above (Fig. 9-3). Those in the second were a more disparate group in the fourth or fifth decade, in whom picking occurred in

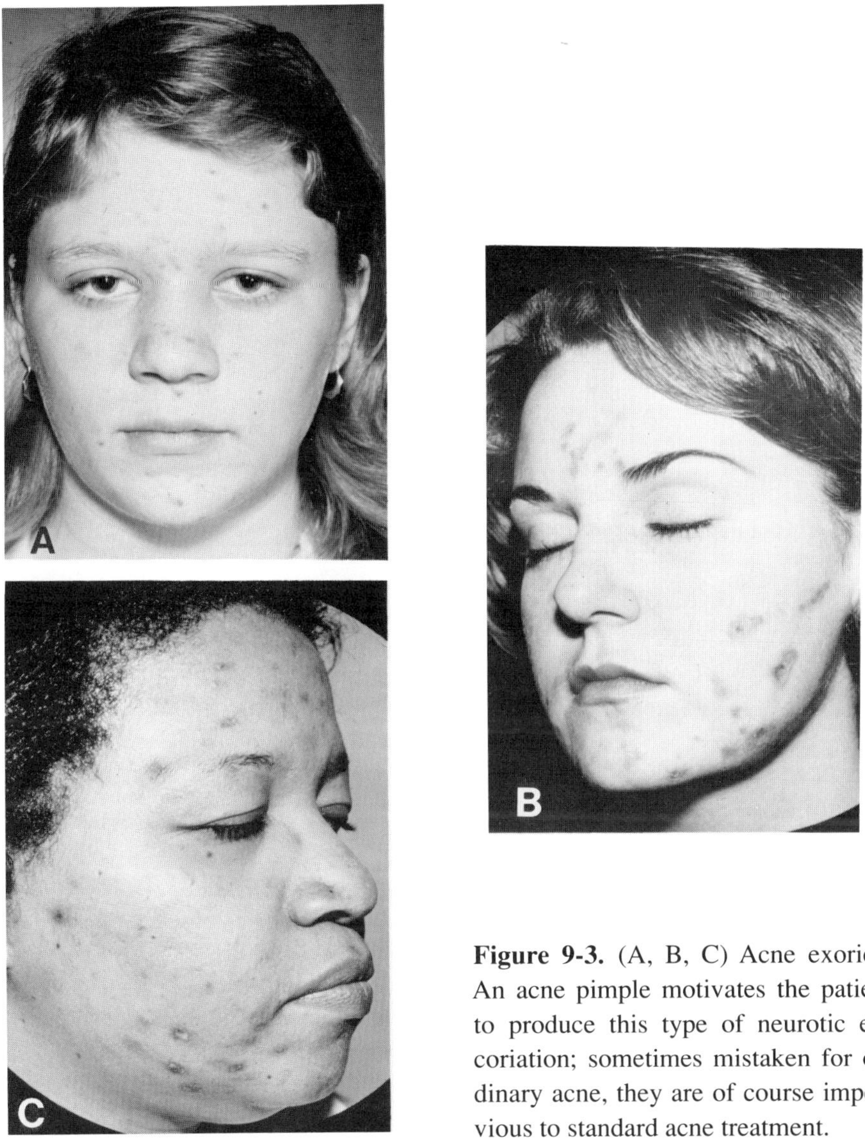

Figure 9-3. (A, B, C) Acne exoriee. An acne pimple motivates the patient to produce this type of neurotic excoriation; sometimes mistaken for ordinary acne, they are of course impervious to standard acne treatment.

sporadic fashion. Zaidens found the prevalence to be greatest in unmarried women in the third and fourth decade.[50] My own experience suggests that neurotic excoriations can be seen at any age, from childhood on, and with a broad spectrum of severity. Some habitually pick any incidental lesion, some experience transient episodes, with intervals free of picking, and there are some with the full-blown syndrome who experience unbearable tension if unable to respond to the compulsion, and whose picking is ritualized. This latter group has its onset usually in the third or fourth decade. In all of these groups women predominate.

Psychodynamics

In each of these groups of patients the underlying personality configuration is obsessive-compulsive and the psychologic defenses against neurotic anxiety will be those characteristically employed by obsessive-compulsive persons (see Chapter 4) Among these defenses are compulsive rituals and obsessional thoughts, which serve to keep aggressive wishes out of consciousness and bind the nascent anxiety as it arises. The tension experienced if the ritual cannot be completed represents the emergence in consciousness of unbound anxiety. These patients tend to be rigid, perfectionistic, indecisive for fear of making a mistake, and judgemental; they have difficulty in handling aggressive strivings, which for them are unacceptable. Frequently their parents are perceived in similar light, as cold, ungiving, and demanding figures whose high standards are impossible for the patient to meet. Much of the unconscious aggression is directed towards these parents or their symbolic substitutes in the current life situation. This aggression, because it is unacceptable to the patient, must be kept unconscious and cannot be expressed directly. Instead, the lesions serve to express the aggressive drive; they serve also as punishment for those unacceptable aggressive strivings. Unconscious guilt is evident both in the punishing aspect, and in the focus on "getting rid of" body products such as crusts, keratin plugs, or pus; there is guilt also in the often expressed concern about contaminating others. In some cases, an auto-erotic function may be served;[12,50] for example, one patient of mine, without prompting, described the build-up of tension, followed by release after picking, as "the same as being sexually satisfied." A hysterical dissociative mechanism is operative in those patients whose picking is done in a trance-like state.

Differential Diagnosis

The clinical history, morphology, and distribution make this an easy diagnosis in the full-blown case. The same lesions can be seen in patients with mental retardation, dementia, and psychosis, but in each of these, other features of the primary diagnosis will be evident. Similarly, delusions of parasitosis can be eliminated in absence of the delusional belief, and dermatitis artfacta is ruled out because there is no denial, secrecy, or overt angry and hostile attitude. In the early stages, dermatitis herpetiformis, papular urticaria and other types of hypersensitivity reaction (i.e., scabies, parapsoriasis lichenoides et varioliformis acuta, lymphomatoid papulosis) might be considered in the differential diagnosis and can be ruled out by biopsy of a relatively early lesion, in which the morphology is not too much distorted by repeated manipulation.

Management

In patients with dementia, mental retardation, or psychosis, the management will be that of the primary diagnosis, with symptomatic treatment only, for the cutaneous lesions. I will discuss management only of the more typical case; this will be both from the dermatologic and the psychiatric perspective.

Dermatologic. The dermatologic managment is symptomatic: (1) compresses, gentle debridement of crusts with moist cotton balls, and application of topical antibiotic ointments all direct the focus of attention to constructive rather than destructive behavior; (2) systemic antibiotics when indicated by the physical findings; (3) supportive dressings such as supportive elastic bandages to relieve discomfort, and if hydrostatic pressure or secondary infection cause local edema.

Psychiatric management in children. In the predisposed child, a compulsion may develop if an environmental stress arouses feelings that seem overwhelming; for example, birth of a sibling, parental strife, or school pressures. Parents may add to this stress by judgemental attitudes and unreasonable demands.

CHILDREN SIX YEARS AND YOUNGER

Compulsive habits in this age group are symptomatic of a childhood neurosis, and cannot be ignored if later emotional, discipline, school, or peer difficulties are to be avoided.

If the condition is of short duration, perhaps 2 or 3 months at most, and if there is some exogenous factor stressful to the child to which the symptoms can be attributed:

1. Help the parents to understand the child's feelings; offer suggestions as to how they may be alleviated.
2. Help them to be supportive and nonpunitive or judgmental.
3. Advise the parents to divert the child's attention if picking is observed.
4. Suggest toys be substituted,[27] absorbing activities arranged, or the day's schedule modified to eliminate opportunity, if there is a pattern to the picking.

If the above measures have not relieved tension and ameliorated the symptom within a period of perhaps 2-3 months; or, if when the child is first seen, picking is already fixed, and has been present for 6 or more months, then, in addition to the above measures, advise the parents that there may be deeper problems that may surface later. Suggest consultation with a child psychoanalyst or analytic psychotherapist. A brief course of therapy at this stage may help the child to handle feelings that would otherwise be repressed, only to surface later.

OLDER CHILDREN AND ADOLESCENTS

Help the parents to adopt a supportive and empathic attitude that recognises the child's wish to give up the habit, and her disappointment at her failure. Educate them as to the part their demanding and punitive attitude plays in aggravating the situation. Help them to be more tolerant and accepting, both of the underlying anger and of the compulsive behavior; help them also to recognize that it is not something that is being done deliberately, maliciously, and consciously against them personally. In such an environment, with increasing maturity the child can learn to master the negative feelings, give up the compulsive behavior, and move forward.[3]

Frequent visits, ostensibly for supervision of topical therapy, provide the best metier; as discussed previously, more can be accomplished in these visits if the child is seen without the parents, after the initial evaluation (see Dermatitis Artefacta in Chapter 6).

If, despite these measures, within a period of 6 months or so the situation remains unchanged: (1) help the parents to recognise other neurotic symptoms that may be present such as depression, discipline or academic problems, or poor peer relationships; (2) on the basis of 1 above, encourage psychiatric referral. Psychoanalysis or psychoanalytic psychotherapy is the treatment of choice. There may be short-term benefit from hypnosis, or from behavioral techniques in conjunction with psychotherapy; and (3) manipulate the environment by parent education, fostering, or hospitalization should the situation warrant these measures.

Psychiatric management in adults. Set up frequent interviews as discussed previously to supervise topical care, and permit the best possible therapeutic relationship to develop. Maintain an optimistic attitude, stressing your belief that the patient can and will master the distressing symptom.[23] Try to ascertain by gentle open-ended questioning, as previously described, whether this is a relatively circumscribed symptom, what circumstance may have precipitated it at this time, and to what extent the neurosis is interfering in other aspects of the patient's life.

If recent and relatively circumscribed, the interested dermatologist may then help the patient to recognise the precipitating factor, understand it in the context of her past life experience, and acknowledge the associated feelings. The patient may then be able to master those feelings and give up the compulsion.

For example: An immature 29-year-old woman depended heavily on her mother for help in running her house and raising her children. She at the same time resented the feeling that she could never satisy her mother's excessively high standards. She felt constantly criticized, and was pleased when her husband was transferred to a town several hours' drive away. However, when she settled into her new home she felt overwhelmed, became depressed and unable to manage the housework. She developed severe obsessive-compulsive symptoms including ritualized excoriation of her legs with the point of a kitchen knife. In this symptom was encapsulated anger and resentment with her mother whom she could not please, who had kept her dependent, and whom the patient experienced as having "abandoned" her when the patient herself left town. It encapsulated also anger with her husband who had bought a house that overwhelmed her, and who "abandoned" her when he travelled on business, and thirdly, there was anger with herself because she was so helpless; a fourth contribution came from the guilt she experienced about these strong negative feelings she held for people whom she needed, and who loved her. As the patient was able to acknowledge, sort out, and work through these feelings, and as she came to understand what the move had meant to her, she was able also, gradually, to give up her self-destructive behavior.

Other measures that may be recommended if they seem indicated include: (1) stress management techniques; (2) hypnosis;[17,49] (3) behavior modification therapy;[4,5] (4) a short course of anxiolytic drugs;[48] and (5) tricyclic-like antidepressants.[21]

If symptoms are long-standing, and there is evidence of a more pervasive neurosis, with interference in interpersonal relationships, job performance, or the capacity for enjoyment, then the treatment of choice is psychoanalysis or psychoanalytic psychotherapy, and an attempt should be made gradually to help the patient to recognise this need, and accept a referral.[40]

In severe cases neuroleptics have been prescribed, as have monoamine oxidase inhibitors.[25]

In patients who are severely incapacitated by symptoms of the obsessive-compulsive disorder, leukotomy has been found by some to lessen the intensity of the compulsive behavior, and relieve suffering.[47] Such a controversial procedure would certainly have to be very much a last resort, and happily such a decision does not fall within the expertise of the practising dermatologist.

Course and Prognosis

Clearly the course and the long-term outlook will depend on the severity of the disorder. Short duration, a supportive environment, and a relatively good psychological adjustment before onset of the symptoms, contribute to a favorable outcome with treatment, in all age groups; but as I have explained, the syndrome is symptomatic of a chronic psychiatric disorder whose course is remitting, so recurrent episodes cannot be discounted.

The prognosis in childhood is good,[48] because of the shorter duration of symptoms and the beneficial effect of increasing maturity, particularly if the environment is favorable; again, recurrences in later life may occur. A similarly satisfactory course is often followed in adult patients under the favorable circumstances mentioned. Cormia, in a series of 13 cases, reported improvement or cure in 66 percent with superficial psychotherapy.[15] Michelson also reported positive results with psychotherapy,[31] while Zaidens' patients did well with psychoanalytic treatment.[50] A general rule in obsessive-compulsive patients after treatments other than leukotomy suggests that 25 percent are cured, 50 percent improved, and 25 percent remain unchanged.[33]

Trichotillomania

Clinical Manifestations

Trichotillomania is the name coined by Hallopeau[20] for the compulsive plucking of scalp hair, eye-brows (Fig. 9-4), eye-lashes, beard, or pubic hair. The scalp is involved more frequently than are the other hair-bearing areas, and the clinical presentation of the lesion is quite characteristic (Fig. 9-5 A, B).

Plucking is accomplished either in wave-like fashion across the scalp, or centrifugally from a single starting point. This results in linear or circular patches with irregular borders containing hairs of varying length, the shortest being those most recently removed, while increasing length with distance from that point signifies the interval between the time of plucking and the time of the clinical evaluation. The process of plucking frequently fractures the hair-shaft above or within the follicle, so that the emerging hair, instead of having the finely tapered silkiness of the new-grown anagen hair, has a fractured end; this gives a stubbly sensation as the hand is passed lightly over the involved area. Plucking is usually confined to a single patch of varying size; this may be quite large, and indeed in rare instances may involve the entire scalp.[22,34] When the process has extended to a point that is no longer comfortable to reach, then the cycle is repeated, starting once again at the point of the beginning.

In many cases, a specific time and location is reserved for the process of plucking, which then takes on a ritualized character. Unlike neurotic excoriations,

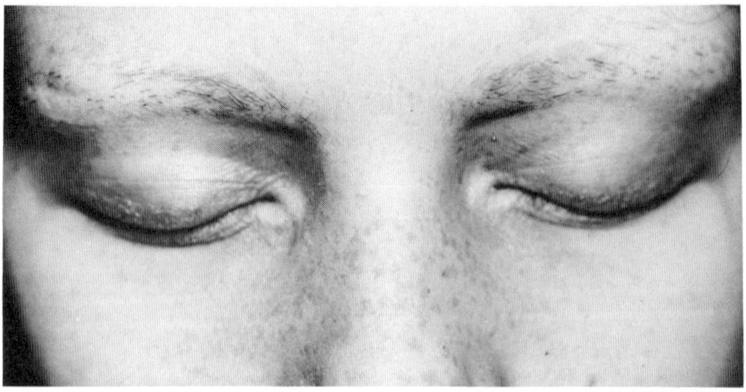

Figure 9-4. Cillotillomania. This patient has epilated both cilia and supercilia. Normally growing hairs of varying length make forcible epilation the only reasonable diagnosis.

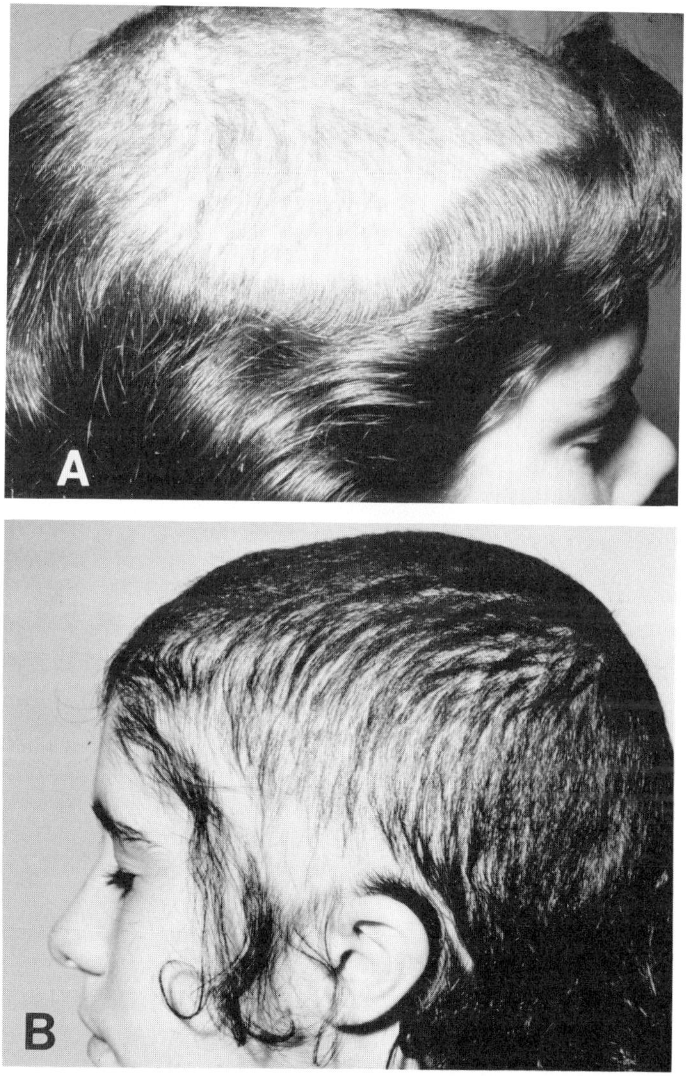

Figure 9-5. *(Continues.)*

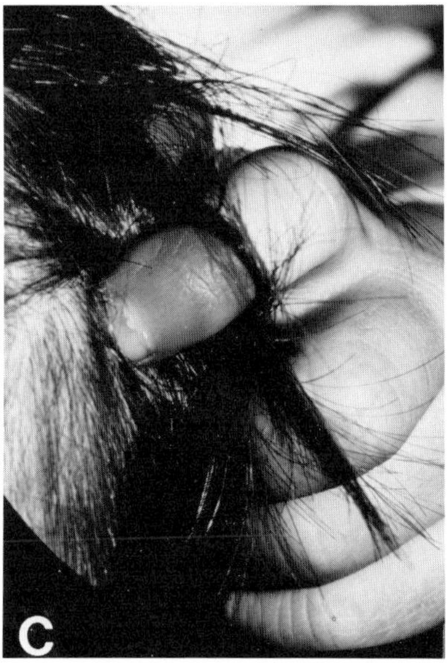

Figure 9-5. *(Continued.)* (A, B, C) Trichotillomania. Normal hair is separated by a narrow band of alopecia from an area in which the hairs become progressively longer, the farther one moves away. There is a characteristic stubbly feel to the regrowing hairs. As seen in the "action picture" (C) considerable force is required; observe the venous suffusion in the index fingertip. Young children may comfort themselves by stroking their skin with the epilated hair (transitional objects; others may ingest them.

however, for reasons of embarrassment or shame, it is more common for the patient not to acknowledge her involvement. Typically she will claim to wake to find balls of hair strewn about the bed, or if she does acknowledge it, she may rationalize her plucking on grounds of some aberrant sensation in the scalp. Parents often will share with the patient in this denial.[19,37]

In infancy and early childhood, the hair may hold an important place in emotional life; it may serve as a transitional object, with a role equivalent to that of a security blanket, and at times even interchangeable with that time-honored source of comfort. Transitional objects are used by the infant to bridge the gap between self and nonself, aiding in separating from the mother, and defining his or her own boundries. While hair is being used in this way, hairpulling may occur, either as a transient episode, or as the onset of true trichotillourania.

The sequence of events depicting an association between security blanket and hair is illustrated in Figures 9-6 A-E. I have often observed in native Africans the phenomenon shown in the 19th-Century Japanese woodcuts (Figs. 9-6 A & B); as the infant nurses at one breast, he or she fondles the contralateral nipple with the free hand. Figures 9-6 C-F illustrate the Western equivalent of this maneuver. As first bottle (Fig. 9-6C) and later thumb (Fig. 9-6D) is sucked, the free hand is used to fondle self (Fig. 9-6D). Mother (Fig. 9-6F) or object (Fig. 9-6E), it is here that security blanket and hair may become interchangeable, and hair-pulling may occur; in the older child there may be a further displacement as in place of sucking breast, bottle, or thumb, the child instead fondles his or her nose or other area of

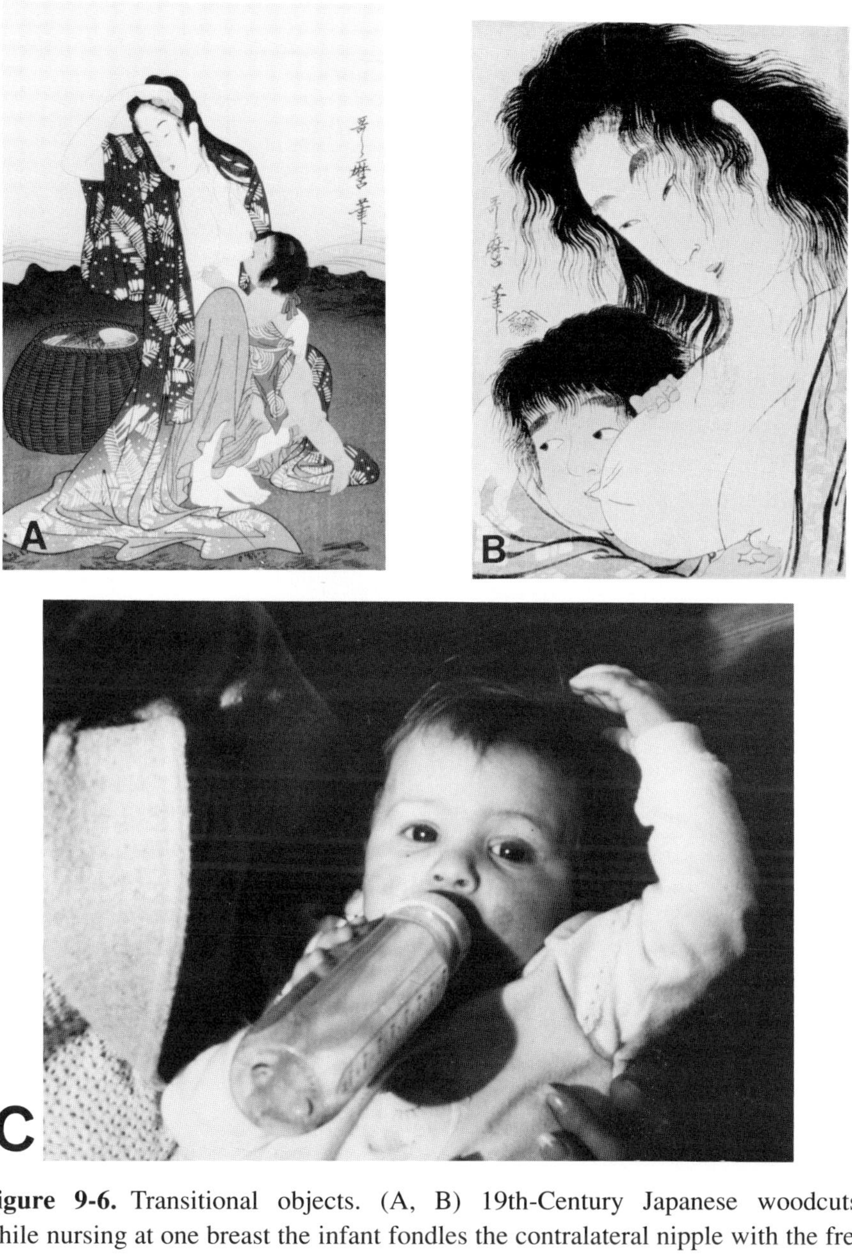

Figure 9-6. Transitional objects. (A, B) 19th-Century Japanese woodcuts; while nursing at one breast the infant fondles the contralateral nipple with the free hand. Figures C, D, and E illustrate the Western equivalent; while taking the bottle (C) or thumb-sucking (D), the opposite hand may fondle self, object (E), or mother (F). *(Continues.)*

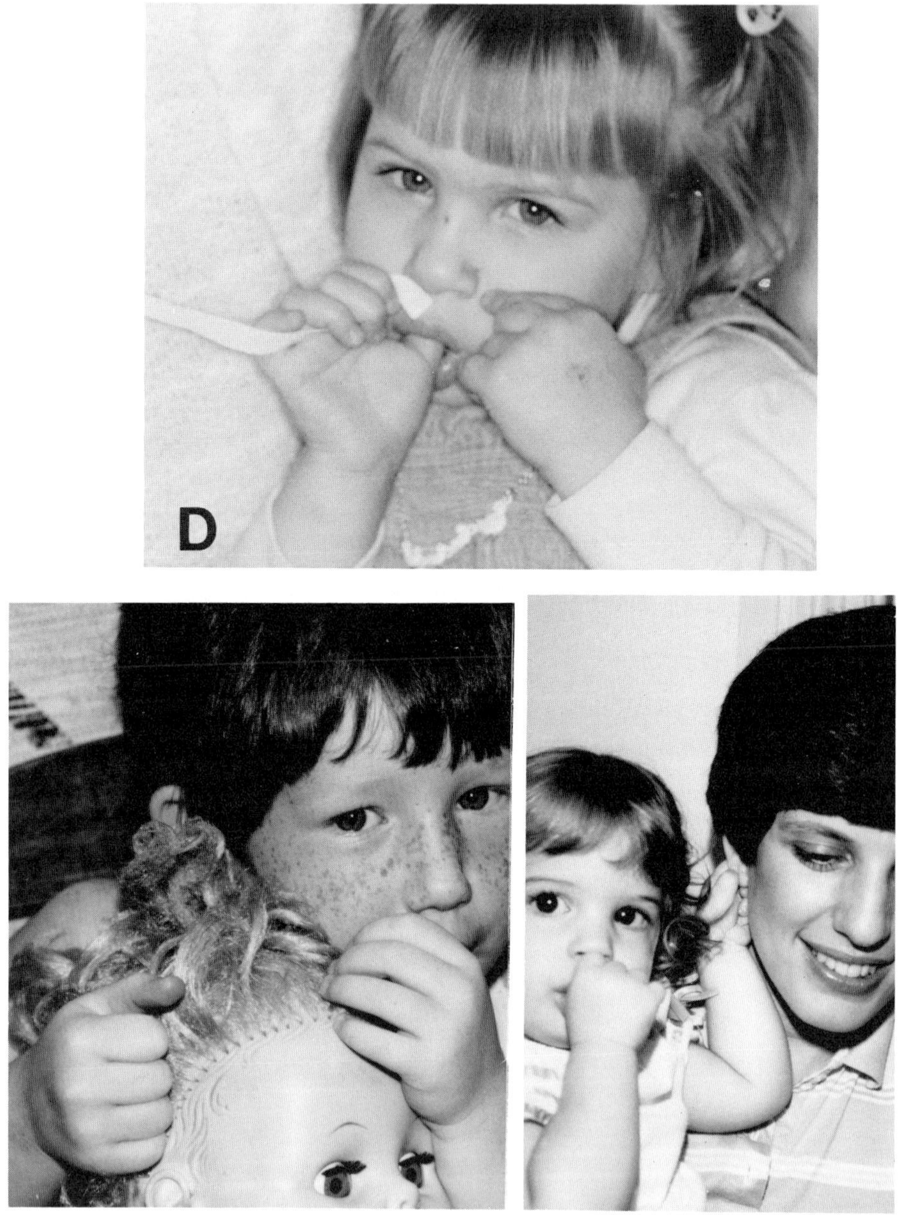

E F

Figure 9-6. *(Continued.)*

skin (Fig. 9-7A) as the hair is manipulated. It is not unusual for the hairs plucked at these times to be chewed, or even eaten as part of the ritual, and occasionally intestinal obstruction may result due to formation of a trichobezoar.[2,22]

Trichotillomania in childhood or adolescence is not often reported in isolation; it is usually associated with other disturbances such as thumb-sucking, nail-biting, nose-picking, poor peer relationships, and academic problems. An associated excessive concern with weight has also been noted, reflecting the opposite aspect of the issue of impulse control.[19,41]

Incidence

Like dermatitis artefacta and neurotic excoriations, patients with trichotillomania present more commonly to dermatologists than to psychiatrists, and the reported incidence and the implication of the symptom reflects inevitably only the particular clinical experience of the individual observer. Spock observed quite normal children sucking one thumb, while simultaneously manipulating the hair with the other hand,[42] a manoever that may go on to epilation of the hair and trichotillomania proper, as I have noted.[23] The symptom has been observed in children as early as 18 months of age. Greenberg and Sarner, reporting on 19 cases from combined dermatologic and psychiatric patient pools, found a male to female ratio of 1:5, with a 68 percent incidence in the adolescent or pre-adolescent age group.[19] Krishnan et al. observed the highest incidence in female adolescents,[24] while other authors found adults to predominate.[19,50] While it is clear that trichotillomania can be seen in either sex and at any time after muscle coordination is sufficiently developed (somewhere about the middle of the second year of life), my own clinical experience supports the findings of Greenberg and Sarner, that females significantly out-number males with the highest incidence occurring in late childhood and adolescence.

Psychopathology and Psychodynamics

Psychopathology. Trichotillomania occurs over a broad spectrum of psychopathology. It may represent a transient compulsive habit in an essentially normal youngster,[30] or it may be symptomatic of a more pervasive neurosis. It may also be seen in more severely disturbed patients either with the borderline personality disorder or with schizophrenia.[6] A secondary depression is a not uncommon finding. When the symptom occurs by itself, or when it persists past childhood without evidence of more serious psychiatric illness, it is like neurotic excoriations, indicative of obsessive-compulsive neurosis.[30,36]

Psychodynamics. Cramer,[14] by attributing trichotillomania to unresolved conflict in the period from age one and a half to the beginning of the fourth year of life, confirms its obsessive-compulsive etiology (see Chapter 4). Family studies have helped to elucidate the character of that conflict.

Greenberg and Sarner[19] found a remarkable consistency in the family constellations and particularly in the quality of mother-daughter interactions in the 19 cases that they reported. Eighty-four percent of the mothers were found to be ambivalent towards their daughters; at once critical, hostile, intolerant of aggression, competitive, and domineering, and at the same time overprotective; they had kept their daughters close, to satisfy their own dependency needs. These mothers alternately infantilized and parentified the patients, projecting onto them their own unfulfilled wishes and ambitions, and at times deriving from them also a degree of erotic gratification. Their relationships were fraught with provocation, hostility, and violent physical quarrels, as the patient sought to resolve her own conflicts over autonomy, her competitive drives, and her dependency needs.

The hair-pulling rapidly became integral to this pathological "symbiotic" relationship, and the focus of a bitter power struggle. These authors postulated that it was the nature of this relationship, depending as it did on the sexual identity of mother and daughter, that determined the significantly higher incidence in girls than in boys. The mother-son relationships, though ambivalent, did not have the same intensity as did those of mothers with their daughters. In most cases the fathers were experienced as passive and ineffectual, incapable of intervening, or of controlling the mothers; alternatively they were experienced as cold, indifferent, and hostile.

In some cases there is evidence to support a genesis at an even earlier period, in the very early struggle of the infant to separate from the mother and achieve her own identity.[18,30] In these cases the syndrome may be precipitated by some event experienced by the child as the real or symbolic loss of an important figure. Here the hair is used as a transitional object, a substitute for the lost person until the feelings of loss, and rage occasioned by that loss, can be mastered and integrated.[11] This view is further supported by clinical experience; for example, in several instances the syndrome has been observed to occur immediately following banishment by the mother of the child's security blanket (Fig. 9-7).*

Other precipitating causes can often be uncovered, and occasionally even the choice of symptom, at least at a superficial level, can be understood. Examples are cases in which the onset of trichotillomania is preceded by disease or trauma to the scalp that made that site a focus of attention; others are cases where the site selected for plucking proves to be identical to the site of pattern alopecia in the father, in unconscious identification with him.[19]

Many authors have discussed the unconscious symbolic meaning of hair, and explicated its suitability for incorporation in neurotic symptomatology; the interested reader is referred to the relevant literature.[8,9,24]

*Koblenzer PJ: Personal communication, 1986.

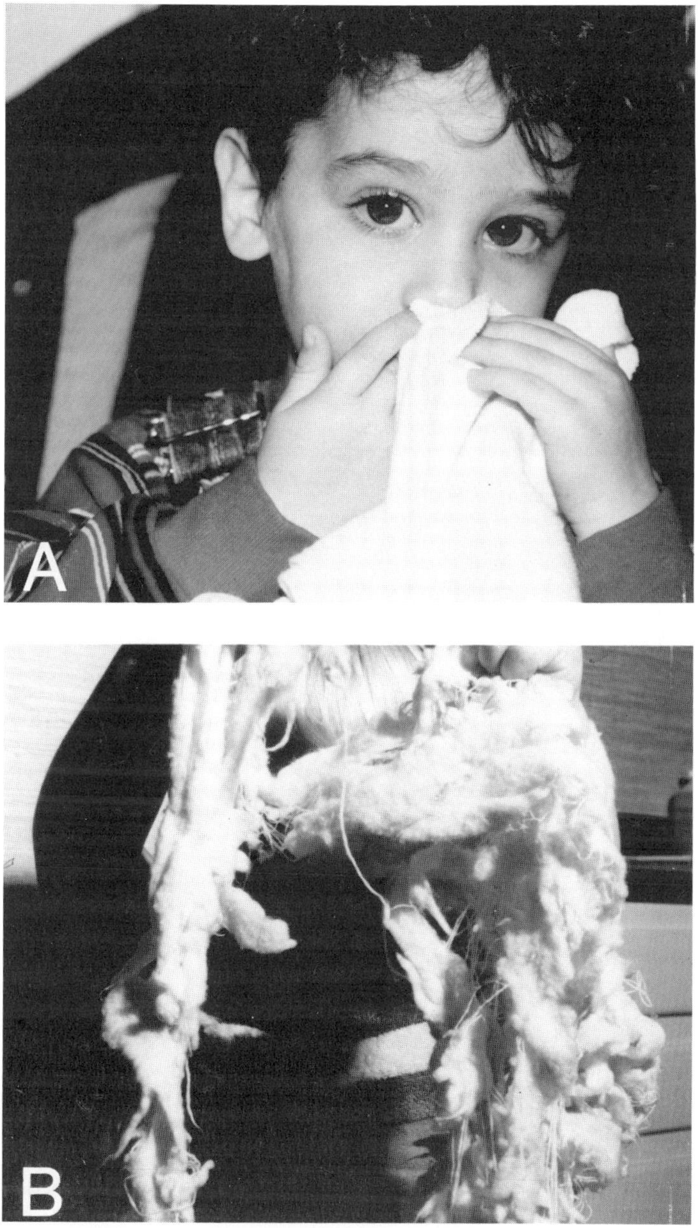

Figure 9-7. Transitional objects. In place of bottle or thumb, the child may fondle nose or other area of skin (A). The children are fiercely possessive of their "security" blanket, which may be reduced to rags (B).

Differential Diagnosis

In a typical case of trichotillomania the clinical features are diagnostic, and biopsy findings characteristic; they show normally growing hairs among empty follicles in a noninflammatory dermis. There may be evidence of damage in the retained portion of partially extracted hairs, and in the follicular epithelium. There may also be a corkscrew appearance to the residual hair shaft in the lower follicular duct.[26]

Fungal infection can be ruled out by Wood's light examination, by microscopic examination of scrapings, culture, and biopsy material; the inflammatory dermatoses are ruled out by absence of the characteristic features of inflammation, observed clinically and microscopically. The most difficult condition to differentiate is alopecia areata, but here the circumscribed margins, the complete absence of hair within the patch, and the fine silky tapered shafts of the regenerating hairs all serve to make the distinction, which can be confirmed by biopsy.[23]

Occasionally, it is necessary to demonstrate that the potential for spontaneous growth exists, if not for one's own edification, at least to convince the family. Orentriech[35a] has devised the "trichotillo test" in which an occlusive dressing is achieved on a small area of the scalp with layers of collodion, while Caserio[13] suggests a rather more cumbersome "growth window."

Management

As with patients with neurotic excoriation, management of the patient with trichotillomania will depend on the severity of the case. This will be determined on the basis of the duration of symptoms, and on the extent to which other neurotic symptoms interfere in the patient's life. Rasmussen[38] confirms that patients with obsessive-compulsive symptomatology frequently present first to their primary physician, and he underlines again the need for us to consider an assessment of the degree of psychiatric impairment as part of our obligation to our patients.

The management is essentially along the same lines as that for neurotic excoriations. The reader is referred to that section and the section on general principles of management for a fuller discussion.

Because these patients are relatively intact psychologically unlike those with dermatitis artefacta and delusional disorders, it is my practice at the outset to confront them with my belief that the lesions are self-induced. This need not be in any way judgemental or challenging, and indeed can be quite vague. For example, "I'm not quite sure why or when it happens, and you even may not know that yourself, but I believe that this is something that you are doing."

Children six years and younger. As with neurotic excoriations, compulsive habits in this age group are symptomatic of a childhood neurosis, and cannot be ignored if later emotional, discipline, school, or peer difficulties are to be avoided. That trichotillomania in children and adolescents is not often reported in isolation supports this view; the thumb-sucking, nail-biting, nose-picking, poor peer relationships, and academic difficulties that often accompany the symptom[30] all signify inner conflict.

If the condition is of short duration, perhaps 2 or 3 months at most, and if there is some exogenous factor stressful to the child to which the symptoms can be attributed, then: (1) educate the parents (see Neurotic Excoriations); and (2) divert attention if the plucking is observed; and (3) provide toys, and modify schedules. Woolly toys that the child can stroke and manipulate are particularly helpful.

If the above measures have not relieved tension and ameliorated the situation within a period of perhaps 2 or 3 months, or if, when the child is first seen, hair-pulling is already fixed and has been present for 6 or more months, then, in addition to the above measures, advise the parents that there may be deeper problems that may surface later; suggest consultation with a child psychoanalyst or analytic psychotherapist. A brief course of therapy at this stage may help the child to handle feelings that would otherwise be repressed, only to surface later.

In cases where the symptom is extensive and of long duration, in addition to the measures listed above, help the parents to acknowledge other areas of difficulty such as nightmares, temper tantrums, or head-banging, and encourage psychiatric referral.

Given the family constellation described for this condition (see Psychodynamics) it is clear that either family therapy, or concurrent psychotherapy for the mother, will be indicated in many cases.

For the patient psychoanalysis or psychoanalytic psychotherapy are the treatments of choice.[19] Beneficial results are reported also from hypnosis,[25] and behavioral techniques[7,44] in conjunction with supportive therapy.

Manipulation of the environment may be indicated, by fostering or by hospitalizing of the patient if parental co-operation cannot be obtained.

Older children and adolescents. The management of trichotillomania in older children and adolescents proceeds essentially along the same lines as outlined for neurotic excoriations. Education of the parents as to the psychodynamics that produce hair-pulling and the need not to provide added stress is important. Important also in long-standing cases is the need to help parents recognize that there are other neurotic symptoms and that psychiatric referral is indicated.

Adults. When trichotillomania persists beyond adolescence in absence of psychosis or borderline personality functioning, it is symptomatic of obsessive-compulsive neurosis,[35] and the treatment must be the treatment of that disorder. This has been discussed previously (see Neurotic Excoriations). The patient must be helped to recognize the underlying neurosis and accept the treatment recommended (see General Principles of Management, and Achieving Successful Referral).

Course and Prognosis

Course and prognosis is essentially similar to that of neurotic excoriations. Cases of short duration, particularly in early childhood, have a good prognosis. Those of longer duration, or with onset in adolescence, without psychiatric treatment tend to take on the characteristics of a chronic illness, subject to remissions and exacerbations throughout life.[19]

Other Common and Less Common Compulsive Habits

A myriad of other types of lesion result from compulsive activities directed against the integument. Among these are included onychotillomania,[39] onychodystrophy with paronychial hypertrophy secondary to rubbing the nail folds, circumscribed areas of lichen simplex chronicus, knuckle pads, prurigo nodularis,[42] and factitious cheilitis due to biting or licking the lips (Figs. 9-8, 9-9, and 9-10).[46]

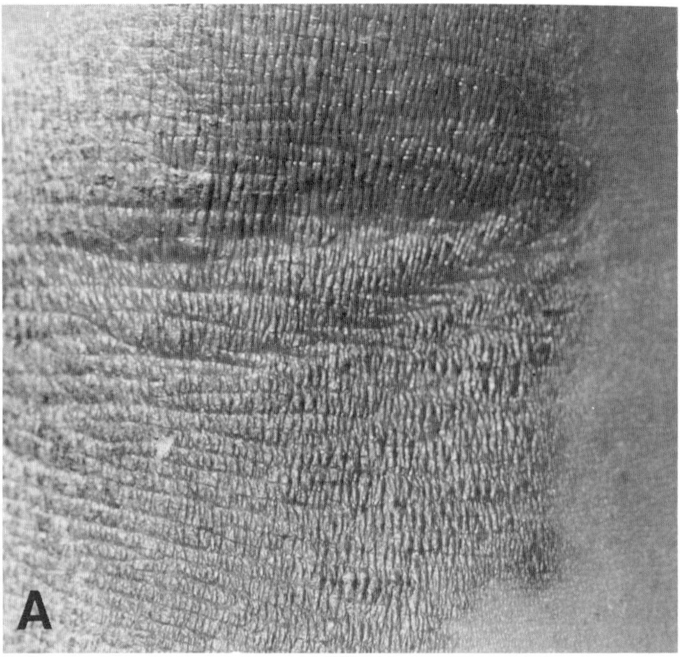

Figure 9-8. (A, B, C) Lichen simplex chronicus (neurodermatitis). Chronic rubbing or scratching may result in lesions of this type, particularly in patients with an atopic background. The appearance is modified by location, but the acanthosis seen microscopically is clearly translated clinically into accentuation of the normal skin markings. Ulcerations and excoriations may be superimposed (B). The lateral malleolus in men, and occiput in women, are common sites.

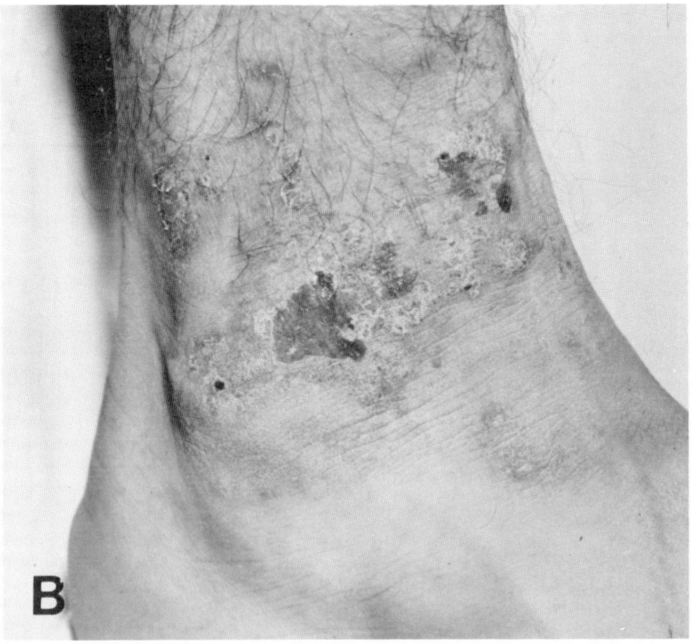
B

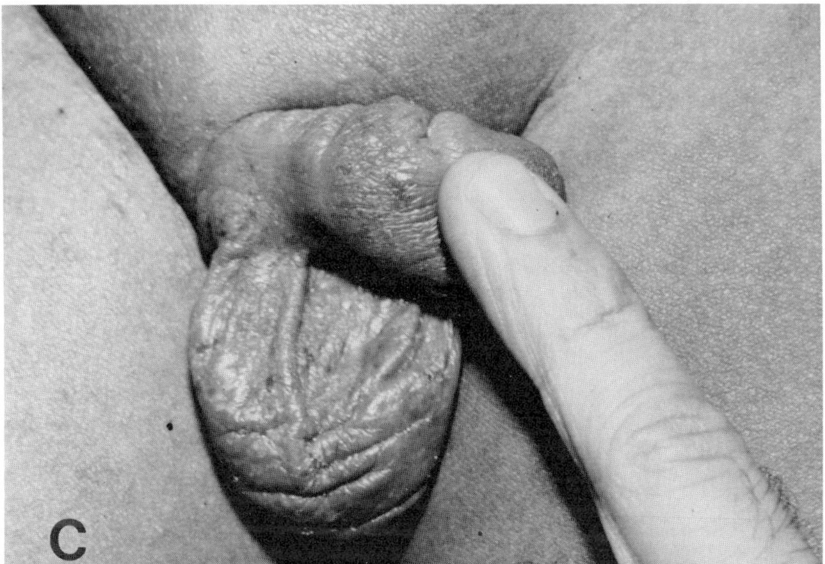
C

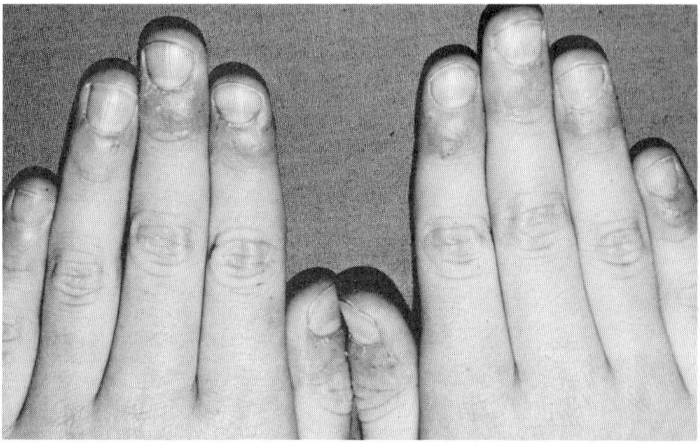

Figure 9-9. Onychotillomania. Nails and cuticles may be compulsively picked, with secondary onychodystrophy; in some cases, recalcitrant periungual warts may result.

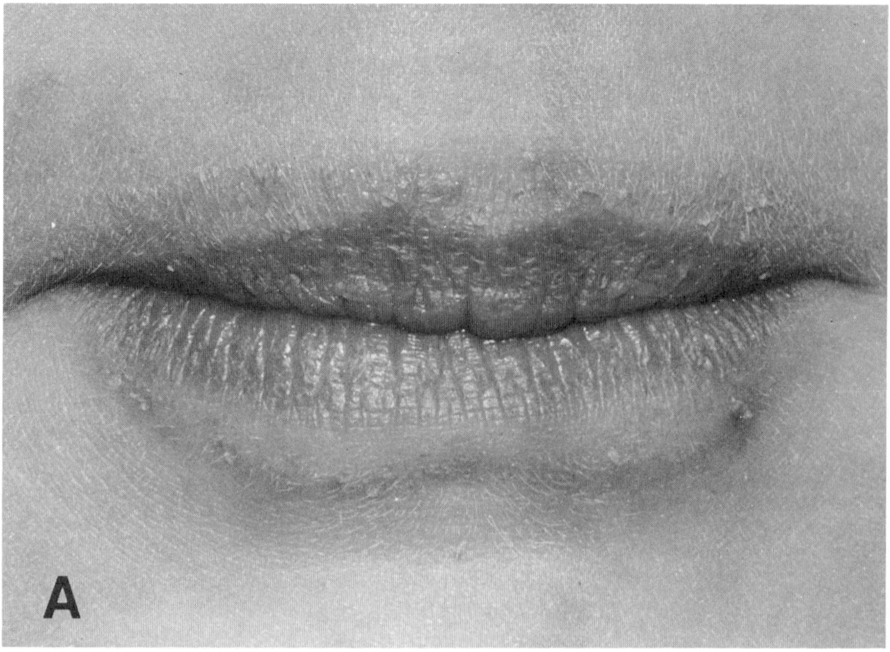

Figure 9-10. *(Continues.)*

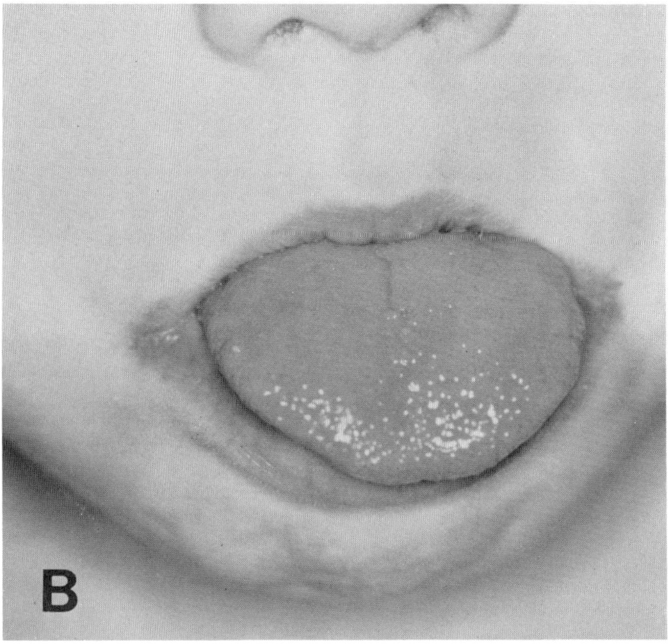

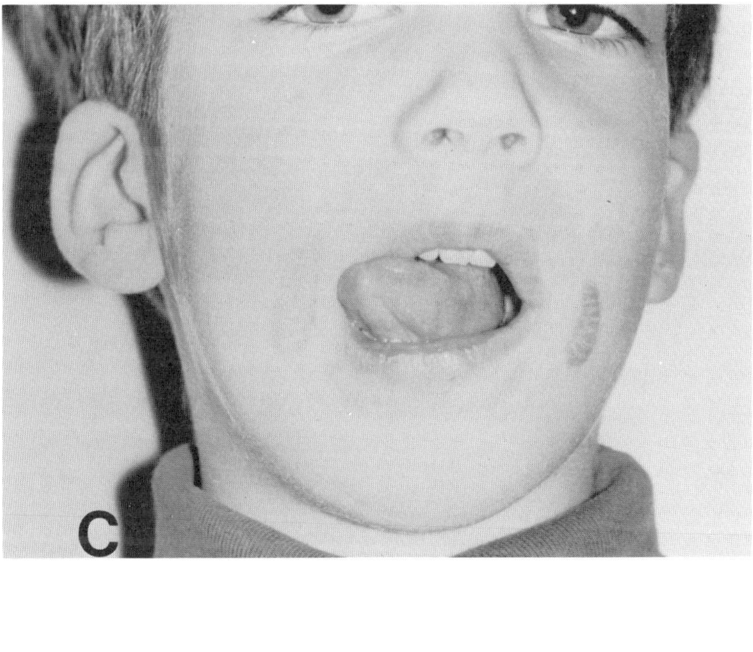

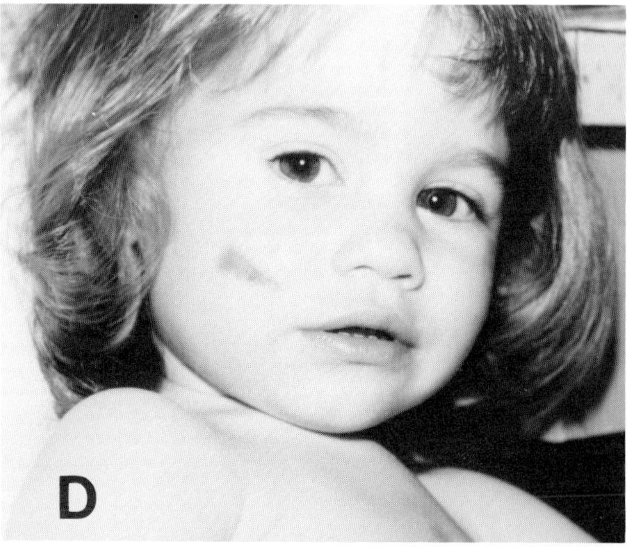

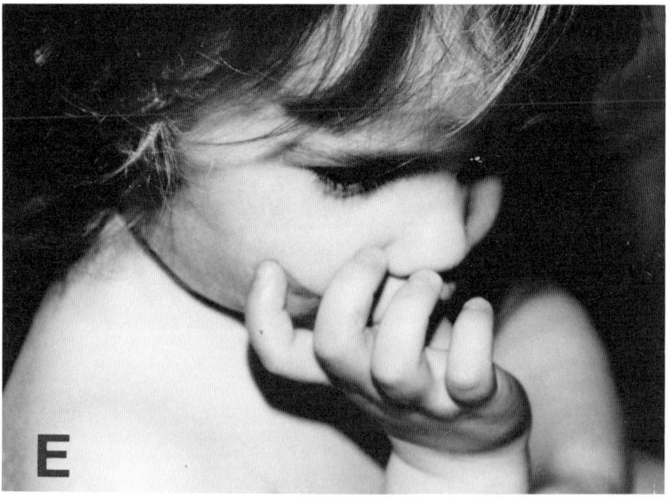

Figure 9-10. *(Continued.)* Compulsive habits. Skin lesions resulting from compulsive habits are particularly common on the face. Chronic cheilitis, pericheilitis (A) and angular cheilitis (B) result from licking and biting. The resultant dryness and irritation stimulates further licking, and a vicious cycle perpetuates the problem. Low humidity in cold weather aggravates further. Lesions quite distant from the mouth can still be caused by licking (C). Little ingenuity was required to elucidate the cause of the lesion in D. The patient (E) ingeniously devised a method to suck her thumb, stroke her nose, and pick her cheek concurrently.

Each of these conditions may result from a relatively transient habit triggered by situational stress, or from a more fixed compulsion that the patient is powerless to resist. Each may be seen over the entire spectrum of psychiatric disease, including mental retardation. As with neurotic excoriations and trichotillomania, however, the underlying psychiatric condition in those whom we see in the office, and who are seeking help for their symptom, is usually an obsessive-compulsive neurosis of varying severity.

There is little documentation concerning incidence or psychodynamic formulation in these conditions, but it is clear that unconscious symbolic meanings will play a part in determining just which site is "chosen" for compulsive manipulation.

Lesions such as prurigo nodularis and lichen simplex chronicus may result from the primary compulsion to rub or scratch, and properly belong in this section. They may also be attributed to the secondary manipulation of an itching lesion. If recurrent episodes of uncontrollable itching are the primary event, then the conditions more properly belong in the section on pruritus, and will be discussed again in that context.

Management will be determined by the duration and severity of the symptom, and the extent to which other neurotic symptoms intrude into the patient's life. It will be along the lines that have been discussed in earlier sections of this chapter.

Obsessional Thoughts

Obsessional thoughts are thoughts that intrude unbidden into the patient's mind, focussing and indeed often totally absorbing attention so that it is diverted from issues that are potentially more distressing, but often also issues that are essential to normal functioning in the everyday world.

These obsessional concerns, like compulsive acts, while in their mildest expression may represent a variant of normal, in a person with obsessive-compulsive personality configuration, in their more extreme expression, interfere in normal functioning and represent rather, an expression of an obsessive-compulsive neurosis.

Although at one level the patient knows that what he or she fears is not in fact a logical or realistic possibility, the patient at the same time believes that it is so. Absent is the conviction of the delusional paranoid psychotic, and these patients are driven to seek, over and over again, reassurance that their fears are without realistic foundation.

Symptoms that fall into this category include many of those that we hear from patients with delusions, but the quality of delusional conviction is missing, and the patient is seeking repeated reassurance rather than therapeutic action. Included here would be obsessional concerns about herpes, AIDS other venereal diseases, hair loss, post-acne scarring, parasitic infestation, malignancy, connective tissue disease, ugliness of varying types, and a pathologic explanation for a variety of normal variants (e.g., fordyce lesions of the labial or buccal mucosa).

Because the overt concern expressed is not the real concern, but rather a compromise that incorporates within it the symbolic expression of both a forbidden unconscious wish, and a psychologic defense against that wish, no reassurance can make the patient feel better, and the patient treks from doctor to doctor, driven inexorably but unfruitfully by the need to relieve his or her neurotic anxiety. As an example, an unmarried man of 22 years consulted me in the course of a long quest for relief of anxiety about the possibility that he might be going bald. I was one of many dermatologists, dermatologic surgeons, plastic surgeons, and also psychiatrists that this handsome young man, with a full head of coarse curly hair, had consulted. He brought pictures from 1 and 2 years ago repeatedly asking whether or not I could perceive any change, and repeatedly during the course of the interview he exhorted me to look at different sites on his scalp, asking if the hair there was thin.

Anxious to attend professional school, this young man was unable to prepare for qualifying examinations because his obsessional fears interrupted his studying. He became depressed, began to avoid social contact, and to lose interest in outside activities. He spent long hours in front of the mirror studying his hair and styling it over and over again for maximal effect.

An only child, his father had left the family during his early infancy and though his step-father, a successful businessman, treated him generously "like a son," the patient never felt that he could satisfy his mother's need for him to please the step-father. He developed an idealized image of his natural father as a swashbuckling he-man, while the more gentle balding step-father was seen as passive and weak.

Relationships were maintained in an uneasy equilibrium until two crises intervened; coincidentally, his girl-friend broke up with him, and several of his friends were accepted into the professional school to which he had not yet even applied. He began to see himself as unattractive and ugly, and also as inferior to his friends. He saw his passive, homely step-father as a loser, and distorted further the idealisation of his natural father: were he more like his father, handsome and macho, he would be in control; he would leave, rather than be left, as he had been left by his father and by his girl-friend, and he would succeed professionally.

Symbolically the hair represented to him good looks, masculinity, and professional and sexual success. Whenever current life circumstances permitted him to see himself unfavorably in any way, he attributed it to the possibility that he was going bald; unconsciously this meant less like the swashbuckling, masculine father, and more like the passive step-father.

What this young man unconsciously was seeking, was confirmation that he was strong, powerful, masculine, and sexually attractive, but these issues were never addressed in his progression from doctor to doctor for consultation about his hair, and he remained unrelieved of his anxiety, and unreassured.

Management

It is important to recognize the symbolic nature of the symptom so that one will not be disappointed by lack of success in addressing only that which is overtly manifest.

While compulsive habits can be controlled by the various approaches enumerated above, the control of a process that is purely internal, such as an obsessional thought, is much more difficult to achieve; treatment to be effective must be that of the underlying psychiatric disorder, the obsessive-compulsive neurosis.

In managing mild cases: (1) Support the patient through the situation that has served to precipitate the symptom, if this can be elucidated. (2) Help the patient to understand that the overt symptom stands for a problem in his or her inner life, and that that is why reassurance does not seem to help. (3) Try to help the patient to focus on inner processes rather than focussing obsessionally on the manifest symtom. (4) Help the patient to see the precipitating cause in the context of his or her past life, and in that context, understand what it might mean to the patient. If indicated, use (5) Stress managment techniques. (6) A short course of anxyiolytic drugs. (7) Tricyclic-like antidepressants.

In managing more severe cases: (1) The treatment of choice for long-term change is psychoanalysis or psychoanalytic psychotherapy.[10] (2) Hypnosis and behavioral techniques are more effective in the treatment of compulsions than of obsessions, but they can be tried.[24,45] (3) Tricyclic antidepressants, monoamine oxidase inhibitors and neuroleptic drugs may be required, preferably in conjunction with psychotherapy.[16]

REFERENCES

1. Adamson HG: Acne urticaria and other forms of "Neurotic excoriations." Br J Dermatol 27:1-12, 1915
2. Aleksandrowicz MK, Mares AJ: Trichotillomania and trichobezoar in an infant. Psychological factors underlying this symptom. Am Acad Child Psychiatry, pp 533-539, 1978
3. Allen KE, Harris FR: Elimination of a child's excessive scratching by training the mother in reinforcement procedures, in Behavior Research and Therapy, Vol 4. England, Pergamon Press Ltd, 1966, pp 79-84

4. Azrin NH, Nunn RG: Habit reversal: A method of eliminating nervous habits and tics. Behavior Research and Therapy 11:619-628, 1973
5. Bab LHJ, Kuypers BRM: Behavior therapy in dermatological practice. Br J Dermatol 88:591-598, 1973
6. Barahal HS: The psychopathology of hair-pulling (Trichotillomania). Psychoanal Rev 27:291-310, 1940
7. Bayer CA: Self monitoring and mild aversion treatment of trichotillomania. J Behav Ther Exp Psychiatry 3:139-141, 1972
8. Berg C: Unconscious significance of hair. Int J Psychoanal 17:73-88, 1936
9. Berg C: The Unconscious Significance of Hair. London, George Allen & Unwin Ltd, 1951
10. Brooke RI: Exfoliative cheilitis. Oral Surg 45:52-55, 1978
11. Buxbaum E: Hair-pulling and fetishism, in Eisler RS, Freud A, Hartman H, Kris M (eds): Psychoanalytic Study of the Child, Vol 15. New York, International Universities Press, 1960, pp 243-260
12. Calnan CD, O'Neill D: Itching in tension states. Br J Dermatol 64:274-280, 1952
13. Caserio RJ: "Growth window" is seen useful aid in hair ills. Dermatol News 19(3):1, 1986
14. Cramer JB: Common neuroses of childhood, in Ariet S (ed): American Handbook of Psychiatry. New York, Basic Books, 1959, pp 797-815
15. Cormia F: Basic concepts in the production and management of the psychosomatic dermatoses 11. Br J Dermatol 63:129-151, 1951
16. Engels WD: Skin disorders, in Kaplan HI, Sadock BJ (eds): Comprehensive Textbook of Psychiatry IV. Baltimore, Williams and Wilkins, 1985, pp 1178-1185
17. Frankel EH: Hypnosis as a treatment method in psychosomatic medicine. Int J Psychiatry Med 6:75-85, 1975
18. Galski T: Hair pulling (Trichotillomania). Psychoanal Rev 70(3):331-346, 1983
19. Greenberg HR, Sarner CA: Trichotillomania—symptom and syndrome. Arch Gen Psychiatry 12:482-489, 1965
20. Hallopeau M: Alopecie par grattage: Trichomanie ou trichotillomanie. Ann Dermatol Syph 10:440, 1959
21. Insel TR, Murphy DL: The psychopharmacological treatment of obsessive-compulsive disorder: A review. J Clin Psychopharmacol 1(5):304-311, 1981
22. Koblenzer CS: Psychosoamtic concepts in dermatology: A dermatologist-psychoanalyst's viewpoint. Arch Dermatol 119:501-512, 1983
23. Koblenzer CS: Neurotic excoriations and other obsessional habits, in Demis, Dobson, McGuire (eds): Clinical Dermatology, Psychocutaneous Disease, Unit 29-7, Vol 4. Harper and Row, 1985, pp 1-14
24. Krishnan DRR, Davidson JRT, Guajardo C: Trichotillomania—a review.

Comp Psychiatry 26:123-128, 1985
25. Krishnan KRR, Davidson JRT, Miller RD: MAO inhibitors in the treatment of trichotillomania associated with depression. J Clin Psychiat 45:267-268, 1984
26. Lever WF, Schaumburg-Lever G: Histopathology of the Skin. Philadelphia, JB Lippincott, 1983, p 203
27. Lockwood K, Bourland G: Reduction of self-injurious behaviors by reinforcement and toy use. Ment Retard 20:169-173, 1982
28. Lyell A: Cutaneous artifactual disease: A review amplified by personal experience. J Am Acad Derm I:391-407, 1979
29. Mackee GM: Neurotic excoriations. Arch Dermatol Syph 1:256-269, 1920
30. Mannino FV, Delgado RA: Trichotillomania in children. A review. Am J Psychiatry 126:505-511, 1969
31. Michelson HE: Psychosomatic studies in dermatology. Arch Dermatol Syph 51:245-250, 1945
32. Musaph H: Itching and Scratching. Philadelphia, FA Davis Co, 1964, pp 1-8
33. Nemiah JC: Obsessive-compulsive disorder, in Daplan HI, Sadock BJ (eds): Comprehensive Textbook of Psychiatry IV. Baltimore, Williams and Wilkins, 1985, p 914
34. Obermeyer ME: Psychocutaneous Medicine. Springfield, IL, Charles C. Thomas, 1955, pp 120-125
35. Oguchi T, Miura S: Trichotillomania: Its psychopathological aspect. Compr Psychiatry 18(2):177-182, 1977
35a. Orentrich N: Disorders of the hair and scalp in childhood. Pediatr Clin N Am 18(3):953-974, 1971
36. Philippopoulos GS: A case of trichotillomania (hair-pulling). Acta Psychother 9:304-312, 1961
37. Pusey WA, Senear FE: Neurotic excoriations with report of cases. Arch Dermatol 1:270-278, 1920
38. Rasmussen SA: Obsessive-compulsive disorder in dermatologic practice. J Am Acad Dermatol 13:965-967, 1985
39. Sait MA, Reddy BSN, Garg BR: Onychotillomania: Two case reports. Dermatologica 171:200-202, 1985
40. Seitz PF: Dynamically-oriented brief psychotherapy: Psychocutaneous excoriation syndromes—an experiment. Psychosom Med 15:200-242, 1953
41. Snyder S: Trichotillomania treated with Amitryptiline. J Nerv Ment Dis 168:505-507, 1980
42. Soter NA, Fitzpatrick TB: Cutaneous changes in disorders of altered reactivity: eczematous dermatitis, in Fitzpatrick TB, Eisen AZ, Wolff K, Freedberg IM, Austen KE (eds): Dermatology in General Medicine (ed 3). New York, McGraw Hill, 1979, pp 507-512
43. Spock B: Baby and Child Care. New York, Pocket Books, 1946, p 138

44. Stabler B, Warren AB: Behavioral contracting in treating trichotillomania: case note. Psychol Rep 34:401-402, 1974
45. Steketee G, Foa EB, Grayson JB: Recent advances in the behavioral treatment of obsessive-compulsives. Arch Gen Psychiatry 39:1365-1371, 1982
46. Thomas JR III, Greene SL, Dicken CH: Factitious cheilitis. J Am Acad Dermatol I:368-372, 1983
47. Vaillant GE, Perry JC: Personality disorders, in Kaplan HI, Sadock BJ (eds): Comprehensive Textbook of Psychiatry IV. Baltimore, Williams and Wilkens, 1985, pp 958-986
48. Van Moffaert M: Factitious affections in dermatology. Arch Belg Dermatol 30:221-224, 1971
49. Wilkinson JB: Hypnotherapy in the psychosomatic approach to illness: a review. J Roy Soc Mcd 74:525-530, 1981
50. Zaidens SH: Self-inflicted dermatoses and their psychodynamics. J Nerv Ment Dis 113:388-395, 1951

Chapter 10

The Psychogenic Purpura Syndromes

Although psychogenic purpura has been associated with the names of Gardner and Diamond since 1955, when four women were reported with a syndrome that consisted of "a form of purpura producing painful bruising, following autosensitisation to red blood cells,"[9] these authors made no mention of psychologic factors in their description. Neither the recognition of spontaneous bleeding within apparently normal skin nor the concept of sensitization to autologous blood products was new at the time of their paper, for medical reports of so-called "hysterical" bleeding go back at least to the middle of the last century,[12,18,48] while Whitfield, in 1921, attributed a generalized erythematous eruption to autosensitization with extravasated blood in two female patients, following traumatic hematomata.[50] The intellectual climate with regard to autoantibodies is very different today from that in 1955, and their role in disease processes is now well established.

Since Gardner and Diamond's landmark paper,[9] over 100 cases have appeared in the literature, with essentially similar clinical features,[17,30,37,39] while reference is made to many other cases, as yet unpublished.[39] On the basis of a careful study of the clinical findings in these cases, and the results of laboratory and clinical tests, Ratnoff has divided them into five separate categories:[39] the autoerythrocyte sensitization syndrome, autosensitivity to DNA, hysterical purpura, factitious bleeding, and religious stigmata. There is considerable overlap between these five categories, as I will explain, and in the pages that follow I will use only three, psychogenic purpura, hysterical purpura (which will include religious stigmatization), and factitious purpura. This latter is mentioned only to be dismissed, as it has been covered adequately already in the section on factitious dermatitis, having as it does the characteristics of the other factitious disorders.

PSYCHOGENIC PURPURA

Clinical Picture

There is a remarkable consistency to the clinical picture of psychogenic purpura. Onset of the specific lesions is preceded almost invariably by weeks or months by a history of one or sometimes a series of physical traumata, or by a surgical procedure; not infrequently the patient can accurately define the date, and sometimes even the hour of onset of their first lesion.[10] Lesions start characteristically with a prodrome that consists of painful stabbing, stinging, or burning sensations, experienced for 1 or 2 hours, before such signs of inflammation as heat, erythema, induration, tenderness, or pain (which may be of great severity) appear. Within succeeding hours to days, this inflammation is followed by the characteristic blue discoloration of the purpuric component, superimposed on or peripheral to the area of inflammation. Usually the pain will gradually diminish, once the bruise has appeared. Devolution of the lesion may then occur, with fading over a period of 1 or 2 weeks, first of the erythema and then the bruise (Fig. 10-1). An alternative course is for the entire process to extend dramatically over succeeding days until a vast area, for example an entire hand and forearm, is involved with painful bruising, before the gradual defervescence begins. Coincident with the onset of cutaneous lesions, systemic symptoms may occur; these consist of fever,

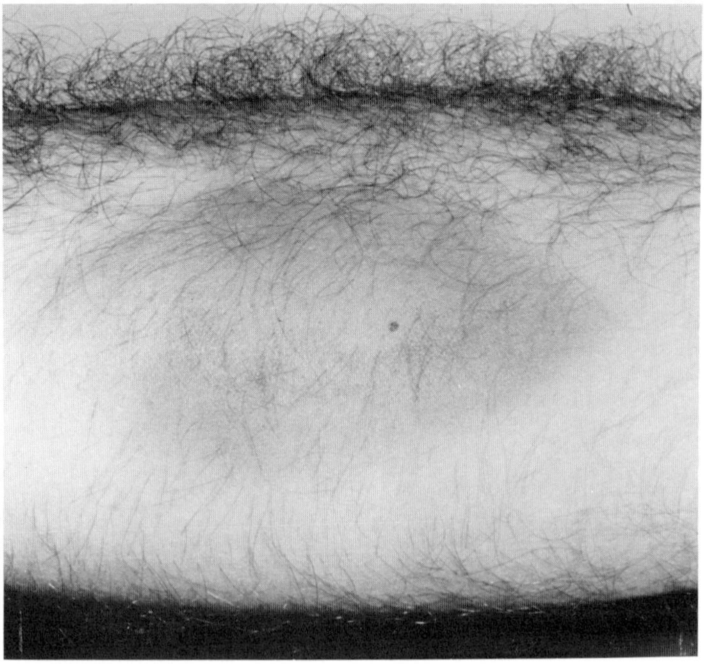

Figure 10-1. Psychogenic purpura. Ill-defined areas of deep bruising are characteristically associated with intense pain; often deforming swelling may be somewhat reminiscent of the swelling sometimes seen in anaphylactoid purpura.

malaise, headaches, chills, vague aches and pains, and occasionally abdominal distress or nausea and vomiting. Interruption of the surface of the skin by abrasion or laceration is not reported.

The size of individual lesions varies from 1-2 cm to large areas such as described above; the pressure within these larger lesions may be so great as to require decompression by aspiration or by incision; yet despite this pressure, permanent disability is unusual.[11,30] Henstell and Kligerman have, however, reported one patient who developed wrist drop.[16] Pain may be prolonged and intense in these more dramatic lesions, and may require narcotics for relief. Interestingly, while a direct blow to the skin may cause a typical lesion at the site of trauma, or a crop of lesions at a distant site, in 50 percent of Ratnoff's patients such a blow resulted only in ordinary bruising;[39] venipuncture too, rarely leads to a typical lesion. Bleeding through the intact skin overlying a lesion has been reported by a number of patients, and in one case was directly observed by Ratnoff and Agle as a welling-up of blood through the follicular orifices.[40]

Like the size, the periodicity of lesions is very variable, and while some patients claim never to be without them, the more common story is of episodic crops, with intervening periods of freedom. The extremities are the sites most frequently involved, but lesions occur also on the anterior trunk, and much less commonly on the back or face.

It is clear that these characteristic cutaneous lesions are only the dramatic and visible component of a much more complex clinical picture. A careful inquiry into the past history will usually reveal that the patient has previously had a variety of other hemorrhagic manifestations that started often years before the onset of the painful bruising; in many cases there is in addition multisystem disease. Many claim that they have "always" bruised easily. Menometrorrhagia leading to hysterectomy; hematuria with often multiple cystoscopies, and normal findings; epistaxis; gastrointestinal bleeding; gingival bleeding; and bleeding after minor surgery, minor cuts, or childbirth are all common findings.[15,37,39]

A plethora of nonhemorrhagic symptoms are also reported. These include very severe headaches, requiring narcotics, as an almost constant component; also neurologic symptoms such as episodic paresis, paresthesias, and anesthesia with no detectable organic cause, frequent syncopal attacks (in up to 50 percent of cases in one series), dyplopia, blurred or tunnel vision, or transient blindness; a variety of abdominal symptoms, requiring often multiple surgical interventions; chest pain and hyperventilation;[31] dysuria and urinary frequency, again with multiple intrusive diagnostic and therapeutic procedures; severe backaches that may or may not have led to laminectomy;[32] arthralgias; lassitude; cutaneous eruptions often attributed to drugs, and urticaria; neuritis secondary to compression by hematomata, and significant fluctuations in body weight, exemplified by unexplained anorexia, or by a sudden significant, but unexplained weight loss.

In each of these ennumerated situations, multiple laboratory studies will have been undertaken and surgical intervention or intrusive examinations will have taken place; but in each case, almost without exception, the objective findings will have been remarkably bland.[37,39] One exception to this rule is the associated immune-complex nephropathy, reported in one case.[31]

Although, as mentioned, Gardner and Diamond[9] did not comment on the emotional state of their four patients, it is clear from their report that at least two had suffered significant emotional stress.[8] The emotional aspect of the syndrome has been further elucidated by Ratnoff and Agle[2,3,5,14,16,39] as well as by Erwin and Granacher,[8] and others.[17,23,30,37,41] Like the physical picture, the emotional status has a remarkable consistency; psychiatric treatment prior to onset of the bruising is not uncommon; hysterical and masochistic personality traits are frequently described, as are anxiety, depression, hostility (particularly towards parents or spouse), and an inability to handle angry feelings. Patients are often characterized as passive-aggressive or passive-dependent, while obsessive traits, low self-esteem, sexual maladjustment, and feelings of guilt are common. Common too is the history of emotional stress immediately preceding the onset of the cutaneous outbreak.

Incidence

Initially thought to be confined to women, the syndrome has more recently been reported in men, with a male to female ratio of 1:20.[37] The age at onset has been anywhere from 9 to 53 years, but in almost 80 percent of patients, it is between 14 and 40. Interestingly, as with factitious dermatitis, there is a higher than expected incidence of patients who are nurses, or other health-care workers, or who have been exposed to family members with physical illness, most especially illness that has lead to such physical deformity as amputation.

Biopsy Findings

The findings at biopsy are variable and in part depend on the age of the lesion; the element most subject to variation is the degree of inflammation. Lever describes numerous extravasated red cells in the dermis and subcutaneous fat, and notes the absence of vasculitis.[25] Ratnoff, in the very early lesion, describes edema and a modest perivascular mononuclear cell infiltrate in the upper dermis; later lesions are characterized by the extravasation of numerous red cells and the absence of significant inflammation is again noted. In contrast are the findings of Hersle and Mobacken, who took biopsies of a developing lesion 3 hours after the intradermal injection of 0.1 ml of an 80 percent suspension of erythocytes.[17] They report a normal epidermis, and in the dermis vasodilation, endothelial cell swelling and a perivascular infiltrate that consists of eosinophils and neutrophils with nuclear damage, findings consistent with an acute vasculitis.[17] Groch et al. describe nuclear dusting at 3 hours,[13] with a massive increase in neutrophils and fibrinoid necrosis at 12 hours. Several authors describe necrosis of subcutaneous fat.

The variations in the degree of inflammation observed by different authors in biopsy specimens, along with inconsistencies in the results of intradermal tests that will be described later, raise a serious question as to whether the psychogenic purpura syndrome is in fact an entity with one pathophysiologic mechanism, or whether we are seeing a single clinical picture that can be produced by a variety of different mechanisms.

Laboratory and Clinical Tests

Despite the flamboyant past medical history that is recounted, and the dramatic clinical picture that is described, results from extensive laboratory tests are reported by most authors to be within normal limits.[9,17] These tests include the coagulation profile, erythocyte sedimentation rate, complete blood count, urinalysis, tests for porphyrins, the liver profile, immunoelectrophoresis, cryoglobulins, antistreptococcal and antistaphylococcal antibodies, febrile agglutinins, C-reactive protein, and tests for the L.E. cell phenomenon. X-ray studies of heart, lung, stomach, colon and abdominal survey to visualize the liver and spleen, likewise have been normal.[17]

Because of the history of preceding trauma in their cases, Gardner and Diamond believed their patients to have developed a sensitivity to autologous blood. In order further to elucidate this, they injected autologous washed red cells in concentrations of 10-80 percent, and also plasma, serum, red-cell stroma, haemoglobin, thrombinogen, fibrin, histamine, and saline colored with phenolphthalein, intradermally into their four patients, and into control subjects. Within 12-26 hours, out of all these different agents, painful ecchymoses developed only after red cells in a concentration of above 20 percent. This ecchymosis mirrored the spontaneous lesions, and was construed as a positive result; positive results were confined to the four patients. Subsequently, similar positive results were obtained also to red cell stroma in these same patients, and in one case to a homologous red cell suspension.

Subsequent workers have undertaken similar testing, but with results that have been inconsistent.[37] Ratnoff and Agle obtained a positive response to injection of whole blood on at least one occasion, in 32 of 57 patients,[39] while others report similar findings variously with hemoglobin,[20] phosphatidyl serine (a component of red cell stroma),[4] trypsin,[44] purified protein derivative of tubercle bacilli (PPD),[13] autologous serum,[28] platelets,[24] and a number of other agents. In two patients, entirely typical lesions have resulted from the intradermal injection of normal saline;[8,23] in others, a positive response was confined to sites only within the patient's field of vision.[40] Suggestibility was evident when the response was positive only where the patient was told it was expected,[47] while suppression of the reaction under hypnosis has also taken place.[40] Biopsy of positive skin tests invariably reveals findings in no way different from those in the spontaneous lesions.

Studies have been undertaken to provide support for immunologically mediated pathogenic mechanisms. For example, Kalden et al. observed that red-cell stroma induced lymphocyte blast transformation;[19] Ratnoff, however, finds the low stimulation indices they report reason for caution;[39] McIntosh found granular deposits of IgG, C_3, C_3PA and erythocyte antigens, deposited in granular fashion along the glomerular basement membrane, in a case of glomerulonephritis associated with psychogenic purpura,[31] and cited evidence for circulating red-cell stromal antigen-containing immune complexes in four other cases; other reports include variations in complement levels, in immunoglobulins, and in the T to B cell ratio.[39] However, Ratnoff has summarized equally impressive negative evidence:[39] for example, serum immunoelectrophoresis, total complement, C_3, C_4, and C_1 esterase inhibitor have repeatedly been found by a number of workers to be normal; tests for circulating antibody to red cell components are consistently negative in many studies, and passive transfer of sensitivity (the Prausnitz-Kustner reaction) has never been achieved. Other abnormalities that have been reported as possible causes of the abnormal bleeding are in one case defective platelet aggregation,[6] and in others, an abnormality in red cell structure observed on electronmicroscopy.[36]

The Anti-DNA Sensitization Syndrome

A group of patients with essentially an identical clinical syndrome has been described by Levin and Pincus,[26] and more recently by Pinnas et al.[38] On the basis of immunologic studies these authors attribute this disease to a sensitivity to autologous DNA. From the published data, these patients apparently come from an identical population with regard to sex, age, social background, and past medical history, as do those with so-called autoerythrocyte sensitization,[5] but in them lesions can be reproduced by intradermal injection of calf thymus DNA, or the stroma of autologous leukocytes,[24,46] rather than erythrocytes. The inflammatory component of the lesions is apparently more intense, and sometimes vesicles or bullae may be observed. The specifity of DNA as the responsible agent is called into question by inconsistencies in the immunologic findings, while positive evidence is again lacking for the presence of humoral or cellular immunity to DNA.[38,43] A decrease in complement titer has been observed, however, during episodes of bruising, and Pinnas et al. were able to demonstrate IgM, C_3, factor B and properdin at the dermo-epidermal junction in a typical lesion, in a patient who had an associated lymphopenia.

In the interest of avoiding repetition, the clinical feature of hysterical purpura and religious stigmatization will be described here. For reasons that will be explained, I will discuss the pathophysiology, psychopathology, differential diagnosis, treatment, and prognosis of all cases together as a single group, later.

HYSTERICAL PURPURA

Clinical Picture

Ratnoff, in his very comprehensive review article,[39] describes hysterical purpura as an entity separate from the autoerythrocyte and autoDNA sensitization syndromes. In some of the cases cited, bleeding is reported to have occurred through normal skin, while in others there were ecchymoses that had been preceded by prodromata of the type described in the autoerythrocyte sensitization syndrome. As with that syndrome, women predominated over men, multisystem symptoms were present, as was evidence of significant psychological disturbance. Frequently, symbolic significance appeared to determine the site chosen for lesions, and suggestibility, and the ability to produce lesions under hypnosis[42] were cited as evidence for hysterical mechanisms.

A case reported by Needles[35] in which a patient developed what were apparently petechiae on the palms in psychoanalytic sessions on three occasions in association with the emergence in consciousness of certain emotionally charged material, certainly fits the requirements of a hysterical conversion, as do cases reported by a number of other authors.[28,33,34]

Religious Stigmatization

There has been some discussion in the literature as to whether or not stigmatization represents a form of hysterical purpura.[22,28,39,49] Stigmatization refers to the spontaneous appearance on the skin of lesions that represent the wounds inflicted on Christ during the Crucifixion. St. Francis of Assisi, the first recorded stigmatist, reputedly developed lesions in September of 1224 after a fast of 40 days, during which he had meditated on "his favorite subject, the Crucifixion";[22] out of the more than 300 cases reported in the literature, only 60-80 have been accepted by the Roman Catholic Church as genuine.

The clinical history is again remarkably consistent; the appearance of lesions is almost invariably preceeded by a long period of physical and psychological ill-health; this ill-health is often "miraculously" cured by onset of the cutaneous bleeding.[52] Frequently the first lesions appear on Good Friday, after prolonged prayer and meditation that terminates in a trance-like state. Religious ecstasy is a frequent component, with visions of the crucified Christ displaying his wounds. The subject (usually female) may herself enact the drama of the Passion, assuming in her trance the posture of Christ on the Cross. On recovering, wounds are observed from which blood is reported to ooze or flow; characteristically these wounds heal rapidly and without infection, only to appear the following week, when the entire drama is reenacted.[52] Lesions are located on hands or wrists, feet, brow (from the Crown of Thorns), and chest (from the lance of the Roman soldier); wheals and ecchymoses may represent the scourging endured by Christ before the walk to Calvary, and bloody tears and sweat are also reported.

Nor is stigmatization confined to mediaeval times, for Siwek reports a case of a woman who developed the wounds of the Passion through hypnotic suggestion and who was investigated in 1932,[45] while Ratnoff too was able to study a recent case, a woman who in addition to the stigmata had many of the somatic complaints, and the psychological make-up that are associated with autoerythrocyte sensitization, though her skin test was negative.

Incidence of Stigmatization

Although the vast majority of subjects are Roman Catholics, the phenomenon is not confined to that group, for it has been reported in Protestants,[52] and also in Moslems, who have developed lesions that mirror those sustained by Mohammed in battle.[35] Geographically, the highest incidence is in Italy, with Catholics from Germany and the Tyrol second, and a few cases from France, Spain, and the Netherlands.

Only four men have been accepted as valid examples. The age at onset is between 20 and 40 years, and the subject most frequently a young, single woman, often a member of a Catholic Order, who has since childhood been preoccupied with the story of the Crucifixion.[52]

Laboratory and Clinical Tests

The only available information as to laboratory or clinical testing is the results of hypnotic studies reported in the clinical findings above. No information is available as to biopsy findings.

PATHOPHYSIOLOGY OF THE PSYCHOGENIC PURPURAS

From the material so far presented, it is clear that a variety of pathophysiologic mechanisms, some of which may be mediated by the immune system and some of which are apparently not, result in a remarkably consistent clinical picture: consistent not only in regard to the past medical history, and the current physical symptoms, but also the psychologic background and make-up. A history of previous psychiatric treatment is not uncommon, psychologic disturbance is the rule, and history of preceding emotional stress, as well as physical trauma can frequently be elicited; this emotional stress is most overt in the case of the stigmatists, but is reported in many other cases also.

Although experimental evidence is lacking in these particular syndromes, the current state of our knowledge in the areas of psychoneuroimmunology and psychoneuroendocrinology (summarized in Chapter 3) does permit us to arrive at a reasonable hypothetical explanation of the pathophysiology. As mentioned in Chapter 3, information is received in the hypothalamus, from external sources such as the various sensory pathways, and from internal sources such as memory, the feeling state, and the vegetative centers; there, it is processed and integrated, and in response hypophysiotrophic hormones are secreted. These hormones are intimately involved in every aspect of pituitary function, including those functions related to the mediation of the immune response, and to inflammation.[29]

Thus it is not unreasonable to suppose that in those cases where immunological findings have been prominent, stress-induced activation of the hypothalmic-pituitary axis has resulted in mobilization of immune mechanisms, while in other cases rather, the disease process has been mediated via B-endorphin, substance P, and the kinins.

PSYCHOPATHOLOGY OF THE PSYCHOGENIC PURPURAS

It does not seem to be productive to describe hysterical purpura as a wholly separate entity for two reasons. First, the concept of hysterical conversion has broadened; the possibility of a symptom serving to resolve conflict, and having a symbolic meaning in the inner life of the patient, is more important than the particular compartment of the nervous system involved in its development.[21] Nor does to designate as hysterical explain pathophysiology; we still must explain how the lesion actually developed, and it is now clear that symptoms with the attributes of a hysterical conversion may be mediated by psychophysiologic processes; thus the distinction between hysterical and psychophysiologic symptoms becomes blurred. Second, the term serves no specific diagnostic function; hysterical conversion symptoms, while they are classically associated with hysterical neurosis, may be seen also in patients with personality disorders or even in patients with psychosis. In carefully reviewing the reported cases, it is clear, for example, that in some of those diagnosed as the autoerythrocyte sensitization syndrome with all its attendant clinical features, lesions psychologically served the function of a hysterical conversion. Put more simply, it becomes clear that while all cases reported as hysterical purpura are hysterical conversion reactions, many of those with the auto-erythrosensitization phenomenon fit those criteria also.

The psychopathology and psychodynamic formulation is hard to evaluate because of the nature of the information provided in many cases; we are given no developmental history, while testing has been confined to such self-administered inventories as the Minnesota Multiphase Personality Inventory (MMPI); these give only superficial information, and deprive us of the unconscious material that projective tests would afford us. Nevertheless, a fairly clear picture emerges.

Patients tend to be the products of unstable homes in which physical and emotional abuse or privation are common. In such a milieu, relationships are ambivalent, and anger with the needed though abusing parent not tolerated. This anger, which cannot be expressed overtly, must then be turned against the self, with unconscious guilt and masochistic tendencies developing as prominent features of the personality, and depression and obsessive traits common. Adult relationships mirror those of the home; they are dependent, ambivalent, unstable, and frequently sadomasochistic, while sexual difficulties are common. The prominent somatization points to difficulties in the very early period, prior to development of speech, but the multiplicity of symptoms, and the frequent surgical interventions sustained, reflect both the masochistic posture and also concerns about physical integrity that are generated by this early abuse.

Many patients have had previous hysterical conversion reactions such as aphonias, paralyses, paresthesias, dissociative episodes, blindness, and hallucinations.[42] Engel has suggested that the form of a conversion symptom will reflect bodily activities or experiences that were involved in the gratifications and conflicts inherent in early important relationships.[7] Agle and Ratnoff question whether the bruises of psychogenic purpura represents abreaction of real truama, as described by Moody,[33,34] or rather, unconscious masochistic beating fantasies.[1] Interestingly, as with patients with factitious disease, suggestibility and a capacity for identification is evident in the high incidence of patients who are in the health care field, or in a Roman Catholic order.

Diagnostically, patients with this syndrome fall primarily into the borderline personality disorder, or severe hysterical neurosis, while a small percentage may be psychotic.

DIFFERENTIAL DIAGNOSIS

The primary consideration, of course, is factitious purpura; this is extraordinarily difficult to rule out in many cases. Occasionally one may be present when a lesion develops, but it may be necessary to demonstrate that new lesions can develop under occlusive dressings such as an Unna boot in order to be convinced. Development of a lesion under such a dressing after intradermal injection of autologous whole blood may also be helpful in ruling out factitious disease.

Other considerations include the various hemorrhagic diatheses, thrombophlebitis, erythema nodosum, and panniculitis. The normal laboratory findings, general good health in face of such dramatic lesions, absence of fever, absence of scarring, and the characteristic biopsy findings, together with the positive intradermal test if this is present, serve to confirm the diagnosis.

TREATMENT

Dermatologic

A vast number of therapeutic agents have been employed either unsuccessfully, or with only occasional success in the treatment of psychogenic purpura. The list cannot hope to be complete, but included are adrenocorticotropic hormone (ACTH), high doses of prednisone, ethinyloestradiol, antimalarials, anticoagulants, antibiotics, antihistamines, and immunosuppressants.[17,39] Splenectomy has been performed,[9] and attempts made at desensitization with autologous blood products,[9] but each has met with signal lack of success; from the information that has been presented about pathophysiology, it is unlikely that in fact any specific dermatologic treatment is available, and indeed Ratnoff and Agle advise that one refrain from giving any medications at all.[40]

Treatment recommendations therefore will be confined to symptomatic measures:

1. Make the patient comfortable with warm soaks and mild analgesics.
2. Avoid narcotics; the potential for addiction exists.[40]
3. Splint when necessary, to mainain good positioning.
4. Maintain mobility; initiate physical therapy early, to relieve anxiety, and to avoid contractures due to immobility caused by anxiety.
5. If edema and interstitial ecchymosis is severe and prolonged, it may occasionally be necessary to aspirate or incise for purposes of decompression. These measures are to be avoided if possible, because: (1) Masochistic traits make these patients seek out such procedures; pressure will be exerted on the physician to have them performed; (2) Dangerous precedents are set by gratifying this masochistic wish; pressures will be strong for more and more extreme procedures, and the possibility of scarring and mutilation is great; (3) It confirms the concept of a physical illness, that requires physical treatments; and (4) It confirms the illness role, and increases dependency.

Psychiatric Treatment of Psychogenic Purpura

That among the plethora of articles describing the psychiatric features of this syndrome, so few authors address the issue of treatment reflects, I think, the discomfort that many workers feel in dealing with these unfortunate patients. Clearly the cutaneous lesions are but one manifestation, albeit a rather overt and flamboyant one, of a more widespread disorder that frequently has multisystem manifestations. It is well to bear this in mind when a treatment plan is formulated.

Treatment should be directed towards the major area of psychopathology, rather than towards symptomatic relief of cutaneous lesions. Avoid repeated laboratory tests and prolonged somatic treatments; these serve to create a mind-set of physical illness and divert focus from psychological issues. Seek psychiatric consultation as soon as the diagnosis is established, resist pressure from patients, family, and colleagues for repeated medical or surgical consultations and somatic therapy.[40] The specific therapeutic modality selected will depend on the level of psychopathology.

Patients with borderline personality disorder are generally not good candidates for insight-oriented psychotherapy; it is to these patients that McDuffie and McGuire refer when they suggest rather that one offer emotional support.[30] This type of supportive psychotherapy in the hands of the interested and empathic dermatologist, particularly in conjunction with a reduction in environmental stress by hospitalization, may permit remission.[32,40] Ratnoff and Agle report a case in which remission was maintained for 1 year, with just such support.[40]

Those patients with borderline personality disorder who are less dependent, who have a more mature ego, and whose general functioning is at a higher level, do in fact have some capacity for insight and may be able to benefit from psychoanalysis or psychoanalytic psychotherapy. Since this is the treatment that can effect structural change within the personality, and lead to long-term gain, it should be offered to those patients able to benefit from it. The treatment of choice for patients whose diagnosis is hysterical neurosis is psychoanalysis or psychoanalytic psychotherapy.

Patients with severe psychopathology, whether it be psychosis or severe borderline symptomatology may require environmental manipulation in order to reduce the stress to which they are subjected. Patients with psychosis should be treated for their primary psychiatric diagnosis by a psychiatrist.

Because depression is a frequent symptom, Settle confirmed clinical depression in one case by the dexamethasone suppression test, and achieved a 10 month remission with amitriptyline hydrochoride in doses of 300 mg daily.[41]

A number of studies demonstrate that patients with the borderline personality disorder also benefit from tricycliclike antidepressants.[27] A trial of such a drug would, therefore, be in order, should progress be unsatisfactory, the response to psychotherapy inadequate, or depressive symptoms prominent.

COURSE AND PROGNOSIS

The course of the psychogenic purpura syndromes is one of remission and exacerbation, interspersed often with episodes of disease in other organ systems. In some cases, the episodic development of crops of lesions over a period of months may alternate with remissions of variable lengths,[17] while in others there may be only very occasional solitary lesions. Very frequently exacerbations are triggered by increasing emotional stress beyond the point of tolerance. Two of Gardner and Diamond's three original cases had had their disease for 17 and 38 years respectively, while the third had a relapse after a remission of 20 years.[9] Out of 56 patients followed by Agle and Ratnoff, at least 13 had typical episodes for at least 10 years, and 1 for 56 years, though others apparently resolved in a matter of months.[39] It was Ratnoff's impression that increasing awareness of the syndrome was permitting earlier diagnosis, and therefore earlier appropriate treatment, and that the prognosis was better in younger patients, particularly if they had had psychiatric therapy.

CLINICAL VIGNETTES

Two brief clinical vignettes from my own practice will serve to exemplify some of the difficulties one may encounter when taking care of patients with psychogenic purpura.

Case 1

On Mother's Day, a 25-year-old married mother of two experienced a throbbing sensation in the left arm. As the whole family sat in her mother-in-law's living room, they watched her left forearm and hand swell spontaneously and become exquisitely painful; thrombophlebitis was diagnosed by the family physician, and heparin and analgesics prescribed. At the moment of swelling, she had been worrying lest she be pregnant again.

A prior episode of bruising, also diagnosed as thrombophlebitis, had occurred in the right arm at age 16, following within hours an angiogram in the same arm, performed to diagnose the cause of "bleeding from the mouth." There had been a second episode in the interim when her infant son was hospitalized for croup. Her past history had been unremarkable except for severe dysmenorrhoea that confined her to bed for several days each month. Neither parent was well; her father had a residual deficit in the left leg following a "stroke" and her mother was under treatment for carcinoma of the cervix, for which a lymphangiogram had recently been performed on the left leg. The patient described a happy childhood in a "wonderful" family, and an excellent marriage. By the time she was seen as a hospital consultation, the swelling had already been replaced by the characteristic bruising. To confirm the diagnosis of auto-erythrocyte sensitization syndrome, 0.1 ml of autologous whole blood was injected into each of three sites on the left anterior thigh, and the patient was advised that a typical lesion was expected to develop at the middle of the three, since that injection was her own blood. Within 24 hours an ecchymosis several centimeters in diameter did indeed appear, at that site only, and a biopsy revealed features of the Gardner-Diamond syndrome.

The patient presented as a rather infantile and dependent personality, with little psychological mindedness. No attempt was made to foster insight, and with strong support and mild analgesics her lesion resolved within 2-3 weeks. She was then lost to follow-up for 4 years, until a new lesion developed on the left arm around the elbow.

With this fourth episode of bruising, the patient seemed much less composed; her strong defensive denial crumbled, and I learned of dependence on alcohol and drugs, and also heavy smoking. Her husband was revealed as a violent man with paranoid ideation, an alcoholic, who abused her physically and verbally, and who was intolerant of her ill-health. He and she were involved in a sexual liason with another couple within which various types of "swapping" took place. Her immediate conflict was related to the relationship with her husband, whose violence she resented, her wish to move in permanently with the male of the second couple, and strong resentment of her children, who, she felt, frustrated her chances for happiness.

Despite the absence of a developmental history it seemed apparent that this woman had major conflict in the area of motherhood and responsibility on the the one hand, and her own dependency needs on the other. Lesions developed variously on Mother's Day as she worried about a possible unwanted pregnancy, while staying in hospital with her sick son, and finally while torn between maintaining her sadomasochistic marriage for the sake of her children, or leaving to be with an older man who would, she believed, take care of her. The abuse of alcohol and drugs, heavy use of tobacco, lack of impulse control in the area of sexuality, and that she had lied to me systematically in the past, all pointed to a personality disorder, and her clinging helpless dependency and unwillingness to look into herself, as well as poor attendance for office visits supported this impression.

I was under no pressure from family or colleagues to intervene actively, so my treatment plan for this patient was to maintain psychological support, prescribe mild analgesics only, and hope to be able to protect her from intrusive treatments and procedures in the future. Under this regimen there was steady resolution again over 2 to 3 weeks, and she has been lost to follow-up for the past 2-½ years.

Case 2

A 17-year-old high school senior had spilt hydrochloric acid on her left hand in school; this was thoroughly washed immediately, and no evident damage occurred. But for 2 days she complained of nausea and vomiting, before the same hand swelled up rather dramatically like a distended rubber glove. Because the pain was unbearable, she was hospitalized on a surgical service with a diagnosis of cellulitis; fruitless attempts at aspiration were made, and intravenous antibiotics started. Over succeeding days the distal portion of the hand developed a blueish discoloration, while the lesion continued to extend proximally, with a sharp drop-off, at the leading edge. X-rays and numerous laboratory studies were within normal limits. Skin tests to autologous whole blood, were negative.

A similar episode of bruising had occurred the previous year under interesting circumstances. The patient's father was hypertensive, and when a course in cardiopulmonary resuscitation was offered at the local hospital, she and her mother enrolled lest they should need to use it to "save father's life." While she was applying chest compression, the patient heard a "pop," felt a severe pain in her left hand, and, looking down, observed her hand swelling up "in front of her eyes." She left immediately for the Emergency Room, never completing the course.

The past medical history was significant in that severe dysmenorrhoea kept her in bed for 1 or 2 days each month and she had had surgery for an ovarian cyst at age 16, allegedly because Mother preferred that she undergo surgery rather than take oral contraceptive pills; she also allegedly had an untreated scoliosis because Father wanted no back-brace. Other than severe headaches and frequent bouts of nausea and vomiting, her health was generally good.

The family background is also interesting; Father, an alcoholic, dropped out of school very early and fended for himself; he described himself as a "loner" and claimed that he married at 30 only because he wanted children. Mother had an 8th grade education and worked till the patient was born. Because Mother did not readily conceive, fertility tests were undertaken and Father was found to have a low sperm count. It was not until 7 years after the marriage and only 3 months after the maternal grandmother's death, apparently a significant association to Mother, that she conceived the patient, her only pregnancy. Father is verbally and physically abusive to the patient, and to Mother, while Mother with complete psychological denial, suggests that the home circumstances are ideal. The patient is subjected to inconsistencies and mixed messages; for example, though Father is loud in his protestations of love to both, he abuses them and frequently fails to obtain for the patient necessary medical treatment; while her performance at school is the subject of close scrutiny, and high expectations, yet no provision has been made for the patient to attend College; the parents are extraordinarily intrusive into her privacy, yet they have had no compunction about sending her away to relatives each summer since the age of 12. Interestingly, until age 8, she was father's constant companion, but from then on, the relationship has been extremely antagonistic.

My relationship with the family started on the second hospital day; initially the patient was angry, demanding, and intolerant of pain. The parents sitting side by side accross the bed from me were overtly hostile, expressing their anxiety and guilt in paranoid complaints about the quality of care, and the ineptitude of the medical profession, and challenging me with unyielding pressure to take some immediate and dramatic action. Each of the three by their attitude and actions fomented the anxiety of the others, and the tension in the hospital room was near panic; the unspoken fear was that the patient would lose her arm, though she herself was struggling with the distortion of her body image created by the swelling, and with frightening feelings of unreality. The deformity was in fact grotesque. The hand, forearm, and distal arm, tense and misshapen by the extreme swelling, were unnaturally white with a patchy mottling of shades of blue and purple.

The degree of swelling fluctuated during the hospital course of 18 days though it never extended beyond the distal one third of the upper arm. The pressure for action from colleagues, both medical and surgical alike, was equally intense, with urgent demands for surgical exploration, heroic drugs, and ever more sophisticated tests. It was only because I had shared Case 1 with the admitting surgeon that we were able to spare this young woman surgery that could well have set a dangerous precedent for the future, as well as causing her scarring or deformity; the pressure to resist took all my fortitude and conviction.

At discharge, only the discoloration remained, but anxiety prevented free mobility, and despite regular physical therapy there was some temporary disuse atrophy. Transient episodes of minor swelling, confined to the hands, took place in association with increased stress during the first 2 or 3 months of her convalescence.

My diagnosis was a hysterical neurosis. The first episode of swelling clearly represented a hysterical conversion reaction and encapsulated conflict over hostile and aggressive wishes towards her father. As I worked with her in psychoanalytic psychotherapy on a once weekly basis, I learned that the second episode was triggered by her conflicted wish to leave home to attend nursing school. The inconsistencies in parental attitudes, Father's violence and intransigence, and Mother's failure to protect the patient from Father's rages, and (in view of the abrupt change in her feelings towards him at age 8) possibly also from his sexuality, all served to foster ambivalent feelings, and a rather hostile dependency. She worked well in therapy and as she got in touch with her negative feelings and worked them through she was able to separate from the parents and form a good relationship with a male fellow-student; she subsequently attended nursing school.

These two vignettes illustrate the range of psychopathology and the differing psychological approaches that they require, but perhaps more importantly, they illustrate the need to make the diagnosis of psychogenic purpura early and with conviction, and the fortitude that may be required to protect the patient from precedent-setting or destructive surgical procedures, and from intensifying the focus on somatic processes.

REFERENCES

1. Agle DP, Ratnoff OD: Purpura as a psychosomatic entity. A psychiatric study of autoerythrocyte sensitization. Arch Intern Med 109:685-694, 1962
2. Alexander F: Conversion hysteria, vegetative neurosis and psychogenic organic disturbance, in Psychosomatic Medicine. New York, WW Morton & Co Inc, 1950, p 39
3. Biot R: The enigma of stigmata, in Daniel-Rops H (ed): Twentieth Century Encyclopedia of Catholicism, Vol 57. New York, Hawthorne Books, 1962
4. Boxley JD (and Alexander S, discussant): Authoerytherocyte sensitization (painful bruising) syndrome. Proc Roy Soc Med 64:1196-1197, 1971
5. Chandler D, Nalbandian RN: DNA autosensitivity. Am J Med Sci 251:145-149, 1966
6. DiGrande E: Psychogenic purpura: Platelet factor 3 deficiency. Arch Dermatol 104:444-445, 1972
7. Engel GL: Somatic consequences of psychological stress. I. Compensated state, conversion reactions, pain, in Psychological Development in Health and Disease. Philadelphia, W B Saunders Co, 1962, p 368
8. Erwin WJ, Granacher RP Jr: New behavioral data concerning the autoerythrocyte sensitization syndrome. South Med J 70:876-878, 1977
9. Gardner FH, Diamond LK: Autoerythrocyte sensitization. A form of purpura producing painful bruising following autosensitization to red blood cells in certain women. Blood X:7:675-690, 1955
10. Ghosh ML, Sandler G: Autoerythrocyte sensitization. J Irish Med Assoc 65:443-444, 1972
11. Gottlieb PM, Stupniker S, Sandberg H, et al.: Erythrocyte auto-sensitization. Am J Med Sci 233:199-203, 1957
12. Gould G, Pyle WL: Anomalies and Curiosities of Medicine. Philadelphia, W B Saunders Co, 1897, pp 388-391
13. Groch GS, Finch SC, Rogoway W, et al.: Studies in the pathogenesis of the autoerythrocyte sensitization syndrome. Blood 28:19-33, 1966
14. Hallstrom T, Hersle K, Mobacken H: Mental symptoms and personality structure in autoerythrocyte sensitization. Br J Psychiatry 115:1269-1276, 1969
15. Heckel GP: Metabolites of steroid hormones and autosensitivity. Proc Staff Conf Rochester Gen Hosp 10:47-55, 1958
16. Henstell HH, Kligerman M: Auto-sensitivity to erythrocytes. A report of a case. Calif Med 87:267-268, 1957
17. Hersle K, Mobacken H: Autoerythrocyte sensitization syndrome (painful bruising syndrome). Report of two cases and review of the literature. Br J Dermatol 81:574-587, 1969

18. Huss M: Cas de maladies rares. II. Hemophilie v serie, tome 10. Arch Gen Medicine 2:165-195, 1857
19. Kalden JR, Hoffken B, Stangel W: Immune mechanism in Gardner-Diamond syndrome. N Eng J Med 297:1350, 1977 (letter)
20. Khan SA, Cash JD: Autoerythrocyte sensitization syndrome. Scott Med J 15:248-249, 1970
21. Koblenzer CS: Psychosomatic concepts in dermatology. A dermatologist-psychoanalyst's viewpoint. Arch Dermatol 119:501-512, 1983
22. Krumbhaar EB: The stigmata of St. Francis of Assisi. Ann Med Hist 9:111-119, 1927
23. Lababidi A, Friedman R: Psychosomatic purpura. Mo Med 68:386-391, 1971
24. Leiba H, Almog C, Kaufman S, et al.: Possible role of bradykinin in a patient with recurrent cutaneous ecchymoses (DNA sensitization). Isr J Med Sci 8:67-74, 1972
25. Lever WF, Schaumberg-Lever G: Histopathology of the skin (ed 6). Philadelphia, J B Lippincott Co, 1983, p 165
26. Levin MB, Pinkus H: Autosensitivity to deoxyribonucleic acid (DNA). Report of a case with inflammatory skin lesions controlled with chloraquine. N Eng J Med 264:533-537, 1961
27. Liebowitz MR: Psychopharmacological intervention in personality disorders, in Frosch JR (ed): Current Perspectives in Personality Disorders. Washington DC, Am Psychiat Press Inc, 1983, pp 68-93
28. Lifshutz JE: Hysterical stigmatization. Am J Psychiatr 114:527-531, 1957
29. Martin JB, Reichlin S, Brown GM: Clinical Neuroenocrology. Philadelphia, FA Davis Co, 1977, p 41
30. McDuffie FC, McGuire FL: Clinical and psychological patterns in autoerythrocyte sensitivity. Ann Intern Med 63:255-265, 1965
31. McIntosh RM, Ozawa T, Persoff M, et al.: Neuropathy associated with Gardner-Diamond syndrome. Autologous erythrocyte antigen-antibody immune-complex disease. N Eng J Med 296:1265-1267, 1977
32. Meister MM, Bodner AC: Autoerythrocyte sensitization—a psychogenic purpura? Cutis 19:221-224, 1977
33. Moody RL: Bodily changes during abreaction. Lancet 2:934-935, 1946
34. Moody RL: Bodily changes during abreaction. Lancet 1:964, 1948 (letter)
35. Needles W: Stigmata occurring in the course of psycoanalysis. Psychoanal Q 12:23-39, 1943
36. Oei SH, deVries E, Cats A, et al.: Abnormal circulating red blood cells in the painful bruising syndrome. Arch Dermatol Res 263:227-233, 1978
37. Pevny I, Metz J, Wernze H, et al.: The erythrocyte sensitization syndrome. Der Hautarzt 33:251-256, 1982

38. Pinnas JL, Eng M, Tan MD, et al.: Autosensitization to DNA: Evidence for an immunologic basis. J Invest Dermatol 72:157-160, 1979
39. Ratnoff OD: The psychogenic purpuras: A review of auto-erythrocyte sensitization, autosensitization to DNA, "hysterical" and factitial bleeding, and the religious stigmata. Semin Hematol 17(3):192-213, 1980
40. Ratnoff OD, Agle DP: Psychogenic purpura: A re-evaluation of the syndrome of autoerythrocyte sensitization. Medicine (Baltimore) 47:475-500, 1968
41. Settle EC Jr: Autoerythrocyte sensitization successfully treated with antidepressants. JAMA 250:1749-1750, 1983
42. Schindler R: Nervensystem und spontane blutungen. Abhandl Neurol Psychiatr Psychol Greuzgebiete 42:1-68, 1927
43. Schwartz RS, Lewis FB, Dameshek W: Hemmorrhagic cutaneous anaphylaxis due to autosensitization to deoxyribonucleic acid. N Engl J Med 267:1105-1111, 1962
44. Shulman NR: The role of histamine in the pathogenesis of a disease characterized by ecchymoses and systemic symptoms. Clin Res 7:216, 1959 (abstr.)
45. Siwek P: The Riddle of Konnersreuth. Dublin, Browne & Nolan, 1954
46. Speira H, Schwartz Al: Autoerythrocyte sensitization reproducible by both autologous red cells and heterologous DNA. Mt Sinai J Med NY 37:108-111, 1970
47. Stocker WW, McIntyre DR, Clendenning WE: Psychogenic purpura. Arch Dermatol 113:606-609, 1977
48. Tuke DH: Illustrations of the influence of the mind upon the body, in Health and Disease. London, J & A Churchill, 1872, p 267
49. Walshe FMR: Stigmatization. Cath Med Guard 16(4):104-114, 1938
50. Whitfield A: Some points in the etiology of skin disease. Lancet 2:122-126, 1921
51. Whitlock FA: Psycophysiological Aspects of Skin Disease. Major Problems in Dermatology 8. Philadelphia, W B Saunders Co, 1976, pp 98-100
52. Whitlock FA, Hynes JV: Religious stigmatization. An historical and psychophysiological enquiry. Psychol Med 8:185-202, 1978

Part 2: Conditions in Which Strong Psychogenic Factors are Imputed

INTRODUCTION

The reader will recollect that in Chapter 3 the current psychosociobiologic view of disease was presented.[2] This view is consistent with current knowledge from many disciplines, and holds that the "choice" of somatic disease, the time of onset of that disease, and the character of its course are determined by the concatenation of a number of nonspecific factors that include genetic make-up, past life-experience, and current life circumstance.

It was noted that "wellness" exists when there is a balance between the stresses to which the organism is exposed on the one hand, and the defensive mechanisms that it is able to employ against those stresses on the other. Any increase in the amount of stress beyond the containing power of the defenses then, will tip the balance and illness will result.

In an encounter with a source of bacterial infection, the bacterial organism constitutes the apparent stress, and though on the surface it seems evident that whether or not the balance will be tipped in its favor will depend on the size of the inocculum, things are not in fact quite that simple. This is because stress is not only external, but may result from internal processes also; the strength of the inflammatory response mobilized will be subject to modification by such factors as the emotional well-being of the patient, the patient's life circumstances, and the unconscious meaning to the patient of illness or infection. This latter, the unconscious meaning of illness, in turn is determined by past life experience; it becomes clear, therefore, that a judgement about the severity of psychological stress cannot be made by an outside observer, unless that observer has access to this inner unconscious information through such means as psychotherapeutic engagement.

And so "stress" in what follows will incorporate all of these various elements and will be used to designate any one of a variety of different nonspecific events, generated externally or internally, that, by making demands on the organism, set in motion a nonspecific bodily response that leads to a variety of temporary or permanent physiologic, psychologic, or structural changes.[1]

The conditions to be discussed in this section, chronic urticaria, the pruritic syndromes, flushing and rosacea, hyperhidrosis and alopecia areata, each are probably caused by a multiplicity of different factors; but in each, psychologic elements have long been thought to play a significant role. It is not suggested that psychogenic mechanisms alone are involved; each condition is multifactorial in etiology, and the question to be kept in mind during the clinical evaluation is: given the history, the clinical findings, the laboratory results, and what is known of the developmental history and past and present lift circumstances, how much of this patient's problem can I attribute to emotional factors?

REFERENCES

1. Lipowski ZJ: Psychosomatic medicine, an overview, in Hill OW (ed): Modern Trends in Psychosomatic Medicine 3. London, Butterworths, pp 7-13
2. Weiner H: Psychobiology and Human Disease. New York, Elsevier, 1977, pp 575-652

Chapter 11

The Urticarias

CLINICAL PICTURE

Urticaria is a reaction pattern that may result from many different stimuli. Most commonly it is characterized by lesions that involve skin or mucosa, but in a percentage of cases the subcutaneous tissue is the affected site, either alone, or in conjunction with skin or mucosa. The reader is referred to the standard texts in dermatology for a full clinical description.

The lesions of urticaria consist of smooth edematous papules or wheals, pink in color, or white with a surrounding pink flare, which vary in size from a few millimeters to large plaques, several centimeters in diameter. Firm to the touch, they present no evidence of epidermal participation in their formation, excepting that the surface is dimpled by rather prominent follicular orifices. Lesions are transient, lasting from 4 to 6 hours, to 1 or 2 days at most, and resolving usually without trace, though occasionally there may be short-lived minimal residual staining. Central clearing within large plaques may result in annular or polycyclic forms.

The distribution is generalized; lesions may be very numerous or quite sparse. Symptoms vary depending on the location; on the trunk and extremeties pruritus may be pronounced, while on hands and feet the tension of accumulated edema fluid may cause, instead, pain and tenderness and difficulty in flexing the digits.

When the subcutaneous tissue is involved, the term angioedema is used (Fig. 11-1); in this condition, erythema and pruritus are absent, but vast and disfiguring swellings may occur; particulary is this so where the tissues are lax, as for example in the eye-lids or lips. Difficulties arise if oesophagus or trachea are involved, when swallowing or respiration may be compromised. Serum sickness refers to a syndrome in which urticaria with or without angioedema occurs together with arthralgias and fever. Acute, chronic, cholinergic, several types of physical urticaria and hereditary angioedema are described, and while chronic urticaria and cholinergic urticaria are those most consistently associated with emotional stress, stress may influence any type of urticaria.

Sparse or profuse lesions may be present continuously during a bout of urticaria (Fig. 11-2), or episodic crops may appear alternating with periods of remission of varying length; the process is somewhat arbitrarily designated as chronic when it

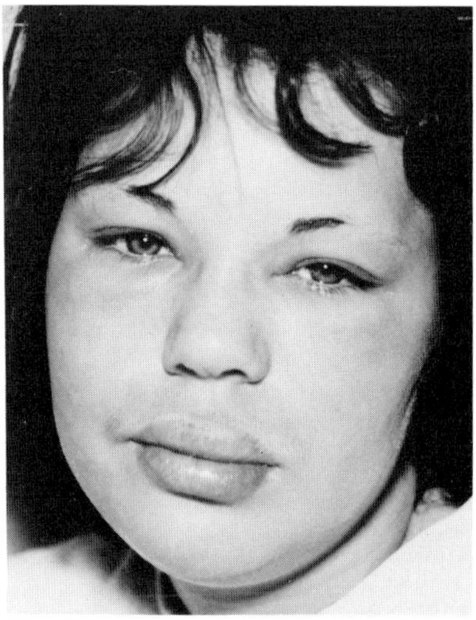

Figure 11-1. Giant urticaria (angioedema). Sudden and severe swelling of the lips and orbits may occasionally be associated with glossal or laryngeal edema.

has persisted for periods variously quoted as anywhere from 4 weeks to 6 months.[15,24,34,57] This distinction is important, because acute and chronic urticaria appear to be different entities

The lesions of cholinergic urticaria are distinctive and consist of intensely pruritic tiny papules each with a large erythematous halo; occasionally only the erythema may be present without papules, but with the characteristic pruritus; large urticarial plaques, angioedema and anaphylaxis may also be part of the syndrome. Urticarial lesions triggered by actinic radiation, water, heat, cold, and pressure are the physical varieties described,[18] and the reader is referred to the standard texts in dermatology for a complete description, as these will only be

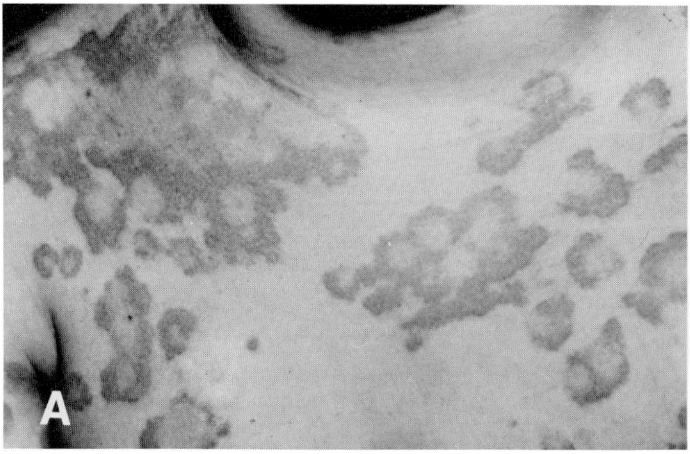

touched on here. Dermographism is one form of physical urticaria where a combination of pressure and traction is required to produce pruritic whealing;[26] it can be demonstrated by firmly drawing the blunt tip of a pen, or cotton swab, down the upper back, where a linear welt will form, surrounded by an erythematous halo. Opinions differ as to the relationship dermographism bears to urticaria.

INCIDENCE

Fifteen to twenty percent of the general population are said to develop hives at some point during their lives.[34,60] Although it may occur at any age, and has been reported as early as the first month of life, the peak incidence is between 20 and 40 years,[59] with equal representation in both sexes in childhood, but a preponderance of females in the adult group.[21,34]

The relative incidence of the different types of urticaria has been determined from the observation of a number of large series of patients. Of 343 patients studied by Juhlin in the course of 1 year, 15 percent were diagnosed as physical

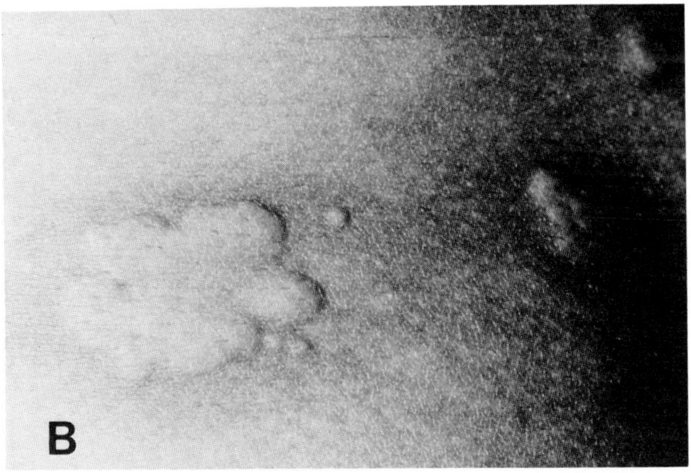

Figure 11-2. (A, B) Urticaria. Lesions of urticaria may consist of aggregated or discrete erythematous or skin-colored papules and plaques, which range in size from a few millimeters to massive gyrate or polycyclic areas. Individual lesions are evanescent but the course of the entire disease may be continuous or phasic, and may last from days to years. Note the nominent follicular orifices (B).

urticaria, 50 percent acute urticaria, 32 percent chronic urticaria, 0.6 percent hereditary angioedema, and 2.4 percent urticaria pigmentosa.[22] Champion et al. analysed the data on 554 out-patients seen over a 10 year period, and report diagnoses of urticaria of unknown etiology in 79 percent, dermographism in 8.5 percent, other types of physical urticaria in 3.4 percent, pregnancy urticaria in 0.5 percent, and hereditary angioedema also in 0.4 percent.[8] Urticaria is reported to occur alone in 40 percent, and with angioedema in 49 percent, while angioedema occurs alone in 11 percent of patients.[1] Dermographism is seen in 5 percent of the population, and of these, more than half also have urticaria.

ETIOLOGY

Clearly the etiology will differ in the different types of urticaria.

Acute Urticaria

Acute Urticaria represents an allergic reaction, and occurs more frequently in atopic patients than in the population at large.[8]

Chronic Urticarla

In contrast, while a small percentage of cases of chronic urticaria are allergic (for example, some reactions to drugs and food additives) chronic urticaria is not more common in atopics than in nonatopics,[8] and other factors may be implicated, such as viral, bacterial, or fungal infections, parasitic infestations of various types, endocrine abnormalities particularly those involving the thyroid gland, collagen vascular disease, a number of drug and chemical direct liberators of histamine, and internal malignancy. Even when these conditions are uncovered in the course of the work-up, however, it is only in as little as 4 percent of cases that their correction results in eradication of the urticaria.[1]

In the vast majority of cases no physical or environmental cause is uncovered and while most authors find emotional factors significant, opinions differ as to the extent that these can be implicated. Champion et al. found emotional disturbance to be the main cause in 11.6 percent of cases, and a contributory factor in a further 23.8 percent.[7] Halpern, in a series of 75 children found chronic urticaria to be psychogenic in at least 27 percent of those with allergies, and in 20 percent of those without;[19] in a further 13 percent of these children the cause was unknown, and we cannot discount the possibility that unrecognized psychogenic forces contributed to their symptomatology also. This may also have been the case in the 70 percent of Green et al.'s 236 patients, whose urticaria was designated idiopathic.[15] Such a possibility would be supported by the fact that Griesemer and Nadelson find an emotional trigger in as high a proportion as 68 percent of cases,[17] and by Panconesi's belief that emotional stressors can act as triggers whether or not another specific etiology is operative.[39] Indeed, this observation with regard to psychogenesis in chronic urticaria has a long and honorable history, having received recognition from Wilson[64] and Hillier,[20] in the middle of the last century, as well as from many more recent observers.

Aspirin and the other salicylates may exacerbate any case of urticaria, regardless of the primary etiology;[19] a number of agents that serve directly to liberate histamine may also induce urticaria in normal individuals as I have noted; these include morphine, curare, polymyxin, codeine, papaverine, and compound 48/80.[34]

Cholinergic urticaria is triggered by cold,[23] heat, exercise, and emotion,[14] and in some cases apparently requires an additional occult contact sensitivity before it can become manifest.[49] Shelley and Shelley have recently reported two cases of a second type of autonomic urticaria, adrenergic in origin, that is also stress-related.[48] The etiology of the physical urticarias is clear in each case from the designated names, while hereditary angioedema is characterized by a genetically transmitted absence or deficiency of the inhibitor of the enzyme C, esterase; the mode of transmission of this defect is autosomal dominant, and attacks of angioedema are triggered by physical trauma and by emotional stress.[58]

BIOPSY FINDINGS

Biopsy material from most urticarial lesions reveals edema and vascular dilation in the upper dermis, with a mild to moderate mononuclear cell infiltrate, and occasionally eosinophils around the small venules; mast cells are reported to be increased in chronic urticaria. Immunofluorescent studies in these lesions fail to demonstrate immunoreactive material.[30,36]

In a small percentage of patients, the biopsy findings are more dramatic, with a perivenular polymorphonuclear cell infiltrate, endothelial cell proliferation, fibrinoid deposits, extravasation of red blood cells, and leukocytoclasis, with nuclear dusting.[30] These vasculitic changes are associated with deposition of immunoglobulin and complement in the vessel walls, and occasionally at the dermo-epidermal junction.[35] In angioedema, the same changes are observed, but located in the deep dermis and subcutaneous tissue.

PATHOPHYSIOLOGY

It is now clear that urticaria can result from one of a number of different mechanisms that may be either immunologic or nonimmunologic, but which in each case will result in the release of vasoactive mediators, primarily histamine from the mast cell. Within the immunologic group, Type I, IgE mediated, or Type III, immune-complex mediated reactions may be responsible. Acute urticaria results from Type I reactions; a small percentage of cases of chronic urticaria may also result from Type I reactions; when an underlying disease is present, however, Type III mechanisms are usually involved.

Immunologic Mediation

Type I Reactions—the IgE Pathway

When a polyvalent antigen bridges two molecules of IgE that are bound to mast cell or basophil membranes, a reaction takes place that results in the reduction of intracellular levels of cyclic AMP (cAMP), and the release of histamine; this reaction is dependent on calcium influx. The increased vascular permeability that results is probably due to direct action of histamine on the vessel walls, equipped as they are with H_1 and H_2 receptors.[32] Whether hyper-responsiveness to IgE of this type results from excessive production of IgE by B cells, or to impaired regulation of helper and suppressor T cells is not clear, but because of the propensity of IgE molecules to bind to cell-membrane receptors in the tissues, serum levels of IgE are not reliable indicators of the degree of reactivity, and indeed a diminished sensitivity to allergen may exist side by side with chronically high serum levels of IgE.

Type III Reactions

Urticaria in Type III reactions is initiated by first an IgM, followed by an IgG response, the end result of which is the formation of immune complexes. Aberrant control mechanisms, due either to inefficient clearing of these complexes or to impaired antibody regulation by helper and suppressor T cells, allows rising titers of immune complexes, and their subsequent deposition in the tissues. This deposition of immune complexes leads in turn to activation of the classical or alternative complement pathways and to histamine release, through the action on the mast cells of the anaphylotoxins C_{3a} and C_{5a} so generated.[32] These are the lesions that may persist for more than just a few hours, and that may on their resolution leave minimal short-lived residual staining.

Nonimmunologic Mechanisms

Nonspecific factors that cause cutaneous vasodilation increase the tendency towards urtication; these include alcohol ingestion, heat, fever, exercise, emotional stress, hyperthyroidism, and estrogens.[1]

B-adrenergic agonists, by increasing the adenylate cyclase activity decrease the intracellular level of cAMP, and so reduce histamine release;[55,56] this reaction is reversed by drugs that block B-adrenergic receptors; these drugs may exacerbate urticaria in some cases.

Kinins have been implicated in cold urticaria, dermographism, and pressure urticaria. That they are involved in some cases of chronic urticaria, also, is suggested by the fact that the intradermal injection of kallikrein will produce a larger than normal reaction in patients with that disorder, and that the urticaria may be improved by aprotinin, a kallikrein inhibitor.[2,34]

Prostaglandins E_1 and E_2 have been implicated in chronic urticaria, both by virtue of their ability to cause vasodilation directly, and also because of their effect on cAMP, and the modulation of histamine release. Intradermal injection of prostaglandin E_2 is reported to produce a more intense response in patients with chronic urticaria than in controls; it has also been suggested that the arachidonic acid cascade may be involved in urticaria caused by aspirin.[32]

Cholinergic urticaria results from the release of acetyl choline by autonomic nerves; this acetyl choline may promote histamine release by increasing the intracellular cyclic GMP (cGMP).[61] Shelley et al. have demonstrated an increased number of acetyl-choline receptors on the mast cells in this disorder, thus explaining the enhanced histamine release from the autonomic discharge of acetyl choline.[19,49]

The "halo-hives" of adrenergic urticaria occur within 10-15 minutes of acute emotional stress. They are associated both with elevated levels of adrenaline and nor-adrenaline, and with mast-cell degranulation; a direct causal relationship is suggested, and supported by the production of lesions by intradermal injection of noradrenalin.[48] The physical urticarias form a heterogeneous group,[18] within which both immunologic and nonimmunologic mechanisms are represented. These entities will not be discussed here further.

The decreased C_1 esterase activity of hereditary angioedema permits activation of the complement system by an increase in plasmin activity;[30] C_{42} kinin, a vasoactive agent, is produced and leads to vascular permeability and edema.[58] Other vasoactive agents probably participate in the production of urticarial lesions; these include substance P, vasoactive intestinal polypeptide, and the enkephalins.[3]

PSYCHOPATHOPHYSIOLOGY

There is evidence to support the participation of psychogenic factors in the clinical expression of each of the above reactions. Nonspecific confirmation of this possibility comes from the classic studies of Graham and Wolf,[13] who, by measuring skin temperature and observing the development of cutaneous vasodilation determined that hives appeared following extreme cutaneous hyperemia; this hyperemia was precipitated by discussing with their patients stressful topics that had in the past caused similiar attacks.

Immunologic Mechanisms

It has been made clear in Chapter 3 that the entire immunologic system is subject to neuroendocrine control by means of a very complex system of interactions. Information in support of this contention from animal studies is summarized by Monjan,[33] and from studies in man, by Palmblad,[38] Maclean and Reichlin,[27] and Stein, Schleifer, and Keller.[52]

Both antibody production and susceptibility to the action of histamine can be enhanced by hypothalamic activity.[28,29,62] In this context, it is important to remember that the hypothalamus is the site for the integration and processing of the information received in the brain from internal and from external sources; internal information regarding vegetative and memory functions, affective level, and emotionality—and external sources via the sense organs from the total environment. As a result of this processing, in the hypothalamus, responses to the integration product are generated, and the hypophysiotropic hormones and neurotransmitters are secreted that will initiate those responses.

By means of this sequence of events, psychic input inevitably will participate in any immunologic response that takes place, and emotional factors will be one of the components that combine to determine the specific character, and the intensity of that response. Much clinical experimental evidence has been adduced in support of this conclusion; for example Black,[4] and also Dennis and Phillipus[12] demonstrated suppression of the IgE mediated pathway by direct suggestion under hypnosis. Black was able to demonstrate a shift in the dose-response curve of the Prausnitz-Kustner reaction,[5] and also suppression of the delayed immune response by the same means.[6] These studies show that not only the degree of sensitivity to histamine but also the level of IgE activity is subject to psychic control; variations in the itch threshold in response to intradermal histamine induced by psychic trauma, as demonstrated by Cormia,[10] further supports this finding. A third source of support comes from clinical situations in which a patient has been deceived into thinking he or she has ingested something to which the patient is allergic, and so developed urticaria.

Nonimmunologic Mechanisms

Vasodilation may be induced by stress-initiated secretion of vasoactive intestinal peptide, substance-P, neurotensin, B-endorphin, bradykinin, and protaglandin

E by the hypothalamus under stress, resulting in the development of urticarial wheals; both cAMP mediated histamine release, and the direct action of the vasoactive peptides themselves on vessel walls are involved. The ability of stress to induce increased secretion of acetyl choline and noradrenaline requires no further comment.

Teshima et al. have demonstrated that emotional stress enhances plasminic activity through the action of adrenalin; and it is by this means that the complement system is activated in hereditary angioedema.[58]

PSYCHODYNAMIC FORMULATIONS

While it is clear that no single personality type or psychodynamic formulation is associated with the various urticarial syndromes, certain trends do emerge.

Acute Urticaria

While it is generally held that "pure" psychogenic urticaria does not exist, occasionally a seemingly clear-cut case is encountered in which no other contributory factors can be identified. Pistiner et al., for example, describe a single, transient, though severe attack in a man with no previous history that occurred within minutes of the realization that he had been defrauded[40] though no attempt is made to understand psychodynamic determinants in the published report. Chue reports a somewhat similar case, but does not fully make clear that allergens may not have been involved.[9]

The Physical Urticarias

Czubalski and Rudzi demonstrated exacerbation of cholinergic urticaria in association with "brief" emotional stress in over 75 percent of 17 patients.[11] The first symptoms of dermographism occurred under conditions of "frustration" in 77 percent of 18 patients, while exacerbations were associated with emotional stress in 83 percent. Although these authors observed no connection between stress and cold urticaria, they quote reports of such from the literature.

Chronic Urticaria

It is in cases of chronic urticaria that we are most likely to consider the emotional component, and a number of constellations crop up with some frequency.

1. Patients trapped in a dilemma to which there appears to be no solution.[63]
2. Driving and competitive individuals, intent in achieving their goals at whatever price.[54]
3. Patients caught in a conflict in which their wish for love and affection is frustrated by sexual and exhibitionistic prohibitions.[31,46,50,65] The symbolic sexual significance of tumescence and detumescence is apt, in this context.
4. Patients who defend against strong dependency wishes, and use activity and acting out, to bind anxiety, may develop urticaria if active expression is frustrated.[50,51] Often unconscious hostility is prominent, and the urticarial wheals have been interpreted as an expression of the conflict between the wish to hurt turned against the self, and the punishment for that wish.[37,64]
5. Patients who harbor resentment about some real or perceived wrong or injustice,[13,37] but cannot overtly express hostility.
6. Anxiety, depression, and obsessive-compulsive features are common findings.[22,25,41,53]

In summary, it seems unlikely that any particular unconscious conflict is specifically expressed in the somatic symptom of urticaria, but rather that idiosyncratic unconscious motivating factors will choose this expression, if hives fit the symbolic needs of the individual conflict, and if genetic and environmental determining factors are in compliance.

DIFFERENTIAL DIAGNOSIS

Differential diagnosis will be directed towards distinguishing between the different forms of urticaria described above, and ruling out urticaria pigmentosum, papular urticaria, and dermatitis herpetiformis.

Most useful is a careful history and review of systems, with special attention to consistent temporal relationships, drugs or other allergens, associated physical symptoms, atopic history, peculiar dietary habits, and also mood, current circumstances, or recent life changes.

A good physical examination will include the distribution of the eruption and the morphology of individual lesions; this latter may point to (1) vasculitic elements; (2) cholinergic, adrenergic or physical etiology; and (3) urticaria pigmentosum, papular urticaria, or dermatitis herpetiformis.

Specific tests will include where indicated, biopsy, with or without immunofluorescence, tests for the various physical urticarias, intradermal injection of mecholyl 1:5000 to rule out cholinergic lesions, intradermal injection of 3-10 nannograms of noradrenalin to rule out adrenergic lesions, tests to rule out infection, infestation, collagen vascular disease or internal malignancy or other internal disease. Tests for food allergies are not generally considered helpful.[34]

MANAGEMENT

Specific management techniques of urticaria include identication and elimination of the specific cause, when possible; reduction of triggering factors; for example, avoidance of the circumstance under which a physical urticaria may develop; and avoidance of nonspecific aggravating factors such as alcohol, aspirin, heat and exertion, and the histamine liberators. Stress management techniques and environmental manipulation designed to reduce stress are also helpful in all types of urticaria. Rarely, elimination diets may be helpful in identifying causes and controlling symptoms.

A number of differenct pharmacologic approaches have been found useful in the different types of urticaria. The six pharmacologic subgroups of antihistamines are summarized by Monroe and Jones, who find hydroxyzine to be the most effective, excepting in cold urticaria, where cyproheptadine appears to be superior.[34]

Some authors find a combination of H_1 and H_2 blockers helpful. H_2 blockers should not be prescribed alone, however, because blockade of the H_2 receptors obstructs the histamine feed-back control mechanism, and a paradoxical increase in tissue histamine may result.[61]

In chronic urticaria the kallikrein inhibitor aprotinin has been shown to be helpful.[2] Aminocaproic acid, and tranexanic acid are valuable in hereditary angioedema.[7,47] Systemic glucocorticosteroids though helpful in acute urticaria have no place in the treatment of chronic urticaria.[34] Topical agents such as menthol or phenol in a simple shake lotion may help to relieve pruritus.

Management schema for chronic urticaria when no specific underlying cause has been identified, or when removal of an identified cause has failed to provide a cure.

These are the cases that are the most frustrating and challenging to manage, and in whom psychogenic factors are most commonly implicated. The following outline is the approach to management that I customarily employ:

- In the course of taking the history and performing the physical examination, particular attention is paid to the way in which the patient presents herself; does she seem to be excessively involved in her symptom? Is there a long history of previous psychosomatic disorders? Is she markedly anxious or depressed? How much does the urticaria interfere in her life, and what does it prevent her from doing?
- Check for dermographism; this reaction can readily be suppressed in most cases with low dose hydroxyzine.
- Explain to the patient that urticaria is a reaction pattern that can be caused by many things, and that although we can usually clear the symptoms readily, we may not discover the actual cause.

- Prescribe hydroxyzine in doses of 10-25 mgm q.i.d.; be positive and reassuring, because 94 percent of patients with chronic urticaria are reported to improve with suggestion and placebo.[45]

If lesions are suppressed, maintain the dose of hydroxyzine for 2 weeks, and then gradually withdraw the drug over a further 2 or 3 weeks. Provided control is maintained, no further steps need be taken.

If control is inadequate, order CBC, U.A., SMA 12 and chest X-ray; double the dose of hydroxyzine, or substitute doxepin, 10 mgm t.i.d.; doxepin is 800 times more potent an antihistamine than is diphenhydramine, and blocks both H_1 and H_2 receptors.[16,44] All tricyclic antidepressants have antihistamine activity that appears to parallel their sedative action; doxepin and amitriptyline are the most effective antihistamines, and desipramine the least.

If lesions are suppressed at this dosage level, and laboratory results are normal, proceed as when using hydroxyzine (described above). Some patients, however, on reassurance may elect to "live" with their hives, and prefer to take no medication of any sort.

If control at this dosage level is inadequate, then a complete work-up is indicated further to rule out a possible physical cause. Doxepin may be increased to a maximum dose of 75 mgm a day, or hydroxyzine to 100 mgm q.i.d. Once control is achieved, an attempt should be made gradually to withdraw the drug after a period of 6 or 8 weeks.

During this step-wise evaluation, you will have had the opportunity to assess the emotional status of the patient. If, despite a negative work-up, and either failure to control the lesions with adequate dosage of doxepin or hydroxyzine, or failure to maintain control on attempting gradually to withdraw the drug, proceed as described below.

Help the patient to recognize the part that urticaria is playing in her life, using the techniques described in Chapter 5. Help her to see her illness in the context of her current situation, and her past life experience, and recommend one of the following; the choice will depend on the circumstances.

1. Continue to see the patient for regular but quite short visits to provide support and reassurance, and to supervise medication; a point may be reached where the lesions lose significance for the patient, who may elect to tolerate them without further medication; for many, this is a satisfactory solution.
2. If urticaria appears to be an isolated symptom in a patient who is neither anxious nor depressed, and who is generally functioning well, behavioral techniques such as biofeedback, autogenic training, or hypnosis might be considered.
3. The patient whose life is clearly significantly affected by her symptoms, who may have had a long history of various somatic difficulties, and who may be

anxious or depressed, should be helped to accept psychiatric referral. For the neurotic patient psychoanalysis or psychoanalytic psychotherapy is the treatment of choice. Those with more severe psychopathology will benefit from a more eclectic approach.

COURSE AND PROGNOSIS OF CHRONIC IDIOPATHIC URTICARIA

Chronic idiopathic urticaria is a disease with great variability of expression, course, and outlook. Patients may have continuous relatively sparse lesions, or episodic flares at intervals of several weeks to several months, and the onset is preceded by an appreciable stressful situation in 51 percent of case.[42] Champion et al. found that the prognosis depended on the duration and severity of the attack, and on the response to treatment with antihistamines. Short duration, a mild attack, and a good response to antihistamines improved the long-term prognosis, but even so, 20 percent of patients can expect still to have their disease after 10 years.[8]

Twarog studied both children and mixed groups of children and adults. In the mixed group 50-60 percent continued to have symptoms for more than 1 year, 34-50 percent for more than 5 years, and 15-40 percent more than 10 years. In the childhood age group girls had an earlier resolution than boys, and those under eight years earlier than those over eight. Fifty-two percent of this group had symptoms for more than 1 year with a median duration of 16 months.[59]

The response to hydroxyzine and doxepin is good in all but 10 percent of patients, but the decision to continue long-term treatment given the chronicity of the disorder, must depend upon the severity of the case and the individual effect on the quality of life for the patient.

No figures are available for the long-term results of hypnosis or biofeedback, but Reinhold reports that 18 of 27 cases improved with psychotherapy.[43]

REFERENCES

1. Beall GN: Urticaria: A review of laboratory and clinical observance. Medicine 43:131-151, 1964
2. Berova N, Petkov I, Andrev VC: Treatment of chronic urticaria with a proteinase (Kallikrein) inhibitor. Br J Dermatol 90:431-434, 1974
3. Bernstein JE: Neuropeptides and the skin, in Goldsmith LA (ed): Biochemistry and Physiology of the Skin. New York, Oxford University Press, 1983, pp 1217-1233
4. Black S: Inhibition of immediate-type hypersensitivity response by direct suggestion under hypnosis. Br Med J 1:925-929, 1963

5. Black S: Shift in dose response curve of Prausnitz-Kustner reaction by direct suggestion under hypnosis. Br Med J 1:990-992, 1963
6. Black S, Humphrey JH, Niven JSF: Inhibition of Mantoux reaction by direct suggestion under hypnosis. Br Med J II:1649-1652, 1963
7. Champion RH, Lachmann PJ: Hereditary angio-edema treated with E-aminocaproic acid. Br J Dermatol 81:763-765, 1969
8. Champion RH, Roberts SOB, Carpenter RG, Roger JH: Urticaria and angio-oedema: A review of 554 patients. Br J Dermatol 81:588-597, 1969
9. Chue PWY: Acute angioneurotic edema of the lips and tongue due to emotional stress. Oral Surg, Oral Med, Oral Path 41(6):734-738, 1976
10. Cormia FE: Experimental histamine pruritus: Influence of physical and psychological factors on threshold reactivity. J Invest Dermatol 19:21-34, 1952
11. Czubalski K, Rudzki E: Neuropsychic factors in physical urticaria. Dermatologica 154:1-4, 1977
12. Dennis M, Philippus MJ: Hypnotic and non-hypnotic suggestion and skin response in atopic patients. Amer J Clin Hynosis 7:342-345, 1965
13. Graham DT, Wolf S: Pathogenesis of urticaria—experimental study of life situations, emotions, and cutaneous vascular reactions. JAMA 143(16):1396-1402, 1950
14. Grant RT, Pearson RSB, Comeau WJ: Observations on urticaria provoked by emotion, by exercise and by warming the body. Clin Sci 2:253-272, 1936
15. Green GR, Koelsche GA, Kierland RR: Etiology and pathogenesis of chronic urticaria. Ann Allergy 23:30-36, 1965
16. Greene SL, Reed CE, Schroeter AL: Double-blind crossover study comparing doxepin with diphenhydramine for the treatment of chronic urticaria. J Am Acad Dermatol 12:669-675, 1985
17. Griesemer RD, Nadelson T: Emotional aspects of cutaneous disease, in Fitzpatrick TM, Eisen AZ, Wolff K (eds): Dermatology in General Medicine (ed 2). New York, McGraw Hill, 1979, pp 1353-1363
18. Gorevic PD, Kaplan AP: The physical urticarias. Int J Dermatol 19(8):417-435, 1980
19. Halpern SR: Chronic hives in children: An analysis of 75 cases. Ann Allergy 23:589-599, 1965
20. Hillier T: Handbook of Skin Diseases for Students and Practitioners. London, Walton and Maberly, 1865, pp 45-55
21. Juhlin L: Clinical studies on the diagnosis and treatment of urticaria. Ann Allergy 39(5):356-361, 1977
22. Juhlin L: Recurrent urticaria: Clinical investigation of 330 patients. Br J Dermatol 104:369-381, 1981
23. Kaplan AP, Garatolo J: Identification of a new physically induced urticaria: Cold induced cholinergic urticaria. J Allergy Clin Immunol 68(16):438-441,

1981

24. Keegan DL: Chronic urticaria: Clinical psychophysiological and therapeutic aspects. Psychosomatics 17(3):160-163, 1976
25. Kenyon FE: A psychiatric survey of a random sample of out-patients attending a dermatologic hospital. J Psychosom Res 6:129-135, 1962
26. Kirby JD, Matthews CNA, James J, et al.: The incidence and other aspects of factitious wealing (dermographism). Br J Dermatol 85:331-335, 1971
27. Maclean D, Reichlin S: Neuroendocrinology and the immune process, in Ader R (ed): Psychoneuroimmunology. New York, Academic Press, 1981, pp 475-520
28. Macris NT, Schiavi RC, Camerino MS, Stein M: Effect of hypothalamic lesions on passive anaphylaxis in the guinea pig. Am J Physiol 222(4):1054-1057, 1972
29. Mathe AA, Yen SS, Sohn RJ, et al.: Effect of hypothalamic lesions on anaphylactic release of prostaglandins from guinea pig lung. Adv Pharm Ther, Proc 7th Int Congr Pharmacol 178:77, 1979
30. Mathews KP: Urticaria and angioedema. J Allergy Clin Dermatol 72(1):1-14, 1983
31. Menninger WC, Kemp J: Psychogenic urticaria. J Allergy 6:467-473, 1935
32. Milliken LE: Urticaria, in Thiers BH, Dobson RL (eds): Pathogenesis of Skin Disease. New York, Churchill Livingstone, 1986, pp 25-31
33. Monjan AA: Stress and immunologic competence: Studies in animals, in Ader R (ed): Psychoneuroimmunology. New York, Academic Press, 1981, pp 185-228
34. Monroe EW, Jones HE: Urticaria: An updated review. Arch Dermatol 113:80-90, 1977
35. Monroe EW, Schulz CI, Maize JC, Jordan RE: Vasculitis in chronic urticaria: an immunopathologic study. J Invest Dermatol 76(2):103-107, 1981
36. Natbony SF, Phillips ME, Elias JM, et al.: Histologic studies of chronic idiopathic urticaria. J Allergy Clin Immunol 71(2):177-183, 1983
37. Obermeyer M: Psychocutaneous Medicine. Springfield, IL, Charles C. Thomas, 1955, pp 271-277
38. Palmblad J: Stress and immunologic competence: Studies in man, in Ader R (ed): Psychoneuroimmunology. New York, Academic Press, 1981, pp 229-257
39. Panconesi E: Psycosomatic dermatology, in Panconesi E (ed): Clinics in Dermatology 2:4 Stress and Skin Diseases: Psychosomatic Dermatology. Philadelphia, J B Lippincott, 1984, pp 105-107
40. Pistiner M, Pitlik S, Rosenfeld J: Psychogenic urticaria. Lancet 2:1383, 1979
41. Preston K: Depression and skin disease. Med J Australia 1:326-329, 1969
42. Rees L: An etiological study of chronic urticaria and angioneurotic edema. J Psychosom Res 2:172-189, 1957

43. Reinhold M: Relationship of stress to the development of symptoms in alopecia areata and chronic urticaria. Br Med J 1:846-849, 1960
44. Richelson E: Tricyclic antidepressants and histamine H1 receptors. Mayo Clin Proc 54:669-674, 1979
45. Rudski E, Borkinski W, Czubalski K: The suggestive effect of placebo on the intensity of chronic urticaria. Acta Allergologica 25:70-73, 1970
46. Saul LJ, Bernstein C Jr: The emotional settings of some attacks of urticaria. Psychosomatic Med III(4):349-369, 1941
47. Sheffer AL, Austen KF, Rosen FS: Tranexamic acid therapy in hereditary angio-neurotic edema. N Eng J Med 287:452-454, 1972
48. Shelley WB, Shelley ED: Adrenergic urticaria: A new form of stress-induced hives. Lancet II (8463):1031-1033, 1985
49. Shelley WB, Shelley ED, Ho AKS: Cholinergic urticaria: Acetylcholine-receptor-dependent immediate-type hypersensitivity reaction to copper. Lancet I (8329):843-846, 1983
50. Shoemaker RJ: A search for the affective determinants of chronic urticaria. Psychosomatics IV(3):125-132, 1963
51. Shoemaker RJ, Levine MI, Shipman WG, et al.: A search for the affective determinants of chronic urticaria. Am J Psychiat 119:358-359, 1962
52. Stein M, Schleifer SJ, Keller SE: Hypothalamic influences on immune response, in Ader R (ed): Psychoneuroimmunology. New York, Academic Press, 1981, pp 429-447
53. Stokes JH, Beerman H: Psychosomatic correlations in allergic conditions. A review of problems and literature. Psychosom Med II:438-458, 1940
54. Stokes JH, Kulchar GV, Pillsbury DM: Effect on the skin of emotional nervous states. Arch Dermatol Syph 31:470-499, 1935
55. Sullivan TJ, Parker KL, Kulczycki A Jr, et al.: Modulation of cyclic AMP in purified rat mast cells. III. Studies on the effects of concanavalin A and cyclic AMP concentrations during histamine release. J Immunol 117:713-716, 1976
56. Sullivan TJ, Parker KL, Stenson W, et al.: Modulation of cyclic AMP in purified rat mast cells. I. Responses to pharmacologic metabolic and physical stimuli. J Immunol 114:1473-1479, 1975
57. Tas J: Chronic urticaria: A survey of one hundred hospitalized cases. Dermatologica 135:90-96, 1967
58. Teshima H, Inove S, Ago Y, Ikemi Y: Plasminic activity and emotional stress. Psychother Psychosom 23:218-228, 1974
59. Twarog FJ: Urticaria in childhood: Pathogenesis and management. Pediat Clin North Am 30(5):887-898, 1983
60. "Urticaria"—commentary. Lancet 2:1344-1345, 1969
61. Wasserman SI: The mast cell and its mediators, in Goldsmith LA (ed): Biochemistry and Physiology of the Skin. New York, Oxford University Press, 1983, 878-898

62. Watson J: The influence of intracellular levels of cyclic neucleotides on cell-proliferation, and the induction of antibody synthesis. J Exp Med 141:96-111, 1975
63. Werth GR: The hives dilemma. Am Fam Phys 17(5):139-143, 1978
64. Wilson E: A Practical and Theoretical Treatise on the Diagnosis, Pathology and Treatment of Diseases of the Skin. London, Churchill Livingston1842, pp 111-117
65. Wittkower BD: Studies of the personality of patients suffering from urticaria. Psychosom Med 15(2):116-126, 1953

Chapter 12

Pruritus: Generalized and Localized

GENERAL CONSIDERATIONS

Pruritus, as we are all aware, is an unpleasant cutaneous sensation that, like pain, is generated in the skin by noxious stimuli. Rather than provoking a reflexive withdrawal, however, pruritus elicits instead the desire to scratch. Although carried by the same sensory fibers as pain, there is good evidence now to suggest that rather than subliminal pain, as was formerly thought, pruritus is a separate and specific sensory function.[46] The site of perception of pruritus, a sensation that is limited to skin and to those mucosal surfaces that are adjacent to skin, is located in the dermo-epidermal junction, and is independent of the epidermis.[3,60,61] Rather than there being specific receptors for the itch stimulus, it is now suggested that the spatial and temporal pattern of neural excitation determines whether itch, pain, touch, or pressure are registered centrally.[8]

The teleological purpose of the scratch response is to protect the organism from injury, by removing noxious substances from the surface of the body; scratching at the same time serendipitously relieves the unpleasant itch sensation; this may be accomplished by creating an interference in the rhythm of transmission of the afferent impulse,[14] or alternatively, relief may result from the impact of scratching on the gate-control mechanism that is thought to mediate transmission within the spinal cord.[22,48]

Two separate types of pruritic sensation are described, each with differing characteristics; epricritic pruritus is sharp, localized, and "pricking" in character, while the protopathic form is a more unpleasant and diffuse sensation, with a burning quality.[29] The former is carried by myelinated A delta fibers, and the latter by the nonmyelinated C fibers that are located peripherally on the cutaneous nerve.

NEURAL PATHWAYS

Although the afferent neural pathways for conduction of the itch sensation have been known for some time, despite much work in this area the chemical mediators that participate in its transmission still remain to be understood fully. These afferent pathways have their origin at free nerve-endings located in the region of the dermo-epidermal junction, from whence the A delta and the C fibers of the peripheral nerve travel to the dorsal horn of the spinal cord via the dorsal root; C fibers travel via the ventral nerve root also.[1] In the cord, the fibers travel in the contralateral and also the ipsilateral spino-thalamic tracts to the thalamus, and thence, via the internal capsule, to the sensory cortex; this arrangement is by no means as simple as it may seem, for complex afferent and efferent neural connections have been identified within the spinal cord, in the periaqueductal gray area of the mid-brain, and perhaps also in other supra-spinal areas not yet identified; these apparently modulate the impulses.[22] The neural pathways that connect the sensory cortex with the hypothalamus and with the other components of the limbic system have been discussed previously in Chapter 3; these are of major significance in the integration of sensory experience, in the generation of affective response, and in somatic reactions to that response.

CHEMICAL MEDIATORS

Inherent in any research on pruritus are the difficulties in quantification imposed by its completely subjective nature, and by the modifying influences of emotional states. These latter will be discussed at length later. A number of ingenious methods have been devised to provide quantifiable reproducible information about experimentally induced pruritus; for example Rajka[53] and Fjellner[22] measured duration, and found it to be rather constant; this method, however, addresses neither the quality nor the severity of the sensation created by electrical stimulation. Edwards et al.[17] followed Shelley and Arthur[60,61] in measuring the level of electrical current required to breach the threshold, while Felix and Shuster[20] recorded the scratch-movements during sleep of patients with pruritic skin disease, using a vibrator transducer attached either to bed or to patient.

Histamine was the central focus of cutaneous mediator research since the publication of Lewis' monograph in 1927,[41] but it was believed that histamine could not be the sole agent mediating pruritus, since histamine-induced itching was known to be accompanied by an erythematous flare; in 1981, however, Greaves et al. demonstrated that histamine could indeed induce itching without causing any visible change in the skin, when they described aquagenic pruritus.[31] A second reason why other mediators were anticipated was the latent period that preceded the onset of the itching that followed histamine injection; this seemed to allow for the activation of an intermediary substance.[22]

Among the pruritogenic substances studied by researchers were a number of endopeptidases. Arthur and Shelley demonstrated that not all of these require the participation of histamine;[3] for example, while kallikrein falls into this nonhistamine dependent category, bradykinin, the peptide end-product of kallikrein activation, is only mildly and indirectly pruritogenic, through the activation of histamine.[33] Another source of possible pruritogens is the proteolytic enzymes liberated by damaged cells,[35] but the focus of much recent attention are the prostaglandins, and the group of polypeptides that are located in the central nervous system and peripherally in the tissues. Prostaglandins of the E series enhance the itch induced by histamine and by papain,[42] perhaps by release of proteases from leukocytes or keratinocytes;[46] if not mediators, therefore, they are certainly modulators of pruritus.[22] Substance P has been identified surrounding cutaneous sensory fibers, and may be released at peripheral nerve endings in the skin; it is presumed to mediate antidromic vasodilation and axon reflex flare;[40] on intradermal injection, substance P is pruritogenic. Pruritogenic also are vasoactive intestinal peptide, secretin and neurotensin, all of them through the mechanism of mast-cell histamine release.[22]

The opioid polypeptides have both central and peripheral effects on the itch sensation. A central effect for these agents can be deduced from the fact that morphine induces itch centrally and enhances centrally itch that is induced peripherally by cutaneous histamine, while the morphine antagonist naloxone relieves intractable itching,[5] and raises the threshold of perception for experimentally-induced itching.[6] Peripherally, met-encaphalin-like immunoreactivity has been identified in the Merkel cell,[34] and intradermal injection of a stable met-encaphilin analogue potentiates histamine-elicited pruritus, as do morphine, and β-endorphin. Despite the known mast-cell degranulating action of morphine, these potentiating effects are not mediated either by histamine, or by prostaglandins.[22] It is postulated that the mechanism may involve the adenylate-cyclase system in a manner analogous to that proposed for pain.[21]

NONSPECIFIC MODULATORS

In addition to the anatomical and chemical mediators and modulators that I have discussed, a number of nonspecific factors will lower the threshold for itching; these include ambient warmth, hyperemia, for whatever cause, and moisture. The circadian rhythm produces a diurnal variation in cutaneous blood flow, with relative hyperemia in the evening; this in part accounts for the increased itching most patients experience at the end of the day. Previous dermatitis or the area surrounding a current dermatitis also will have a lowered itch threshold.[29]

CLINICAL ASPECTS

Pruritus is the most frequent complaint of the patient with skin disease, and also the most distressing; pruritus may also be symptomatic of a variety of systemic disorders in which frequently no primary cutaneous lesion is detected (Fig. 12-1). The individual itch threshold is subject to great variation, and while some skin diseases are almost universally pruritic, there are others that are usually relatively free of symptoms, but that nevertheless in certain patients may cause intolerable itching. In similar fashion there is variability in the visible manifestations of itching dermatoses; though some have eminently visible and characteristic clinical findings, in others the cutaneous signs may be very subtle, and must be scrupulously searched for, if the correct diagnosis is not to be missed.[43]

Disorders Associated with Pruritus

The list of *cutaneous* disorders associated with pruritus can only be partial at best, because essentially the entire spectrum of dermatologic disease can probably under some circumstances be associated with pruritus; the common offenders, however, are listed in Table 12-1. Table 12-2 lists the *systemic* disorders associated with pruritus.

INCIDENCE

In a series of 74 patients with pruritus, Lyell found that 31 percent were due to cutaneous disease, 31 percent were psychogenic, 25 percent had underlying systemic illnesses, and in 10 percent no cause could be identified.[43]

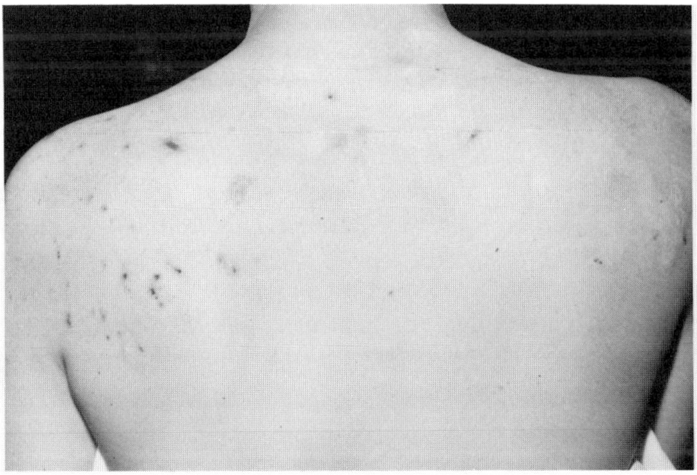

Figure 12-1. Generalized pruritus. The paucity of clinical findings is in stark contrast to the symptoms. Lesions are accessible to the dominant hand, and consist of linear excoriations and crusted papules. Pruritus on the back is common.

Table 12-1
Cutaneous Disorders Associated with Pruritus

Sensitivity reactions
Insect bites
Infestations
Urticaria
Some drug eruptions
Infections
Bacterial
Yeast
Fungal, particularly dermatophytes
Viral
Environmental
Sunburn
Miliaria
Polymorphous light eruption
Photocontact dermatitis
Phototoxic eruptions
Pernio
Xerosis
Fiberglass
Mucuna pruriens (itch powder) and other proteolytic enzyme-containing substances.
Irritant dermatoses (e.g., industrial or domestic contactants, etc.)
The Eczemas
Atopic dermatitis
Dyshidrotic eczema
Allergic contact dermatitis
Bullous Dermatoses
Dermatitis herpetiformis
Bullous impetigo
Papulosquamous Eruptions
Seborrheic dermatitis
Lichen planus
Psoriasis
Cutaneous Neoplasia
Mycosis fungoides
Mastocytosis

Table 12-2
Systemic Disorders Associated with Pruritus

Renal disease
Chronic renal failure
Hepatic Disease
Primary biliary cirrhosis
Cholestasis of pregnancy
Extrahepatic biliary obstruction
Hepatitis
Certain drugs
Central Nervous System
Drug toxicity (e.g., opiates, alcohol, cocaine)
Psychogenic
Hematopoetic
Polycythemia
Hodgkin's disease
Lymphomas and leukemias
Systemic mast cell disease
Iron deficiency anemia
Endocrine Disorders
Hyperthyroidism
Carcinoid syndrome
Diabetes mellitus
Miscellaneous
Malignant neoplasms
Neurological syndromes (e.g., multiple sclerosis)
Advanced age
Internal parasites
Viremia (Viral exanthemata)

In a series of 43 cases of pruritus without skin signs, Beare found an equal sex incidence, and all age groups to be susceptible,[4] although clinical experience would seem to suggest a higher incidence in the elderly. In approximately 40 percent of these patients, no cause could be identified, 10 percent of the adults were believed to be of psychogenic origin, and in 16 percent, an underlying systemic disease was the cause. Eleven of the 43 cases were children, and in all of these the diagnosis was psychogenic; indeed it is Beare's opinion that in childhood, this is the invariable cause.

In a breakdown of patients whose pruritus is associated with systemic disease, some information is available about specific incidences; for example, 80-90 percent of patients with renal failure itch.[67] Pruritus in patients with liver disease is rare, unless there is cholestasis; it is present in 20-25 percent of jaundiced patients, virtually 100 percent of patients with primary biliary cirrhosis, and up to 50 percent of patients with carcinoma of the ampulla of Vater; it is also present in 1.5-3.0 percent of pregnant women, and in patients taking drugs that cause cholestasis, such as the phenothiazines, tolbutamide, erythromycin estolate, anabolic steriods, estrogens, and progestins.[28] Thirty to fifty percent of patients with polycythemia complain of pruritus, as do 30 percent with Hodgkin's disease, and 4-11 percent with thyrotoxicosis.[28] While diabetes mellitus is frequently quoted as an occult cause of itching, in my clinical experience it is extremely rare; Gilchrest quotes a figure of 3 percent,[28] while Vallance-Owen believes the two to be unrelated.[52] In contrast to these rather low figures for systemic disease, Rajka found an association in 50 percent of 34 patients.[52]

PSYCHOGENIC PRURITUS

As will become clear in the discussion of pathophysiology that follows, emotional factors can prolong and intensify the sensation of pruritus, whatever the etiology. While authors differ as to whether or not it is possible for pruritus to be purely psychogenic, clinical experience leaves me in no doubt that there are patients in whom psychogenic factors if not the sole cause, play by far the major role, with only rather trivial and nonspecific agents serving as auxiliary initiating or contributory factors.

Generalized Psychogenic Pruritus

Clinical Characteristics

Psychogenic pruritus may be generalized or localized to a specific area. Certain areas are involved with a relatively greater frequency; these, which include the perianal, the vulva, the scrotum, and scalp, are areas that have special symbolic psychological implications; they will be addressed individually later. Only cases in which visible lesions are confined to those that result from scratching or rubbing, and in which no cutaneous or underlying systemic disease can be identified, should be included under this rubric.

Although by no means exclusive to psychogenic pruritus, certain features are characteristic: rather than a constant level of discomfort, paroxysmal attacks of itching occur; these parallel rather faithfully the emotional state, and are often at their worst on retiring; attacks of itching, however, seldom prevent sleep, and appear to be less disturbing if the attention is diverted; the evidence of scratching is frequently less marked than the florid and exaggerated description of severity would seem to warrant.

Pathophysiology

The wealth of clinical material suggesting that pruritus may be precipitated or exacerbated by emotional stress[9,12,17,38,47] is supported by impressive experimental evidence. Studies include those of Cormia, who in 1952 demonstrated a lowering of the itch threshold following psychic trauma, and a prolongation of the duration of histamine-induced itching in patients with psychogenic pruritus;[12] Calnan and O'Neill confirmed an association between chronic emotional tension and itching,[9] while Cornbleet showed an increase in the intensity of itching, with fatigue.[13]

Recent elegant and sophisticated studies have been directed towards a clearer understanding of the mechanisms whereby these changes in perception take place. The physiologic response to stress results from activation of the neuroendocrine system, with a complex interaction between the sympatho-adrenomedullary and the pituitary-adrenocortical axes.[2] One result of this activation is the release of adrenalin from the adrenal medulla. Increased adrenalin levels have been shown to cause a decrease in the itch response and an increase in the flare response to histamine.[24] Under experimental conditions, using standardized stressors, Fjellner and Arnetz showed that psychosocial factors and neurotic character traits both affect the itch and flare responses, and that these variations in response in turn are related to the adrenalin response pattern. Greater increases in adrenalin over pretest levels were recorded in subjects who felt in control of the experimental situation, and who were better adjusted psychologically, with a parallel increase in the flare response, while those who were described as experiencing "moodiness" instead demonstrated an increase in the duration of itching.[25]

A second link in this complex chain is the opioid peptides. Stress-induced analgesia involves the activation of both opioid and nonopioid pathways; selective activation of the former is associated with situations that are uncontrollable, while the latter are involved in those that are controllable.[24] Opioid peptides enhance itching, while decreasing the perception of pain,[23] and Fjellner et al. suggest that it is therefore reasonable to assume that stressful, uncontrollable, and unpredictable life situations, in analogous fashion, may potentiate pruritus through activation of opioid pathways.[24] In support of this suggestion is the finding that β-endorphin is secreted simultaneously with adrenocorticotropic hormone (ACTH) in stressful situation.[32] Substance P, which is also liberated in response to stress, is also pruritogenic.

So it is clear that although many questions remain to be answered about the pathophysiology of psychological influences on the perception of the itch sensation, age-old clinical observations are validated by recent laboratory confirmation, and partial answers are available that point to the possibility of exciting findings in the future.

Psychopathology

Pruritus is most frequently symptomatic of psychoneurosis, but may occasionally occur in patients with psychosis. While it may be a symptom of overt neurotic depression in all types of neurosis it is frequently seen as a depressive equivalent in a patient who is quite unaware of feeling depressed; particularly is this so in older patients, in whom characteristic depressive symptomatology can often be uncovered on careful questioning. Whitlock is of the opinion that most patients with psychogenic pruritus are depressed.[64] Edwards reported six depressed patients with severe and intractable itching, all of whom were cured when their depression was successfully treated,[18] and Cormia too found depression to be prominent.[64]

Pruritus may occur also as a hysterical conversion symptom; in this context Robinson et al. report an epidemic of hysterical itching and rash in a rural elementary school; itching was the initial symptom in an epidemic that involved 57 of 159 children.[54]

Psychodynamic Formulations

A number of authors have addressed the question of psychodynamic mechanisms in psychogenic pruritus. Musaph, noting that orangutans scratch themselves when thwarted in their desires, interprets the state of itching and the scratch response that automatically follows in terms of a "derived activity," a means of permitting the displaced expression of unacceptable feelings such as embarrassment, rage, impatience, or sexual excitement.[49]

Because scratching relieves the sensation of itch, the behaviorists feel that it becomes a reinforced behavior, that leads to development of the itch-scratch cycle; through reinforcement scratching becomes a habit. Another interesting "use" of itching is described by Elberlik in patients engaged in the task of restructuring their body-image, following loss of an organ; here itching helps define boundaries for the patient,[19] in a fashion analogous to the way in which some borderline patients use factitious lesions.

Cormia's patients demonstrated the psychologic characteristics so often reported in those who somatize; patients from neurotic and unstable families who have sustained psychological trauma very early in life, whose own relationships are unstable and whose adult adjustment is poor; in these patients, Cormia often was unable to identify a precipitating event.[2]

In contrast, both Calnan and O'Neill,[9] and Musaph[49] describe patients less severely impaired, with neurotic conflict in the area of aggression, who, for fear of loss of love, are unable to express anger or resentment directly. In these patients, as a partial solution to the neurotic conflict, itching expresses both the aggressive or resentful feelings and punishment for the guilt that these unacceptable feelings arouse. Musaph described 10 such patients in whom aggression was aroused in situations they felt powerless to alter. This finding is particularly interesting, in light of the fact that the opioid-mediated itch pathways are thought to be activated by "uncontrollable" situations.[24] Seitz studied 120 patients but it is not clear that they did not have underlying skin disease.[59] For him too, the unconscious conflict is over aggression, the scratch response representing a masochistic hysterical conversion reaction to release the tension of suppressed rage through muscular activity; this Seitz believes, atones for guilt through mutilating self-punishment, and provides through cutaneous pleasure some gratification of the need for love.

In addition, such functions as the avoidance of anxiety-provoking situations, gratification of dependency needs, perpetuation of "illness" behavior, and litigiousness may be served by pruritus, just as they may by any psychogenic symptom.

Diagnosis

The diagnosis is based on positive and negative findings. In both generalized and localized pruritus, the index of suspicion is raised when the diagnostic characteristics mentioned at the beginning of this section are present. Other suspicious findings, particularly in the localized forms, are either localization to a single area of skin, frequently one that is inconsistent with the sensory innervation of the part, or wild and idiosyncratic theories as to the pathologic process responsible. Often there is a long history of other psychosomatic illness, and not infrequently a precipitating event, or difficult psychosocial circumstances over which the patient has no control, may be evident in the recent history.

Clearly the negative findings must be the absence of cutaneous disease, or an underlying somatic condition.

Management

Discussion in this section will be confined to the management of generalized psychogenic pruritus, and those localized forms that do not involve the genitalia or perianal areas.

Dermatologic management. Recommend measures to assure adequate hydration, and to avoid moist, warm ambient conditions that may provoke sweating, irritation, or hyperemia (i.e., neutral soaps, avoid hot water, avoid wool next to the skin, avoid synthetic fabrics, apply dusting powder to absorb perspiration, etc.). Cool open compresses soothe, because evaporation produces cooling and reduces hyperemia; these should be followed by emollients; creams are more effective generally than lotions; white vaseline is excellent. Phenol 0.3 percent, menthol 0.1-0.2 percent, or camphor 0.2 percent incorporated into the emollient creams relieve itching by a similar cooling mechanism. Topical steroids are of no benefit, if no visible lesions are present. UVB may be very helpful in recalcitrant cases. Where lichenification is a feature: (1) Topical steroids, applied after the compresses, and before the emollient cream. (2) Tar gel or ointment (e.g., Fototar Cream, Elder Pharmaceuticals, Inc., Bryan, OH or Estar Gel, Westwood Pharmaceuticals Inc., Buffalo, NY) may be used in conjunction with topical steroids as in 1 above. (3) Two percent pine tar may be incorporated in steroid cream or ointment, as in 1 above. (4) Tar compresses or soaks (e.g., Balnetar, Westwood Pharmaceuticals Inc., Buffalo, NY or Zetar Emulsion, Dermik Laboratories Inc., Swarthmore, PA) may be substitued in 2 above. Where excoriations are prominent, the topical treatment will be as for neurotic excoriations (see Neurotic Excoriations in Chapter 9).

Hydroxyzine, in doses of 10-25 mg three or four times daily may be prescribed as an antipruritic; promethazine hydrochloride in doses of 12.5-15 mg three or four times daily, is often helpful, if hydroxyzine is ineffective. Doxepin is perhaps the most effective drug (see treatment for urticaria); the dose of doxepin for use as an antihistamine or antipruritic is 10-25 mg three or four times daily.

Such prostaglandin antagonists as acetyl salicylic acid or ibuprofen may occasionally be helpful. While an opioid antagonist, were a practible one available, might well relieve the physical symptom, the emotional factors would, of course, remain to be addressed.

When the scalp is involved: (1) any dandruff shampoo is satisfactory; my own preference is for those containing salicylic acid, sulfur, or tar, rather than the heavy metals zinc or selenium; I find them more soothing and less irritating; (2) topical steroid lotions—for example, 1 percent hydrocortisone, or a mid-potency preparation, if scratching and lichenification are pronounced or if mild seborrheic capitis is associated; and (3) lotions containing tar and salicylic acid or sulfur may be substituted or incorporated in 2 above.

Psychiatric management. The psychiatric management, as in all situations, is most appropriate and most effective if it is based on the psychiatric diagnosis. It will be along the lines as described for psychogenic urticaria, and in Chapter 5—the general principles of management. Explain to the patient the studies that have been done and the negative findings, pointing out that no dermatologic or underlying physical disease has been uncovered. Warded off aggressive feelings most frequently underlie the symptom of pruritus.[49] Be aware of the possible effect of these on the blossoming doctor-patient relationship. Do not permit yourself to be made angry; do not mobilize angry feelings too rapidly, address them, and diffuse them gently. Try to educate the patient in the current psychosociobiologic view of disease. In so far as the patient can accept it, explain the part played in the mind-body relationship by chemical mediators, in a way that fits his or her particular needs. Point out that many times we are not consciously aware of stresses that are affecting our lives. Set up regular, if short, visits to provide support and reassurance, and to supervise medications as suggested in the above section on dermatologic management. Use these short visits to assess the patient psychiatrically:

1. If on careful questioning, obvious depression is present, increase the doxepin dosage to therapeutic levels.
2. Gradually prepare the patient for psychiatric referral along the lines previously suggested, if this is indicated.
3. Short term use of tranquillizers may be indicated in conjunction with doxepin, or while preparing the patient for psychiatric referral if psychosocial circumstances warrant it.
4. Environmental manipulation to reduce stress and stress-management techniques may be indicated in some cases.

Course and Prognosis

The course and prognosis will depend on an interaction between the psychiatric status of the patient, and the patient's individual life circumstances. Beare reports spontaneous resolution over 2 years, in 13 of 33 cases of psychogenic urticaria, but there is no question that without appropriate psychiatric, as well as dermatologic treatment, many such cases become chronic, These develop the secondary features of often extensive lichenification and excoriations, and pursue a fluctuating course characterized by remissions and exacerbations that parallel the exegesis of life's ups and downs.

Many patients whose symptoms are of relatively short duration, and where situational factors are operative, will do well with simple measures and a supportive therapy that is well within the competence of a dermatologist; they may give up their symptom, or learn to live with it without real distress, or need for further treatment.

Patients with overt depression, or in whom pruritus is a depressive equivalent do well with doxepin, prescribed within the context of a positive doctor-patient relationship. Complete relief is usually achieved within a period of about 4-6 weeks, and the drug can gradually be withdrawn, when relief has been maintained for 2-3 months. Recurrences may be anticipated during subsequent periods of depression, or unusual psychosocial stress. Both Edwards[18] and Wright[66] report resolution with appropriate and effective treatment for depression; both used electroconvulsive therapy (ECT)

Where underlying neurotic conflict is the major psychopathology, psychoanalysis or psychoanalytic psychotherapy is the appropriate treatment, and though the outcome is less favorable if fixed characterologic features are present, Calnan and O'Neal,[9] Seitz,[59a] and Sonneck[63] all report good results.

In my own experience even quite short-term psychoanalytically-oriented psychotherapy in conjunction wtih dermatologic measures often resolve the problem, though recurrences may be anticipated at times of particular stress.

Pruritus Ani

Clinical Characteristics

Prolonged intractable perianal pruritus is set apart from generalized psychogenic pruritus for two major reasons: first, the unconscious symbolic psychologic significance of the area, and second, ambient conditions that subject the skin to warmth, moisture, and fecal contamination. As with generalized pruritus, cutaneous, systemic, psychogenic, and idiopathic variants are described. My discussion will be confined to those cases where cutaneous or systemic disease is of minor importance and the pruritus primarily perpetuated by psychological forces (Fig. 12-2).

According to Cunliffe, the patient with pruritus ani seldom has localized pruritus at other sites,[14] though in my own experience symptoms in the scalp or other seborrhoeic areas are not unusual. The spasms of itching are often acute, and remarkably violent in their intensity, and accompanied by anxiety because of the proscription of perianal scratching. Worse at night, and when the attention is not occupied, unlike generalized pruritus, pruritus ani may prevent sleep and the patient often awakens scratching during the night. Maceration, fissuring, excoriations and lichenification frequently supervene, with colonization by yeast organisms, and saprophytic skin or intestinal bacteria.

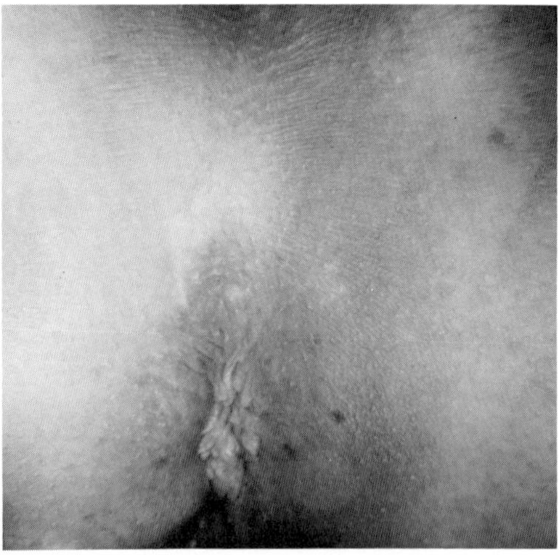

Figure 12-2. Pruritus ani. The symptoms often are not consonant with the physical findings. This lady, who complained of ferocious itching inducing wakefulness, had only mild lichenification (on the right side of the picture).

Incidence

Males predominate over females in a ratio of 2 to 4:1,[7,11,65] and though occurring at virtually any age, a peak is reported in the fifth decade. Though authors vary in the percentages they attribute to different causes, some do not mention psychogenic as one of these,[15,26] and few regard it as of primary etiologic significance; many refer to it as an aggravating or perpetuating factor.[10,30] Hunt reported 8 of 300 cases to be psychogenic,[36] and Bowyer only 1 percent in a series of 200 patients,[7] while Fromer considered 45 percent to be idiopathic, or "essential."[27]

My own clinical experience suggests that significant psychogenic factors have a much higher incidence than these figures seem to indicate.

Etiology

Par excellence, pruritus ani is an entity of multifactoral etiology. A seborrheic diathesis may render the perianal skin particularly susceptible to maceration and irritation; obesity, tight clothing, synthetic fabrics or plastic seat covers, and increased sweating secondary to stress or high ambient temperatures contribute to maceration, as the opportunity for evaporation of sweat is limited. Mucous leakage from a lax anal sphincter, fecal soiling, inadequate perianal hygiene, or excessive cleansing, all may contribute to local irritation. Dietary indiscretions such as spicy food or loose stools render the feces irritating. Chronically macerated skin is readily colonized by yeast and bacteria, and finally as in any chronic and irritating condition, the contribution of iatrogenic factors cannot be ignored. Once the itch-scratch cycle is established it takes on a momentum of its own.

Pathophysiology

The pathophysiology of itching is as described for generalized pruritus; however, the ambient moisture and the local irritants peculiar to the perianal area cause tissue damage, and generate hyperemia, thus lowering the itch threshold. Anxiety and loss of sleep secondary to these factors add to this effect, and the itch-scratch cycle becomes a spiral.

The usual sequence of events in the evolution of chronicity is as follows:

1. Attention is focused on the area by an often inconsequential or transient physical problem, or anxiety about a possible problem.
2. Feelings of guilt or shame, often unconscious and experienced only as anxiety or embarrassment, lead the patient to over-cleanse and over-medicate, with resultant irritation.
3. Increased sweating, triggered by anxiety increases maceration and irritation.

4. A lowering of self-esteem begins to occur.
5. Anxieties continue to escalate, as a multitude of therapeutic modalities fail to produce the desired relief; thus the itch-scratch cycle is firmly established.

Psychopathology

The majority of patients with prolonged and intractable pruritus ani have an obsessional personality configuration;[50,65] depression or depressive equivalence is not uncommon.[11] Occasionally those with mental retardation or psychosis may produce hypertrophic changes in the area from rubbing, but seldom do they complain of pruritus.[39]

Psychodynamic Formulation

It is perhaps not surprising that intractable pruritus in the perianal area is most commonly seen in persons whose psychological difficulties are those difficulties that have their origins in the period when anal function has particular significance to the developing child. This is the period when the child is striving to separate and achieve autonomy from the mother on whom the child is still dependent. Since bowel function is one of the few things over which a child can exert control, it readily becomes an arena for playing out this struggle for autonomy; as such, the psychological significance is enhanced, and a fixation point developed, "priming" the area for later somatic compliance (see Chapter 2).

Unacceptable unconscious aggression and ambivalent feelings towards important figures are characteristic. The defenses employed against these unacceptable feelings include submissiveness and passive dependency;[11,62] mild paranoia and fears of persecution are not uncommon, and exacerbation of symptoms may occur in situations where persecution might be anticipated.[65] Although a submissive posture protects the patient from the possible damaging effects of the patient's unconscious aggressive and sadistic feelings, it at the same time renders the patient vulnerable. That latent unconscious homosexual fears may result from this defensive passive stance is supported by the fact that in one series, all sexually active male patients were premature ejaculators.[45]

Sexual preoccupation, autoeroticism, and exhibitionism are other characteristics mentioned by a number of authors relative to pruritus ani; one may speculate as to possible underlying psychodynamic forces leading to these traits.

Panconesi studied 26 patients using projective tests and psychosomatic questionnaires.[51] His results showed patients to be in conflict about ambition and wish for social contact on the one hand, and an underlying sense of inadequacy on the other. They compensated for this inadequacy with self-aggrandizement and were querulous, intolerant, and resentful of an environment that appeared to thwart their wishes. Pleasure and shame were derived from scratching. The management of pruritus ani will be discussed in the next section, along with pruritus vulvae et scroti.

Pruritus Vulvae et Scroti

Clinical Characteristics, Incidence, Etiology, and Pathophysiology

Less attention has been paid to genital pruritus in the literature, than to anal (Fig. 12-3). Ambient conditions, systemic illness, and unconscious symbolic significance play the same part here, and the clinical picture is similar. Information as to the overall incidence is sketchy, but as with pruritus ani, the percentage attributed to psychogenic causes in those series of cases reported, is small. For example, Rumpianski and Shiskin quote 6 out of 952, and an additional 6 with neurodermatitis,[57] and Jeffcoate, 18 out of 254.[37]

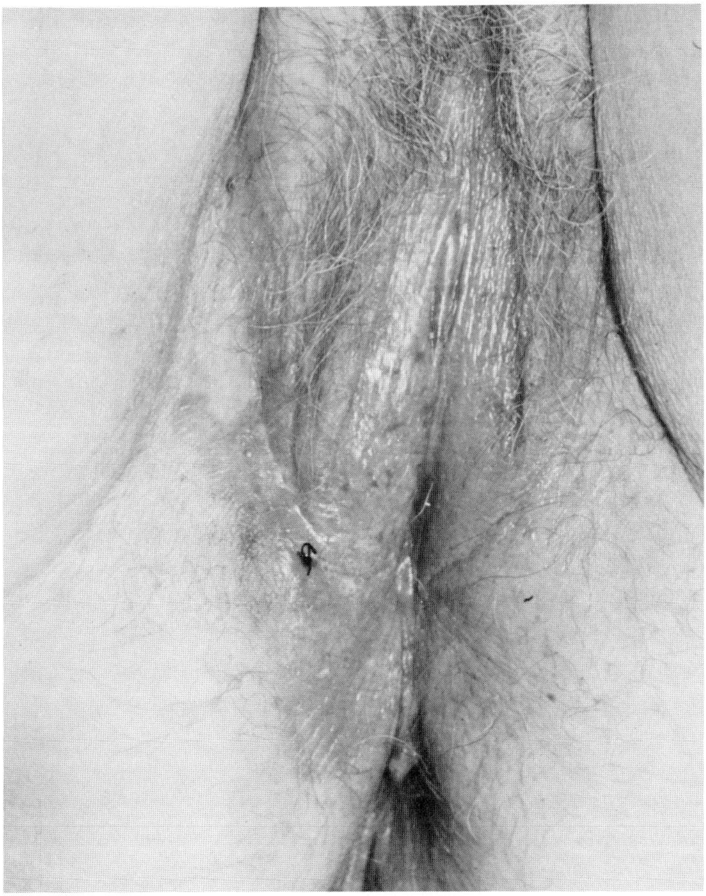

Figure 12-3. Pruritus vulvae. Changes are often minor and in no way consonant with severity of the symptoms. In this rather severe case, there is erythema and lichenification on labia and perineum.

Etiologic factors and pathophysiology too are similar, though vaginitis with or without discharge in women, takes the place of rectal mucous leakage, and dietary indiscretions have a lesser significance. The evolution of the cycle frequently follows a course similar to that of chronic pruritus ani.

Psychopathology

Rather than obsessional personality configuration or neurosis, hysterical features are more common in genital pruritus.[44,56,65] The incidence in psychotics and those with mental retardation is as for pruritus ani, and depression or depressive equivalence is again stressed by many authors, particularly in older women.[65]

Psychodynamic Formulations

Frustration of the sexual drive, whether it be for neurotic conflictual reasons, or for realistic reasons, figures prominently in the literature and is referred to by Cormia, Jeffcoate,[11,37] and Druneck[16] amongst others, while Lynch reports a higher incidence in separated and divorced women, suggesting a similar psychodynamic. Guilt about forbidden sexual wishes in some cases may lead to a defensive displacement of drive expression from masturbation to pruritus and scratching;[11] both the needs of drive and conscience are gratified, in the combination of pleasure and pain. Clinical experience, particularly in psychoanalytic practice suggests that it is simplistic to suggest that such conflicts have less relevance in this more overtly sexually permissive day and age, than in the past.[64] In 41 patients reported by Wittkower and Russel, 30 percent were experiencing frustration at the time of onset of their symptoms, frustration that though not necessarily sexual in nature often could be recognized to have its origins in childhood.[65] Some of these women were overtly impaired psychologically, and were thought to be dealing with such unconscious issues as resentment of their female status, and unresolved difficulties in interfamily relationships. Hostile feelings may also be involved, but as Whitlock notes, the relationship of this to disturbed sexuality needs no emphasis.[64]

The tendency among more recent authors has been to downplay the etiologic influence of psychogenic factors and to ignore the possible influence of dynamic unconscious factors; there is a rather simplistic focus on overt linear direct causal relationships.[55,64]

This verbalized and conscious denial is belied, however, by the therapeutic measures that some of these authors suggest, which clearly address psychogenic factors.[55]

Managment of Anogenital Pruritus, Course and Prognosis

Dermatological management. The dermatological managment of anogenital pruritus is directed towards restoring the ecological balance of the area by keeping warmth and moisture down to a minimum, reducing irritation, and eradicating infection. Patients should be instructed as follows:

1. Wear loose, all-cotton underwear (e.g., boxer rather than jockey shorts, and panties without leg-elastic).
2. Avoid tight clothing and synthetic fabrics; for women, skirts are preferable to pants, and pantygirdles and pantyhose should be avoided.
3. Avoid plastic or leather-covered seats; use air-flow seats for the car; take absorbent cushion, air-ring, or terry-cloth pad to work, if necessary.
4. Avoid toilet paper; cotton swabs impregnated with 50 percent witch-hazel (Tucks Cream, Parke-Davis, Santurce, PR) or soothing emollient cleanser such as Balneol (Rowell Laboratories, Inc., Baudette, MN) and cottonballs for perianal hygiene if soap and water and a soft washcloth are impractical.
5. Treat infection with antibacterial, antifungal, or antiyeast agents where indicated. Ensure that diabetes has been ruled out, in resistant or recurrent infections.
6. There is no contraindication to high potency glucocorticoid creams for short periods, to eradicate lichenification and to achieve rapid resolution of inflammation. Once control is achieved these should be replaced by low potency agents. Cool compresses before application of creams, by hydrating the skin both soothes, and increases absorption of topical medications.
7. Treatment is otherwise along the lines outlined for generalized pruritus, with antipruritics and psychotropic drugs where indicated.
8. A light dusting of talcum powder reduces friction and absorbs perspiration; if too much is used it forms irritating little balls.
9. When severe irritation is present, bland but protective pastes such as zinc oxide may be necessary on top of the steroid cream until the worst of the inflammation is resolved.

Psychological management. Psychological management of anogenital pruritus should follow the general principles, as set out in Chapter 5. Allay unspoken anxiety about cancer, infection, or the physical integrity of the area involved. Be alert to unspoken feelings of shame, guilt, dirtyness, fear of contaminating others, and unacceptability; empathize with these, and permit their expression. Allow the patient to know that you do not find such feelings realistic or appropriate to the physical situation. Be supportive, encouraging, and reassuring; positivity is important. Other measures as outlined in the section on generalized pruritus may be employed when necessary.

Course and prognosis. It has been my experience that as a dermatologist I am asked to see patients with anogenital pruritus after a course of as long as 6 months to perhaps 10 or 20 years, and after failure at the hand of proctologist or gynecologist. Usually this provides confirmation that the dermatologist is the appropriate specialist, because in the vast majority of cases, the measures outlined above provide resolution within a reasonable period of time, to the total amazement of the patient.

Only in a very small percentage of cases is there resistance to treatment, and in these psychiatric referral may be indicated. Even prior to the advent of effective topical glucocorticoids, Cormia reported a 25 percent cure rate, with a further 25 percent improving[11] while a number of authors report cure of pruritus paripassu with improvement in depression.[56,58]

REFERENCES

1. Applebaum ML, Clifton GL, Coggeshall RE, et al.: Unmyelinated fibers in the sacral 3 and caudal 1 ventral roots of the cat. J Physiol 256:557-72, 1976
2. Arnetz BB, Fjellner BO, Eneroth P, Kallner A: Stress and psoriasis. Psychoendocrine and metabolic reactions in psoriatic patients during standardized stressor exposure. Psychosom Med 47(6):528-541, 1985
3. Arthur RP, Shelley WB: The role of proteolytic enzymes in the production of pruritus in man. J Invest Dermatol 25:341-346, 1955
4. Beare JM: Generalized pruritus. A study of 43 cases. Clin Exper Dermatol 1:343-359, 1976
5. Bernstein JE, Swift R: Relief of intractable pruritus with naloxone. Arch Dermatol 115:1366-1367, 1979
6. Bernstein JE, Swift RM, Soltani K, Lorinez AL: Antipruritic effect of an opiate antagonist, naloxone hydrochloride. J Invest Dermatol 78:82-83, 1983
7. Bowyer A, McColl I: A study of 200 patients with pruritus ani. Proc Roy Soc Med 63:96-97, 1970
8. Brodal A: Neruological Anatomy (ed 3). New York, Oxford University Press, 1981, pp 48-50
9. Calnan GD, O'Neill D: Itching in tension states. Br J Dermatol 64:274-280, 1952
10. Copland SM: Management of pruritus ani. JAMA 194(2):164-166, 1965
11. Cormia FE: Basic concepts in the production and management of the psychosomatic dermatoses. Br J Dermatol Syph 63:83-92, 1951
12. Cormia FE: Experimental histamine pruritus. J Invest Dermatol 19:21-34, 1952
13. Cornbleet T: Scratching patterns: influence of site. J Invest Dermatol 20:105-110, 1953
14. Cunliffe WJ: The skin and the nervous system, in Rook A, Wilkinson DS, Ebling FJG (eds): Textbook of Dermatology (ed 2). Oxford, Blackwell, 1979, pp 1993-2022
15. Dailey TH: Pruritus ani. Practical Gastroenterology IV:7, 1980

16. Drueck CJ: Pruritus vulvae and repressed sexual urge. Neurolog Cutaneous Rev 49:306-308, 1945
17. Edwards AE, Shellow W, Wright ET, Dignam TF: Pruritic skin disease, psychological stress, and the itch sensation. Arch Dermatol 112:339-343, 1976
18. Edwards KCS: Pruritus in melancholia. Br Med J, Vol II:1527-1529, 1954
19. Elberlik K: Organ loss, grieving and itching. Am J Psychother 34(4):523-533, 1980
20. Felix R, Shuster S: A new method for the measurement of itch and the response to treatment. Br J Dermatol 93:303-312, 1975
21. Ferreira SH, Nakamura M: II-Prostaglandinhyperalgesia the peripheral analgesic activity of morphine, enkephaline and opioid antagonists. Prostaglandins 18:191-200, 1979
22. Fjellner B: Experimental and clinical pruritus. Acta Dermatol Venereol 97(suppl):1-34, 1981
23. Fjellner B, Hagermark O: Potentiation of histamine-induced itch and flare responses in human skin by the enkephalin analogue FK 33-824, B-endorphin and morphine. Arch Dermatol Res 274:29-37, 1982
24. Fjellner B, Arnetz BB, Eneroth P, Kallner A: Pruritus during standardized mental stress. Relationship to psychoneuroendocrine and metabolic parameters. Acta Dermatol Venereol 65:199-205, 1985
25. Fjellner B, Arnetz BB: Psychological predictors of pruritus during mental stress. Acta Dermatol Venereol 65:504-508, 1985
26. Friend WG: The cause and treatment of idiopathic pruritus ani. Dis Col Rect 20(1):40-42, 1977
27. Fromer JL: Dermatologic concepts, and management of pruritus ani. Am J Surg 90(11):805-815, 1955
28. Gilchrest BA: Pruritus. Review article. Arch Intern Med 142:101-105, 1982
29. Graham DT, Goodell H, Wolff NG: Neural mechanisms involved in itch, "itchy skin", and tickle sensations. J Clin Invest 30:37-49, 1951
30. Granet E: Pruritus ani. G P 36(1):89-93, 1967
31. Greaves MW, Black AK, Eady RAJ, Coutts A: Aquagenic pruritus. Br Med J 282:2008-2010, 1981
32. Guillemin R, Vargot T, Rossier J, et al.: B-endorphin and adrenocorticotropin are secreted concommitantly by the pituitary gland. Science 197:1367-1369, 1977
33. Hagermark O: Studies on experimental itch induced by kallikrein and bradykinin. Acta Dermatovener 54:397-400, 1974
34. Hartschuh W, Weihe E, Buchler M, et al.: Met-enkephalin-like immunoreactivity in Merkel cells. Cell Tissue Res 201:343-348, 1979
35. Hopsu-Havu VK, Fraki JE: Proteinases and their inhibitors in skin disease. Int J Dermatol 20:159-163, 1981

36. Hunt E: Skin affections underlying pruritus of the vulva and anus. Lancet, March 14:592-594, 1936
37. Jeffcoate TNA: Pruritus vulvae. Br Med J ii:1197, 1949
38. Koblenzer CS: Psychosomatic concepts in dermatology. A dermatologist-psychoanalyst's viewpoint. Arch Dermatol 119:501-512, 1983
39. Ladee GA: Hypochondriacal Syndromes. Amsterdam, Elsevier, 1966
40. Lembeck G, Holzer P: Substance P as neuronenic mediator of antidromic vasodilatation and neurogenic plasma extravasation. Naunyn-Schmiedeberg's Arch Pharmacol 310:175-183, 1979
41. Lewis T: The Blood Vessels of the Human Skin, and their Responses. London, Shaw & Sons, 1927
42. Lovell CR, Burton PA, Duncan EHL, Burton JL: Prostaglandins and pruritus. Br J Dermatol 94:273-275, 1976
43. Lyell A: The itching patient: A review of the causes of pruritus. Scot Med J 17:334-347, 1972
44. Lynch FW: Pruritus vulvae as seen in dermatologic practice. JAMA 150:14-18,1952
45. Macalpine I: Pruritus ani. Psychosom Med 15:499-508, 1953
46. Martin J: Pruritus. Int J Dermatol 24:634-639, 1985
47. Medansky RS, Handler RM: Dermatopsychosomatics: Classification, physiology, and therapeutic approaches. J Am Acad Dermatol 5:125-136, 1981
48. Melzack R, Wall PD: Pain mechanisms: a new theory. Science 150:971-979, 1965
49. Musaph H: Psychodynamics in itching states. Int J Psychoanal 49:336-339, 1968
50. Musaph H: Psychodermatology, in Hill OW (ed): Modern Trends in Psychosomatic Medicine. London, Butterworths, 1976, p 358
51. Panconesi E: Psychosomatic dermatology, in Panconesi E (ed): Stress and Skin Disease: Clinics in Dermatology 2(4). Philadelphia, JB Lippincott, 1984, pp 98-99
52. Rajka G: Investigation of patients suffering from generalized pruritus, with special reference to systemic disease. Acta Dermatovener 46:190-194, 1966
53. Rajka G: Evaluation of drug influence on the itch duration in the skin of patients with atopic dermatitis, various eczemas, and psoriasis. Acta Dermatovener 48:98-102, 1968
54. Robinson P, Szewczyk M, Haddy L, et al.: Outbreak of itching and rash. Epidemic hysteria in an elementary school. Arch Intern Med 144:1959-1962, 1984
55. Rook A, Wilkinson DS: Psychocutaneous disorders, in Rook A, Wilkinson DS, Ebling FJG (eds): Textbook of Dermatology (ed 3). Oxford, Blackwell, 1979, pp 2023-2035

56. Rosenbaum M: Psychosomatic factors in pruritus. Psychosom Med 7:52-57, 1945
57. Rumpianski R, Shiskin J: Pruritus vulvae: a five-year survey. Dermatologica 131:146, 1965
58. Salerno EV: A case of pruritus vulvae treated by psychotherapy. Exc Med 4:368, Abst.1579, 1950
59. Seitz PFD: Psychocutaneous aspects of persistant pruritus and excessive excoriation. Arch Dermatol Syph 64:136-141, 1951
59a. Seitz PFD: Dynamically oriented brief psychotherapy: Psychocutaneous excoriation syndromes. An experiment. Pyschosomatic Med 15(3):200-242, 1953
60. Shelley WB, Arthur RP: Studies on cowhage (mucuna prurieus) and its pruritogenic proteinase, Mucanain. Arch Dermatol 72:399-406, 1955
61. Shelley WB, Arthur RP: The neurohistology and neurophysiology of the itch sensation in man. Arch Dermatol 76:296-323, 1957
62. Smith LE, Henrichs D, McCullah RD: Prospective studies on the etiology and treatment of pruritus ani. J Col Rect Surg 5:358-363, 1982
63. Sonneck HJ: Psychotherapy for psychogenic pruritus. Dermat Wehnshr 124:693, 1951. Exc Med XIII 6:93, Abst 416, 1952
64. Whitlock FA: Psychophysiological Aspects of Skin Disease. Major Problems in Dermatology (8). Philadelphia, WB Saunders Co, 1976, pp 110-129
65. Wittkower E, Russell B: Emotional Factors in Skin Disease. London, Cassell, 1953, pp 74-83
66. Wright CS: Psychosomatic factors in dermatology. South Med J 42:951-958, 1949
67. Young AW Jr, Sweeney EW, David D, et al.: Dermatologic evaluation of pruritus in patients on hemodialysis. NY State J Med 73:2670-2674, 1973

Chapter 13

Flushing Reactions, and Rosacea

GENERAL CONSIDERATIONS

Historically, rosacea was considered to be one of the dermatoses significantly influenced by emotional factors.[14,25] In recent years, perhaps because of improved treatment methods and the relative readiness with which it can be controlled since the advent of modern therapeutics, and most particularly the tetracyclines, this facet has received less attention. Recent information on the pathodynamics of the flushing mechanism, however, support the possibility that stress is one of the triggers in the phenomenon of flushing, and that rosacea results from flushing; for this reason, it will be discussed briefly here.

PATHODYNAMICS OF FLUSHING

Flushing results from transient vasodilatation. Although most evident in the skin, the flush is apparently an expression of a generalized hemodynamic alteration in the vasomotor system, because at laparotomy hyperemia of the abdominal vessels can be observed, coincident with facial flushing.[2] The "flush areas" of the face, which include the convexities of the cheeks, nose, mid-brow, chin, and ears, and also the neck and chest, are those areas most markedly involved; this is because they have more numerous blood vessels,[20] and a greater cutaneous blood flow than do other areas of skin.[22]

Hemodynamic control is by means of specific vasoconstrictor and vasodilator autonomic fibers, and by the direct effect of chemical mediators on the smooth muscle of the vessel walls; evidence to suggest that opioid peptides may be among those chemical mediators will be discussed later. The control varies in different areas of the body, but the autonomic control of the cutaneous vessels in the flush areas rather than resulting from inhibition of vasoconstriction is by means of active vasodilator fibers.[6] These fibers have their origin in the brain stem, and perhaps also higher cerebral centers, and travel to the cutaneous blood vessels together with the cutaneous nerves.[7] The color of the flush varies with the size of the venules in the sub-papillary plexus; considerable volumes of blood may be shunted to these venules during flushing, and this shunting of blood may, with frequent and intense dilation, lead to loss of vascular tone and to the development of permanent telangiectasis, and facial edema.[29] Actinic damage to dermal connective tissue may further add to these effects, through diminished external support of venule walls.[11]

Facial flushing takes place under a variety of different circumstances; physical exertion, emotional disturbance, defecation, high ambient temperatures, alcohol ingestion, and ingestion of hot or spicy foods are some of these. Flushing is also a feature of the menopause and of the carcinoid syndrome, and the flush in these conditions has the same distribution and is qualitatively no different than that in the conditions previously mentioned.[28] Evidence from study of alcohol-induced flushing[3] and menopausal flushing suggests endogeous opioid mediation; naloxone, an opioid antagonist, controls the "hot flash" of the menopausal patient, while alcohol-induced flushing can be triggered by an enkephalin analogue, and inhibited by naloxone. Many authors suggest that most but not all flushing is in fact mediated in this way.[8] One exception is the alcohol flushing that occurs in a high percentage of Orientals; this appears to involve high concentrations of acetaldehyde. As I have noted previously β-endorphin and met-enkephalin both are secreted centrally in response to stress; they may be involved, in addition to the autonomic innervation of the cutaneous vessels, and peripheral mediators, in the flushing that occurs in response to psychosocial stress in some individuals.

Flushing due to drugs, systemic disease, and genetically determined enzymatic anomalies will not be discussed further here; the interested reader is referred to the recent and comprehensive review by Wilkin.[28]

ROSACEA

Clinical Description

Rosacea is a chronic inflammatory disorder of insidious onset, that involves primarily the flush areas of the face (Fig. 13-1). The earliest changes consist of transient episodes of vasodilatation and facial erythema that resolve spontaneously in a matter of minutes. As the condition progresses, the erythema becomes more fixed, and telangiectases appear against the background of an erythema that blanches on diascopy. Varying numbers of dome-shaped papules of a deep shade of erythema, and less commonly pustules stud the involved areas in the fully developed case; these may merge together to form boggy deeply erythematous, granulomatous plaques. Occasionally extrafacial but entirely typical lesions may be seen on the neck, bald head, or extremities, in a case that is otherwise typical.

Complicating the characteristic picture may be involvement of the blepharal margins, and conjunctiva, and rarely, the sclera. Other complications are

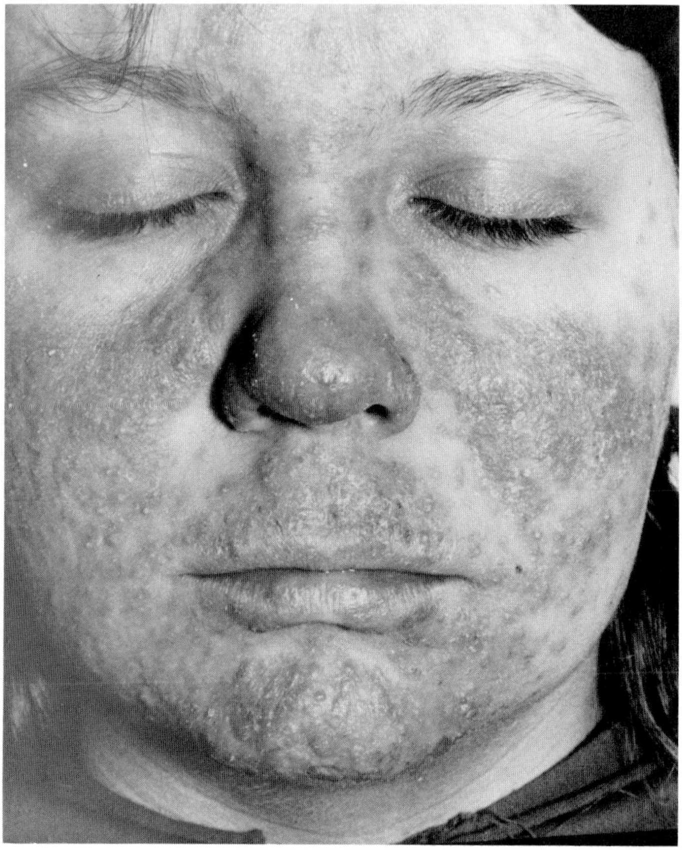

Figure 13-1. Rosacea. This severe case shows the erythema, brawny swelling and numerous inflammatory papules and pustules in a characteristic distribution.

rhinophyma, characterized by a boggy hypertrophy of the soft tissues of the nose; localized facial lymphedema is also reported; this is firm, only slightly reddened and remarkably resistant to treatment;[5] unilateral or bilateral, it may involve forehead, periorbital areas, or cheeks.

Incidence

The onset most commonly is between 30 and 50 years, though rosacea is reported both in the elderly and in childhood.[21] Opinions differ as to whether the sex incidence is equal,[9] or women predominate, but men appear to be more severely involved.[26] Racial differences are observed. Northern Europeans and Celts having a higher incidence than do those with darker skin; Marks and Wilkinson observe also a higher incidence in persons of lower socioeconomic status.[12]

Etiology

Historically four factors have been blamed in the etiology of rosacea. These are gastrointestinal disturbances, psychogenic causes, infection with the mite demodex folliculorum, and climatic conditions. While the evidence to support gastrointestinal disturbances[9] or infection with the demodex mite[18] is in each case less than impressive, both climatic conditions and psychogenic factors remain in contention. There is impressive evidence to demonstrate that in the predisposed individual flushing leads to development of rosacea;[9,23] this being the case, the contribution of actinic elastosis to the development of telangiectasia through passive vasodilatation[11] on the one hand, and the effects of emotional flushing on the other cannot be discounted.

Pathophysiology

The basic premise with regard to pathophysiology is that flushing is important in the genesis of all of the stigmata of rosacea.[11] As noted earlier, frequent flushing leads to shunting of blood into the subpapillary venous plexus, and to a progressive loss of vascular tone that results in permanent vasodilatation. This provides the background erythema, the permanent flush of the patient with rosacea.[29] In support of this premise, a number of facts can be adduced. Flushing is the first sign of early disease.[16] Marks found an increase in flushing in patients with rosacea,[9] and Starr and MacDonald, a correlation between the severity of ocular rosacea and the tendency to strong flushing.[24] In further support, patients with flushing due to the carcinoid syndrome develop all of the stigmata of rosacea including ocular lesions, facial telangiectasia, and tissue hypertrophy,[24] and the disease is exacerbated during treatment with vasodilators that cause flushing.[27] With persistence of tissue edema, there is disorganization of the connective tissue, the inflammatory components of the condition appear, and the hypertrophic changes follow.

Histopathology

Histologic findings will vary with the lesion biopsied, and are characteristic rather than pathognomonic. The features of vascular ectasia, dermal edema, and disorganization of the dermal connective tissue are constant,[11] but inflammation varies from a perivascular lymphohystiocytic infiltrate to a more typical granulomatous picture. Where pustules are present, polymorphonuclear leukocytes are situated in and around follicular structures; comedones are absent.

Differential Diagnosis

In the early erythematous stage, other causes of facial congestion must be considered, including the carcinoid syndrome, polycythemia, superior vena cava syndrome, or the heliotrope periocular lesions of dermatomysitis. Once papules, pustules and granulomatous plaques, or the characteristic changes of rhinophyma have appeared, the diagnosis is relatively simple; in some cases lupus erythematosus, seborrhoeic dermatitis, perioral dermatitis, and acne vulgaris may be considered. It is likely that cases of the rosacea-like tuberculid of Lewandowski and Lutz are in fact examples of rosacea.[26]

Psychopathology and Psychodynamics

Despite the evidence cited, that repeated and intense flushing is the primary event in the development of rosacea, all subsequent lesions being secondary to that effect, and despite a common perception that flushing is frequently emotional in origin, there is a remarkable reluctance in the standard texts to consider psychogenesis among the possible causes of rosacea.

Bar and Kuypers describe the patient troubled by chronic blushing as timid and socially inhibited, with emotions bottled up lest they earn disapproval by expressing them.[1] These patients have diminished self-worth and both a central[19] and an autonomic response to social anxiety that includes facial flushing.[1] The flush in turn generates its own embarrassment and anxiety (erythrophobia) so that there is even greater inhibition, the patient avoiding the social situations that are perceived as dangerous, and developing poor social and sometimes poor family relationships.[15]

Obermeyer,[13] Cormia,[4] Wittkower and Russel,[30] and Panconesi,[15] each on the basis of studies on a number of rosacea patients describe similar personality types; their patients were rather immature anxious individuals, with diminished self-worth, who were troubled by feelings of guilt and shame. In some of these patients, Panconesi was able to trace the evolution from easy blushing in adolescence, through the stage of permanent erythema, to frank rosacea.[15] Several authors stress identifiable psychic trauma prior to the onset of acute rosacea, and Cormia more specifically found patients to be overwhelmed by their life circumstances.[4]

In no case was an attempt made to uncover the unconscious determinants of the neurotic symptoms in these patients. Clearly they are psychoneurotic, with features suggestive more of a hysterical configuration than an obsessive-compulsive one.

Treatment

Dermatologic Treatment

Measures to reduce flushing. Several measures to follow in order to reduce flushing include avoidance of ambient heat, extreme cold, hot foods or liquids, alcohol, sunlight, and spicy foods. If possible avoid also vasodilator drugs, and where indicated, treat menopausal flushing.

Systemic antibiotics. Longterm administration of tetracycline is the mainstay of treatment and will improve inflammatory lesions, ocular lesions, and to a lesser extent rhinophyma. A reasonable regimen is to start with 500 mg b.i.d. and after one month reduce to 250 mg b.i.d. until the condition is quiescent. The dose can then gradually be reduced until a maintenance dose is determined, or complete withdrawal achieved.

Metronidazole is reported to be effective, and erythomycin also, though to a lesser degree than tetracycline.[17]

Topical measures. Both topical tetracycline and erythromycin are to some extent effective. Precipitated sulfur 2 percent or sulfur with salicylic acid 2 percent in a cream base help to reduce inflammation, and permit the avoidance of topical glucocorticods. Glucocorticoids are best avoided because of the possibility of increased telangiectasia, and the development of steroid dependent dermatitis. Two percent metronidazole in a cream base mey also prove effective.

Physical measures. A number of physical measures may help reduce the effects of flushing; these include electrocoagulation for residual telangiectases once the inflammatory component is under control, surgical procedures to produce cosmetic improvement in rhinophyma, and facial massage therapy to mobilize the edema.[9,23]

Psychiatric Treatment

Indications for psychiatric treatment will depend on the severity of the physical symptoms, the response to conventional therapy, and the extent to which neurotic symptoms interfere in other aspects of the patient's life. It is particularly important to suggest psychotherapy if flushing is extreme, since the full-blown picture of rosacea, with all of its potential disfigurement might then be aborted.

When flushing is pronounced, and when shyness, embarrassment, and erythrophobia interfere in social and professional interaction, significant neurosis is present, and the treatment of choice is psychoanalysis or psychoanalytic psychotherapy. Stress management techniques and assertiveness training are reported to be effective,[1] and biofeedback may be helpful.

Course and Prognosis

In some cases there may be only a single episode, but usually the disease tends to be chronic, and although the response to treatment is usually excellent, future episodes are likely to occur.

Rhinophyma may recur even after surgical correction, while the reponse to treatment of localized edema is poor.

REFERENCES

1. Bar LHJ, Kuypers BRM: Behavior therapy in dermatologic practice. Br J Dermatol 88:591-598, 1973
2. Bernstein JE: Neuropeptides and the skin, in Goldsmith LA (ed): Biochemistry and Physiology of the Skin, Vol II. New York, Oxford University Press, 1983, pp 1217-1233
3. Bernstein JE, Soltani K: Naloxone inhibition of alcohol-induced flushing in rosacea. Clin Res 28:718A, 1980
4. Cormia FE: Basic concepts in the production and management of the psychosomatic dermatoses—II. Br J Dermatol 63:129-151, 1951
5. Domonkos AM, Arnold HL, Odam RR: Acne, in Diseases of the Skin. Philadelphia, WB Saunders, 1981, pp 275-295
6. Fox RH, Goldsmith R, Kidd DJ: Cutaneous vasomotor control in the human head, neck and upper chest. J Physiol 161:298-312, 1962
7. Gonzalez G, Onofrio BM, Kerr FWC: Vasodilator system for the face. J Neurosurg 42:696-703, 1975
8. Lightman SL, Jacobs HS: Naloxone: Non-steroidal treatment for postmenopausal flushing. Lancet 2:1071, 1979
9. Marks R: Concepts in the pathogenesis of rosacea. Br J Dermatol 80:170-177, 1968
10. Marks R, Ellis J: Comparative effectiveness of Tetracycline and ampicillin in rosacea; a controlled study. Lancet 2:1049-1052, 1971
11. Marks R, Harcourt-Webster JN: Histopathology of rosacea. Arch Dermatol 100: 683-691, 1969
12. Marks R, Wilkinson DS: Rosacea and perioral dermatitis, in Rook A, Wilkinson DS, Ebling FJB (eds): Textbook of Dermatology (ed 3). Oxford, Blackwell Scientific Publications, 1979, pp 1433-1440
13. Obermeyer ML: Psychocutaneous Medicine. Springfield, IL, Charles C. Thomas, 1955, pp 280-287
14. O'Donovan WJ: Dermatoses with important emotional factors, in Obermeyer ML: Psychocutaneous Medicine. Springfield, IL, Charles C. Thomas, 1955, p 282

15. Panconesi E: Psychosomatic dermatology, in Panconesi E (ed): Clinics in Dermatology, Vol 2(4): Stress and Skin Diseases: Psychosomatic Dermatology. Philadelphia, JB Lippincott, 1984, pp 131-133
16. Plewig G, Kligman AM: Acne: Morphogenesis and Treatment. New York, Springer-Verlag, 1975, p 261
17. Pye RJ, Burton JL: Treatment of rosacea by metronidazole. Lancet, June 5, 1:1211-2, 1971
18. Robinson TWE: Demodex folliculorum and rosacea. Arch Dermatol 92:542-544, 1965
19. Rosenbaum JF: The drug treatment of anxiety. NEJM 306:401-404, 1982
20. Ryan TJ: Structure, pattern and shape of the blood vessels of the skin, in Jarrett A (ed): The Physiology and Pathophysiology of the Skin, Vol II. The Nerve and Blook Vessels. London, Academic Press, 1973, p 619
21. Savin JA, Alexander S, Marks R: A rosacea-like eruption of children. Br J Dermatol 87:425-429, 1972
22. Sjersen P: Cutaneous blood flow and tissue blood exchange, in Montagna W, Van Scott ES, Stoughton RB (eds): Advances in Biology of the Skin, Vol 12. Pharmacology and the Skin. New York, Appleton-Century-Crofts, 1972, pp 191-205
23. Sobye P: Aetiology and pathogenesis of rosacea. Acta Dermatovener 30:137-158, 1950
24. Starr PAJ, Macdonald A: Oculocutaneous aspects of rosacea. Proc Roy Soc Med 62:9-11, 1969
25. Stokes JH, Beerman H: Effect on the skin of emotional and nervous states, IV The rosacea complex; a reappraisal, with special reference to the constitutional background and the rationale of treatment. Arch Dermatol Syph 26:478-494, 1932
26. Strauss JS: Sebaceous glands, in Fitzpatrick TB, Eisen AZ, Wolff K, et al. (eds): Dermatology in General Medicine. New York, McGraw Hill, 1971, pp 666-685
27. Wilkin JK: Vasodilator rosacea. Arch Derm 116:598, 1980
28. Wilkin JK: Flushing reactions: Consequences and mechanism. Ann Intern Med 95:468-476, 1981
29. Wilkin JK, Josephs JA: Infrared photographic studies of rosacea. Arch Dermatol 116:676-678, 1980
30. Wittkower E, Russell B: Emotional Factors in Skin Disease. New York, Paul B Hoeber, 1953, pp155-158

Chapter 14

Psychogenic Disorders of the Sweat Glands

ECCRINE SWEATING AND HYPERHIDROSIS

General Considerations

The conditions to be considered here are hyperhidrosis and bromidrosis; the former involves the eccrine sweat gland system, and the latter primarily the apocrine.

The normal role of the eccrine sweat gland is to produce evaporative heat loss for thermoregulation. Eccrine glands are distributed over the entire cutaneous surface, with a density that varies in different areas. Sweat secretion is intermittent and depends on the need for evaporative cooling, except on the palms and soles where emotional as well as thermoregulatory sweating occurs and where secretion may be either intermittent or continuous. Under maximal stimulation as much as 12 liters can be secreted in 24 hours,[4] with a composition that is subject to modification in terms of the concentrations of electrolyte, urea, lactate, and a variety of excretion products, as it passes through the duct.[4]

Although much has been learned about the control of eccrine sweating in recent years, the process has not yet fully been elucidated. Innervation of the eccrine glands is primarily by sympathetic post-ganglionic cholinergic fibers, but a loose network of adrenergic fibers also surrounds the gland, and the secretory cells are equipped with α- and β-adrenergic receptors in addition to those for acetyl choline.[29] While physiologic sweating is primarily cholinergic, β-adrenergic stimulation in some circumstances apparently has an additive effect; the exact role of adrenalin is unclear, however, since both thermal and emotional sweating are completely inhibited by atropine.[29] Sympathetic stimulation results in the release not only of acetyl choline at the nerve endings, but also a number of vasoactive peptides; these, by causing vasodilatation permit an efflux of fluid from the blood into the eccrine gland, to supplement secretion.[21] Vasoactive intestinal peptide and substance P have both been identified at sudomotor nerve-endings,[14] and when sweating is heat-induced, a kinin-like substance can be detected within the secretion itself;[10] all of these, through vasodilatation add to the volume of sweat secreted.

The volume of sweat depends also on the size of the gland, and on the relative number of acetyl choline receptors with which it is equipped; acclimation to higher ambient temperatures is accomplished through an increase in these two factors. An increase in the size of the glands takes place at puberty also, in response to androgenic stimulation.[29]

Three types of eccrine sweating are recognized: thermoregulatory, gustatory, and emotional.

Thermoregulatory Sweating

The center for temperature regulation is located in the preoptic portion of the hypothalamus. This center is activated by increases in the temperature of the blood that perfuses it, and by afferent stimuli from the skin; in response to these stimuli, the mechanism described above is set in motion, vasodilatation and generalized sweat secretion take place,[29] followed by evaporative cooling. The mechanism is the same whether the temperature increase be exogenous, or endogenous from such causes as systemic infections, hyperthyroidism, obesity, cholinergic drugs, or febrile illnesses. Thermoregulatory sweating is frequently more severe at night, and an instability of the thermoregulatory center may permit it to continue for some time after the resolution of febrile conditions.

Gustatory Sweating

Gustatory sweating may be physiologic or pathologic. Physiologic gustatory sweating occurs in many people on the lips, brow, and nose, after eating spicy foods. The gustatory sweating is pathologic, however, if false connections are made between sympathetic and parasympathetic fibers, as nerves regenerate following injury to sympathetic nerves, in the head and neck area.[25] As a result, vasodilatation and sweating may occur on the area of skin served by a damaged nerve, rather than, for example, the expected parotid secretion, in response to the stimulus of taste or chewing. A number of other anatomical variants are described,[13,22] from traumata at other sites, a similar situation may occur spontaneously, for reasons that are not understood.

Emotional Sweating and Hyperhidrosis

Clinical Picture

That sweating can be psychogenic is generally accepted (Fig. 14-1). The location of origin of the sudomotor pathways in the hypothalamus, their sympathetic character, the part played by vasoactive peptides, the fact that these vasoactive agents are known to be released under stress, and the mechanism of sweat secre-

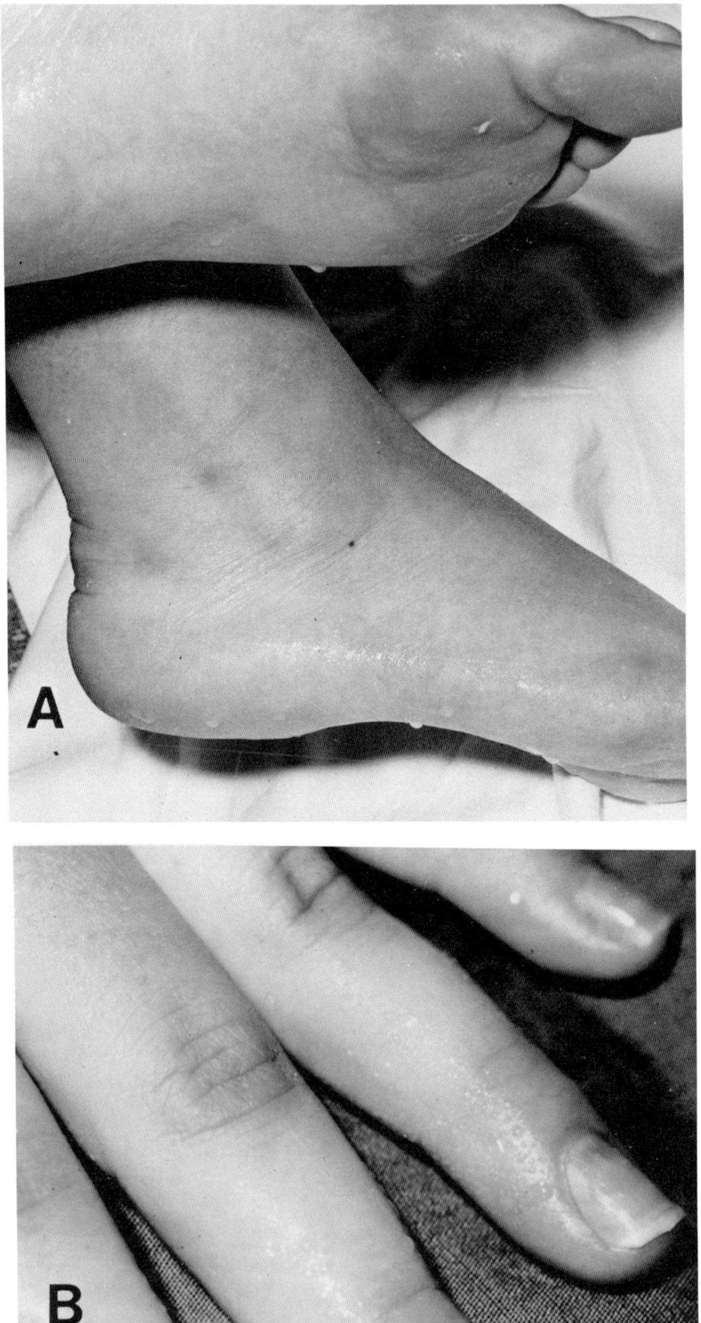

Figure 14-1. (A, B) Hyperhidrosis of the hands and feet. Moments before this photograph, the hands and feet were quite dry. Note the beads of eccrine sweat produced at such a rate as to cause actual dripping.

tion, all make this acceptance understandable. Psychogenic sweating may be generalized, although it is most frequently bilateral, and localized to the palms, soles, and axillae either individually or in any combination; occasionally the anogenital area is also involved; sweat-secretion is triggered by fear, anger, excitement, or mental effort, and it may be exacerbated by heat.

There are broad individual variations in the amount of physiologic emotional sweating, and it is hard to determine the cut-off point, where it becomes pathologic, but hyperhidrosis can be considered to be present if clothing is consistently stained and spoiled in the axilla, or if the hands or feet are constantly wet. Occasionally the condition is so extreme that sweat literally drips from the extremities, to pool on the floor (Fig. 14-1). As with flushing, patients are usually painfully embarrassed, and a secondary phobic anxiety about the sweating itself may develop, to add further to the stress, causing the patient diminished self-esteem and a wish to retreat from social contact,[4] and from physical activites that generate heat.

Japanese patients have a much higher incidence than do Caucasians or other Orientals,[10] and a family history is not uncommon. The condition may start in childhood, but onset or exacerbation in adolescence is common, and the added embarrassment at an age of already heightened social sensitivity may lead the youngster to avoid important adolescent experiences such as athletics, dancing, and dating. As an example, a young patient of mine found herself unable to continue in gymnastics because in spite of liberal amounts of powder, her hands were too slippery to hold the equipment safely; home economics was closed to her, because her work in sewing was always damp, dirty, and a source of shame, and she gave up typing because her fingers slipped off the keys and she was scolded for papers that were damp and grubby. A fastidious young woman, socially she became reclusive and dropped out of all extra-curricular school activities.

Some patients are aware of the problem only at times of particular stress, while in others the condition is constant, the result perhaps of a deeper-seated conflict. There is a tendency for the condition in most cases to improve after the age of 25.

Complications

Complications of hyperhidrosis in addition to the psychosocial ones mentioned above, are those that result from the constantly moist and macerated skin; these include:

1. Contact dermatitis from shoes, clothing, or other contactants.
2. Dyshidrotic eczema.
3. Seborrhoeic dermatitis of the axilla in the genetically predisposed.
4. Secondary infections; yeast, trichomycosis axillaris, or bacterial folliculitis in

the axilla; pitted keratolysis or dermatophytosis of the feet; secondary bacterial infection of eczema.

5. Eccrine bromidrosis. This refers to the offensive odor, most commonly of the feet, that results from bacterial action on sweat, and on macerated keratin. Axillary odor is most commonly apocrine in origin, and in fact tends to be less pronounced when eccrine hyperhidrosis is present, as the excessive eccrine sweat dilutes and flushes away the apocrine secretion.

Psychopathology and Psychodynamics

There is very little documentary evidence concerning the psychology of hyperhidrosis, but it has generally been considered to be a physiologic expression of anxiety.[9] Many authors have stressed that aspect[33,36,37] while Davis and Bick found patients to be restless, sensitive, and resentful.[6] In contrast, Lerer et al. in a comprehensive and well-controlled study of 23 randomly selected patients[20] found that not only were anxiety levels no higher in hyperhidrosis patients than in controls, but in 25 percent of cases they were in fact lower. Their study showed hyperhidrosis patients to have a high need to avoid potentially dangerous, depreciating, or rejecting situations, to be passive and lacking in ambition, with poor coping skills and a tendency to withdraw from difficulties. Caution and selectivity in relationships reflected their feelings of inferiority and insecurity; projective tests revealed impulsivity, poorly integrated emotional responses, and a preoccupation with sex at a fantasy level. Diagnostically these patients fit the picture of psychoneurosis, and clearly their use of avoidance as a defense works well for them as it permits them to avoid the unpleasant experience of anxiety. Though we do not have adequate anamnestic information to permit a psychodynamic understanding of the neurosis in these patients, other reports in the literature describe hyperhidrosis as a hysterical conversion symptom, and certainly that is not impossible here.[8]

Dermatologic Management

Topical measures. There are several topical measures to be considered: (1) the use of glutaraldelyde and formaldehyde for the palms or soles has essentially been given up because of the disadvantages of skin discoloration, contact sensitization, and altered skin texture; (2) 25 percent aluminum chloride hexahydrate (Drysol, Person & Covey, Inc., Glendale, CA) under an occlusive wrap can be used effectively for axilla, palms, and soles;[31] and (3) cotton clothing and the judicious use of dusting powder will absorb the excessive secretion.

Systemic measures. Anticholinergic drugs such as probantheline bromide (Pro-Banthine Tablets, Searle & Co., San Juan, PR) in doses of 15-50 mg three times daily as tolerated, may be effective, but side effects are often troublesome; these include dryness of the mouth, blurred vision, and occasionally glaucoma, hyperthermia, and convulsions.

Iontophoresis. Either tap water or anticholinergic drugs may be used with good effect. Recently an iontophoresis unit has become available for home use at reasonable cost; marketed as Drionic (General Medical Company, Los Angeles, CA) it has gained excellent patient acceptance.

Surgical measures. There are two surgical procedures to consider. The first is sympathectomy,[5] which has the disadvantage that the effects frequently are not permanent, and sweating tends to recur after a period of years. A further disadvantage is the possibility of a compensatory hyperhidrosis on the trunk, if more than one limb is treated.[11]

The second consideration is local excision of the axillary vault, a relatively simple and very successful procedure.[3,16,24]

Treatment of the complications of excessive sweating. Treatment of such complications as dyshidrotic eczema and secondary infections will naturally follow on conventional lines. Bromidrosis of the feet requires frequent changes of cotton or pure wool socks, absorbent shoes rather than those made of rubber or plastics, dusting powder for sweat absorption, and antibacterial soaps and topical antibiotics.

Psychiatric Management

As has repeatedly been stressed throughout this volume, the psychiatric managment of hyperhidrosis as with all other conditons discussed will depend on a psychiatric assessment of the patient, as well as on the severity of the somatic symptoms and the response achieved with conventional treatment methods. Lerer's study[20] indicates that hyperhidrosis patients frequently manifest psychopathology of a degree greater than one might anticipate from the manifest symptom, and urges that controlled psychiatric evaluations be undertaken to allow the development of effective psychotherapeutic approaches. These, he feels, may obviate the need for surgical intervention.

Anxiolytic drugs. Anxiolytic drugs may be prescribed for judicious use at times when stress is anticipated, in those patients with manifest anxiety.[7]

Psychotherapy. Psychotherapy for hyperhidrosis may include psychoanalysis, supportive psychotherapy, or gestalt therapy. Since the reported patients have been psychoneurotic,[8,18,20] and since hyperhidrosis frequently has the characteristics of a hysterical conversion symptom, psychoanalysis or psychoanalytic psychotherapy are the treatments of choice. There are a number of reports in the literature of patients successfully treated by these means.[8,18,19]

Supportive psychotherapy is an alternative, for patients who are unwilling or unable to commit themselves to psychoanalysis;[2] however, the prospects for long-term benefit are less favorable.

Gestalt therapy has been reported successful;[32] this method relies heavily on psychoanalytic theory.[34]

Hypnosis.[12] Hyperhidrosis is one of the conditions for which hypnosis has been reported successful.

Behavioral therapy. Behavioral therapy includes: (1) assertiveness training and desensitization;[2] (2) conditioning;[17] and (3) biofeedback.[23]

Each of the above techniques have been reported successful in very small numbers of cases, but clearly the prospects for long-term benefit with the possibility of structural change within the personality can most realistically be anticipated from insight-oriented approaches (psychoanalysis or psychoanalytic psychotherapy).

APOCRINE SWEAT AND BROMIDROSIS

General Considerations

Aprocrine sweat glands are found predominantly in the axilla; small, relatively inactive glands are also located in the perineal area, and modified glands in the areola of the breast, the glands of Moll around the eyes, and the ceruminous glands of the auditory canal. Rather than thermoregulation, as is their function in many species, in people apocrine glands serve primarily as scent organs, and produce their secretion in response only to strong emotions and to pain.[4] The secretory portion does not develop until puberty, and so apocrine glands become functional only at that time.[26]

Both adrenergic and cholinergic fibers are identified around apocrine glands, but in contrast to eccrine glands, the former predominate, and the secretory response to adrenergic stimulation is greater than it is to cholinergic.[1,27] Denervation does not inhibit emotive sweating, so that although nerve fibers containing catecholamines and adrenergic nerve terminals have been identified around apocrine glands,[35] the response is apparently largely humoral and due to circulating epinephrine or norepinephrine.[30]

Apocrine sweat is rich in electrolytes, but also in protein fragments,[28] and short-chain fatty acids.[15] Although sterile and odorless when secreted, there is rapid break-down by gram-positive surface bacteria, primarily staphylococci,[15] once it reaches the skin surface, with the development of characteristic apocrine odors. The moist and warm ambient conditions in the axilla, and the presence of hair that traps and holds the secretion, serve to enhance the odor generated.

BROMIDROSIS

Normal Situations

Some degree of axillary odor is physiologic, but our society, with the able assistance of the advertising community, has made it a crime. For this reason antibacterial soaps, antiperspirant, and deoderant preparations are in general use, and by and large are effective.

Pathologic Bromidrosis

Bromidrosis that is both subjective and objective. Objective verifiable axillary odor is an occasional complaint in patients who generally demonstrate less than perfect personal hygiene. Once the examiner is satisfied that there is indeed an odor present, attention can be given to reducing the circumstances that favor bacterial growth and entrapment of secreted sweat:

1. Carefully shave axillary hair.
2. Use antibacterial soaps for all cleansing purposes, or such agents as chlorhexidine gluconate (Hibiclens Antimicrobial Skin Cleanser, Stuart, Wilmington, DE).
3. Apply twice daily a topical antibiotic preparation, such as 2 percent erythromycin cream or lotion or 1 percent neomycin cream.
4. Use effective antiperspirants; there are many on the market, but 25 percent aluminum chloride hexahydrate (Drysol®) is the most potent.
5. Use dusting powder to absorb secretion.
6. Occasional anxiolytics, stress-management techniques, or psychotherapy may be indicated, as for hyperhidrosis, if the problem is incapacitating; adequate dermatologic managment should obviate the need for this.

Subjective bromidrosis. There are some patients who claim to have severe problems with body odor, but in whom, on careful objective examination, no odor can be detected. The claims for potency or for toxic effect of the odor on others are extreme and often bizarre; ideas of reference may be evident, the patient believing that others are constantly talking about or shunning him or her because of the offensive and often dangerous nature of his or her sweat.

These patients fall into one of two categories; they suffer either from an obsessive-compulsive neurosis, with obsessional concerns that they might be causing offense to others, or from a paranoid psychosis or monsymptomatic hypochondriasis, with disordered perception and hallucinatory odor. The reader is referred to the appropriate sections for further discussion of these two groups of patients.

REFERENCES

1. Aoki T: Stimulation of human axillary apocrine sweat glands by cholinergic agents. J Invest Dermatol 38:41-44, 1962

2. Bar LHJ, Kuypers BRM: Behavior therapy in dermatological practice. Br J Dermatol 88:591-598, 1973
3. Bretteville-Jensen G, Mossing N, Albrechtsen R: Surgical treatment of axillary hyperhidrosis in 123 patients. Acta Dermatovener (Stockholm) 55:73-77, 1975
4. Champion RH: Disorders of sweat glands, in Rook A, Wilkinson DS, Ebling FJG (eds): Textbook of Dermatology (ed 2). Oxford, Blackwell Scientific Publications, 1979, pp 1675-1731
5. Cloward RB: Hyperhidrosis. J Neurosurg 30:545-551, 1969
6. Davis DB, Beck JW Jr: Skin reactions observed under wartime stress. J Nerv Ment Dis 103:503, 1946
7. Dobson RL: Hyperhidrosis said to be usually emotional in nature. Skin and Allergy News, Jan 1986, p 28
8. Dosuzkov T: Idrosophobia: a form of pre-genital conversion. Psychoanalytic Q 44:235-265, 1975
9. Engels WD: Skin disorders, in Kaplan HI, Sadock BJ (eds): Comprehensive Textbook of Psychiatry IV, Vol 2. Baltimore, Williams and Wilkins, 1985, pp 1178-1185
10. Fox RH, Hilton SM: Bradykinin formation in human skin as a factor in heat vasodilatation. J Physiol 142:219-232, 1958
11. Gillespie JA: Extent and permanence of denervation produced by lumbar sympathectomy: An investigation of its effects on sudomotor activity. Br Med J i:79-83, 1961
12. Grant G: Essential hyperhidrosis. (correspondence) Med J Aust 2:390, 1971
13. Herxheimer A: Gustatory sweating and pilomotion. Br Med J i:688-689, 1958
14. Hokfelt T, Ogohansson J, Kellerth GO, et al.: Immunohistochemical distribution of Substance P, in von Euler US, et al. (eds): Substance P. New York, Raven Press, 1977, pp 117-145
15. Hurley HJ: Apocrine glands, in Fitzpatrick TB, Elsen AZ, Wolff F, et al. (eds): Dermatology in General Medicine (ed 2), New York, McGraw-Hill, 1979, pp 473-484
16. Hurley HJ, Shelley WB: Axillary hyperhidrosis: Clinical features and local surgical managment. Br J Dermatol 78:127-140, 1966
17. Kuypers BRM, Cotton DWK: Conditioning of sweating: A preliminary report. Br J Dermatol 87:154-160, 1972
18. Lerer B: Hyperhidrosis: A review of its psychological aspects. Psychosomatics 18:28-31, 1977
19. Lerer B, Jacobowitz J: Treatment of essential hyperhidrosis by psychotherapy. Psychosomatics 22(6):536-538, 1981
20. Lerer J, Jacobowitz J, Wahba A: Personality features in essential hyperhidrosis. Int J Psych in Med 10(1):59-67, 1980-81
21. Lundberg JM, Anders A, Fahrenkrug J, et al.: Vasoactive intestinal polypep-

tides in cholinergic neurons of exocrine glands: Functional significance of coexisting transmitters for vasodilation and secretion. Proc Nat Acad Sci (USA) 77:1651-1655, 1980

22. McGibbon BM, Paletta FX: Further concepts in gustatory sweating. Plast Reconstr Surg 49:639-642, 1972
23. Miller RM: Biofeedback and dermatology, in Rickles WH, Sandweiss JH, Jacobs DW, et al. (eds): Biofeedback and Family Practice Medicine. New York, Plenum Press, 1983, 145-153
24. Munro DD, Verbov JL, O'Gorman DJ, DuVivier A: Axillary hyperhidrosis: Its quantification and surgical treatment. Br J Dermatol 90:325-329, 1974
25. Murray JG, Thompson JW: The occurrence and function of collateral sprouting in the sympathetic nervous system of the cat. J Physiol (London) 135:133-162, 1957
26. Pinkus H: Anatomy and Histology of Skin, in Graham JH, Johnson WC, Helwig ED (eds): Dermal Pathology. Hagerstown, Maryland, Harper and Row, 1972, pp 1-24
27. Robertshaw D: Catecholamines and the control of sweat glands, in Handbook of Physiology, Endocrinology Section 7, Vol VI. Washington D.C., American Physiology Society, 1975, pp 591-603
28. Robertshaw D: Apocrine sweat glands, in Goldsmith LA (ed): Biochemistry and Physiology of the Skin, Vol I. New York, Oxford University Press, 1983, pp 642-653
29. Sato K: The physiology and pharmacology of the eccrine sweat gland, in Goldsmith LA (ed): Biochemistry and Physiology of the Skin, Vol I. New York, Oxford University Press, 1983, pp 596-641
30. Shelley WB, Hurley HJ: Methods of exploring human apocrine sweat gland physiology. Arch Dermatol Syph 66:156-161, 1952
31. Shelley WB, Hurley HJ: Studies of topical antiperspirant control of axillary hyperhidrosis. Acta Dermatovener (Stockholm)55:241-260, 1975
32. Siemens H: "Gestalt" therapy in blushing and sweating. Symposium on Pathological Blushing and Sweating. Acta Neurochir 74(3-4):154-155, 1985
33. Sneddon IB: The mind and the skin. Br Med J i:472-475, 1949
34. Strupp HH, Blackwood GL Jr: Recent methods of psychotherapy, in Kaplan HI, Sadock BJ (eds): Comprehensive Textbook of Psychiatry IV, Vol 2. Baltimore, Williams and Wilkins, 1985, pp 1450-1460
35. Uno H: Sympathetic innervation of the sweat glands and piloerector muscles of macacques and human beings. J Invest Dermatol 69:112-120, 1979
36. Whitlock FA: Psychophysiological Aspects of Skin Disease. London, WB Saunders Company Ltd, 1976, pp 166-167
37. Wittkower E: Emotional Factors in Skin Disease. New York, Paul B. Hoeber Inc, 1953, pp 20-21

Chapter 15

Alopecia Areata, Telogen Effluvium, and Hirsutism

ALOPECIA AREATA

Clinical Picture

The initial lesion of alopecia areata is usually asymptomatic and noted quite by chance as a small circumscribed smooth white patch completely devoid of hair, located anywhere on the scalp. Occasionally it may be preceded by local irritation, tenderness or pruritus and, early in its course, there may be mild surface erythema or edema.

If the process is active and the lesion is continuing to extend, hairs around the periphery will epilate readily, or broken "exclamation point" hairs may be seen; if the patient is graying, occasionally a few strong white terminal hairs may remain, within the alopecic patch. This initial lesion may resolve spontaneously in a period of weeks to months, or it may be succeeded by a sequence of similiar lesions, separated by varying intervals of time. As lesions extend peripherally they may coalesce to form large areas, or assume a reticulate patterning; while one area is shedding, a fine peach-fuzz of lanugo hair may appear in another as the process of regrowth begins; these fine white downy hairs increase in diameter and acquire pigment gradually with time.

Occasionally instead of the slow progression described above, there may be explosive and extensive shedding with loss of the entire pelage in a matter of days, or it may start as a diffuse process, with typical patches appearing only later. Nor is the process confined to the scalp; brows, lashes, beard, and body hair may be involved, either in isolation or as part of a more extensive process. Characteristic nail changes too are recognized; these consist of a cross-hatched pitting, longitudinal ridging, irregular thickening or friability of the nail plate. These changes are more common in severe cases; in some cases they may precede the hair loss, or even occur alone. A distinctive form, ophiasis, is more common in children, and starts at the occipital hair line from whence it spreads laterally and antero- superiorly, following the hair-line, sometimes throughout its entire length. When the condition involves the entire scalp it is termed alopecia totalis, while universalis is used to describe the same condition involving scalp, facial, and body hair (Fig.

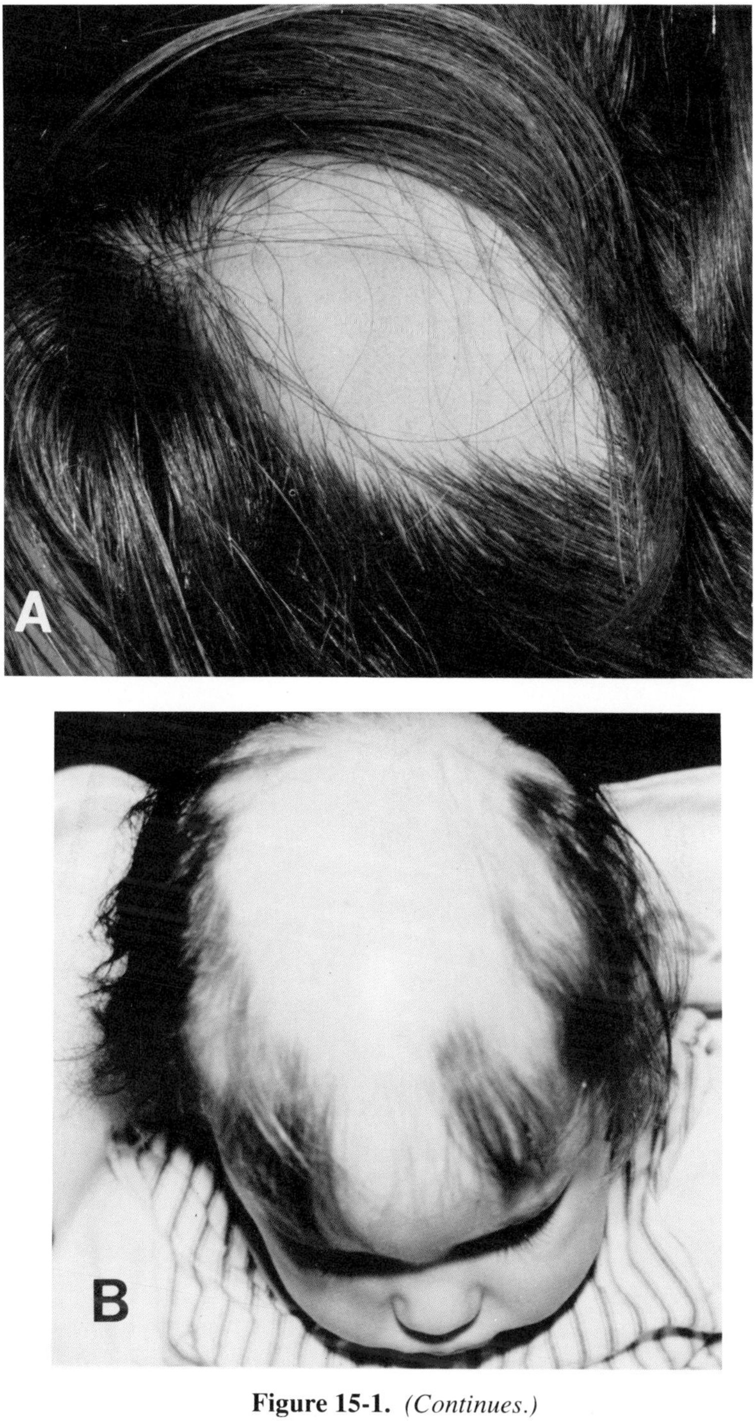

Figure 15-1. *(Continues.)*

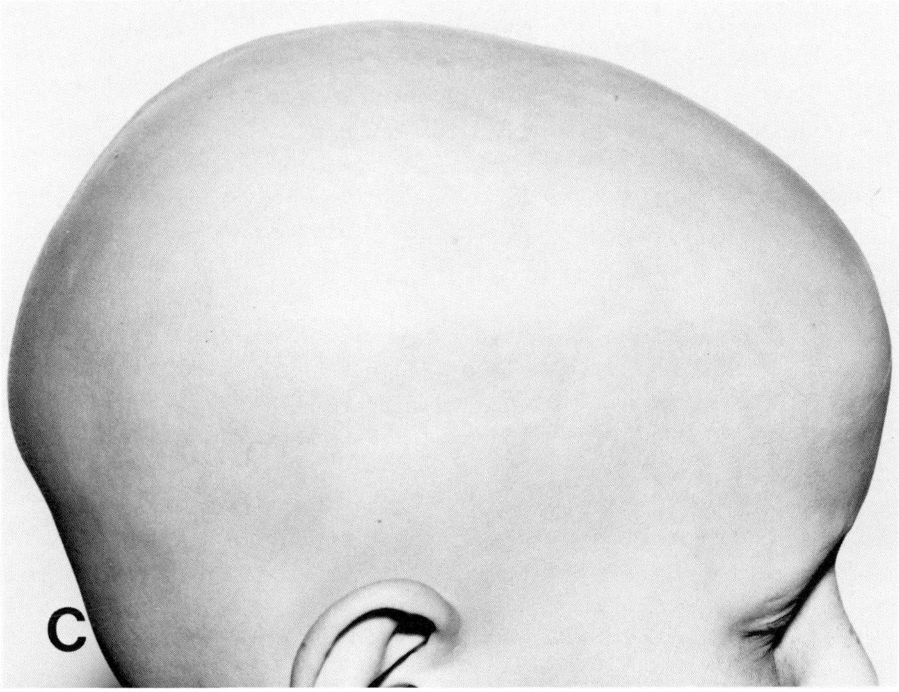

Figure 15-1. *(Continued.)* Alopecia areata. Lesions may be single or multiple, and small (A) or extensive (B); the entire scalp (totalis), or scalp and body hair may be lost (alopecia universalis) (C). Lesions are circumscribed, glazed, and free of hair. In contrast to trichotillomania newly regrown hairs are fine, tapered, and often hypopigmented and of uniform length. The father of patient C was imprisoned just prior to her loss of hair.

Associated Conditions

A number of other physical conditions are associated with alopecia areata with a frequency greater than in the population at large. Their relevance to etiologic considerations will be discussed later, but Thiers and Galbraith suggest that these factors act as a permissive influence rather than a directly causal one.[42] These conditions include heredity, atopic diathesis, autoimmune disorders, and psychologic factors.

Heredity

There are extraordinary variations in the reports of familial incidence from different countries; these vary from around 20 percent in France and England,[5] to 10-17 percent in the United States,[29] only 4 percent in Italy, and zero percent in Spain. Reports of twin involvement exist, though not necessarily concurrently, and an autosomal dominant transmission with variable penetrance has been suggested.[39] Gm types (1gG heavy-chain allotype determinants) have proved more helpful than HLA typing,[15] in pointing to disease susceptibility and these studies suggest that while some individuals have genes that predispose them towards the condition, there are others whose genes protect them. The observation that persons with dark hair are more susceptible remains to be proven, and while the reportedly higher incidence among the Japanese in Hawaii suggest racial differences, this too awaits further elucidation.[2]

The Atopic Diathesis

As with heredity, great variation exists in the reported coexistence of atopy with alopecia areata; while in Holland a 50 percent coexistence is reported,[33] the figure for Denmark is but 1 percent,[17] and in Japan, 10 percent.[21] A study from the United States quotes 9 percent for adults and 18 percent for children, but of those 18 percent, 23 percent had alopecia totalis.[29] Several other authors have suggested that alopecia areata has an earlier onset, and a more prolonged and resistant course in atopic individuals.[37]

Autoimmune Disorders

Reportedly, vitiligo has an incidence four times greater in patient with alopecia areata than in the population at large. One must wonder whether this finding may not reflect a biased patient population, because in a large and busy general dermatology practice and one to which many severe cases of alopecia areata are referred, I have not seen such a patient in 20 years. An increased incidence is reported also with thyroid disease,[9] Down's Syndrome,[11] and in Turner's Syndrome. Other autoimmune conditions with which alopecia areata has been associated are autoimmune testicular disease,[4] lupus erythematosus[23] and ulcerative colitis.[1] Association with lichen sclerosus et ateophious, polymyalgia rheumatica,[13] lichen planus, and nail distrophy are also reported.[38] It might be mentioned here that an association with polymyalgia rheumatica or ulcerative colitis speaks at least as eloquently for a psychogenic etiology as for an autoimmune one, since both have strong psychosomatic features, though of course the two, autoimmune etiolgy and psychogenesis, are in no way mutually exclusive.

Psychological Factors

The role of psychologic factors in the development of alopecia areata is of considerble importance and has been a subject of dispute for many years. It will be discussed in detail below.

Incidence

Alopecia areata accounts for about 2 percent of new dermatologic out-patient attendances in Britain and the United States.[12] The onset may be at any time from infancy to old age, with a maximal incidence between 5 and 40 years, and a gradual decline after that time. There is equal sex distribution in the United States, but in some southern European countries, males predominate by a ratio of 2:1. Alopecia totalis results in 10 percent of patients, and involves children more frequently than adults. In another 10 percent of cases, only sites other than the scalp are involved.[12]

Histopathology

Microscopic examination of tissue from an early lesion shows a perivascular lymphocytic infiltrate around the hair bulb and the follicular openings, with some spongiosis of the overlying epidermis. As the condition progresses, the infiltrate becomes more sparse and the epidermal changes less prominent. Degeneration of the connective tissue around vessels and hair papilla follow, with dystrophic changes in the matrix. Follicles are small and situated mid-way up in the dermis. In early cases, up to 75 percent of these are dystrophic anagen follicles, while in those of long-standing dystrophic telogen follicles predominate; a thin cord of epithelial cells extends downwards from the base of the follicle. The root sheath is thickened and as the disease progresses gradual diminution in the size of sebaceous glands follows.[38]

Around the periphery of a patch of alopecia areata the proportion of telogen follicles is increased above normal, and dystrophic anagen follicles are present. Similar but less severe changes have been reported on the contralateral uninvolved scalp, and lymphocytic infiltrates have been identified in the apparently normal skin of the upper arm.[38]

Pathophysiology

It is suggested that the sequence of events in the development of a patch of alopecia is as follows: trauma to the follicle (the possible nature of which will be addressed below) may, if severe, precipitate the hair into catagen, and weaken the shaft in the keratogenous zone; subsequent fracture will occur at this point, with development of an exclamation point hair.[38] A less severe trauma precipitates the hair into normal catagen, with the subsequent shedding of a club hair, while mild trauma results merely in a dystrophic anagen follicle that will continue to grow.

What of the trauma that triggers this sequence of events? Historically, local and focal sepsis, trophoneurotic influences, vascular insufficiency, and psychogenesis, all have been inculpated, but to date the theory that begins to address all aspects most satisfactorily is that which invokes an autoimmune process. The question of psychogenesis will be discussed in the next section, and it must be stressed again that psychogenesis and autoimmunity are in no way mutually exclusive.

Although attempts to demonstrate autoimmune phenomena against follicular constituents have not met with success to date,[14] a number of alterations in T cell function are documented. In nearly all cases of alopecia areata absolute numbers of circulating lymphocyes are reported to be decreased,[39] the peribulbar inflammatory infiltrate is found to contain a predominance of helper T cells,[44] and in severe cases, reduced numbers of interactive T cells have been observed.[16] These interactive T cells are cells that are reduced in recurrent severe viral infections; they are thought to be involved in the interaction between T and B lymphocytes.[18] It has been suggested that perhaps damage to hair follicle structures by an agent such as a virus might provide an autoantigen against which autoantibodies might be directed although such an autoantigen remains to be demonstrated. The only immunoreactive material detected in biopsy specimens is C_3,[20] and the majority of studies have been negative.

Psychiatric Aspects

Par excellence, diverse opinions about the cause of alopecia areata over the years have exemplified the polarization of our understanding of disease etiology in terms of psyche and soma. The literature seems to stress a dichotomy between the two, suggesting a mutual exclusivity so that disease must be due either to one or to the other, rather than the result of an interaction between the two, as we now believe.

For early observers the cause was psychogenic and the literature is replete with dramatic stories of sudden hair-loss at times of unusual stress, and of the high incidence of concomitant psychiatric illness among alopecia areata patients.[30] More recently, opinion sits rather firmly at the opposite pole, and in an information leaflet published by the National Alopecia Areata Foundation, it is stated rather firmly that "nerves" are not the cause,[36] and that "those who have it, have not caused it and have no control over its course." This interesting statement not only suggests that those who suffer from psychogenic conditions do so wilfully, but also that to do so is in some way shameful or naughty, and worthy of reprimand. From the preceding pages it would seem evident that the etiology of alopecia areata, as is the case in so many conditions, is multifactorial. Genetic permissivity is demonstrated,[15] a possible contribution from an infective agent has been suggested,[18] and the mediating pathway, from all available evidence, seems to point to autoimmune mechanisms. The complex interactions between the psychoneuroendocrine system and the immune system have been discussed more fully in Chapter 3. That the immune system is influenced by psychologic factors has been clearly demonstrated by numerous workers, both in humans[31] and in animals,[28] and disease processes mediated by autoimmune mechanisms are recognized to be exacerbated by stress.[41] Further, considerable clinical evidence can be adduced to support the probability that psychogenic factors are a frequent precipitant of alopecia areata.[8,30,32]

It is sometimes difficult to interpret meaningfully, reported findings, because of the different ways in which the concept of "stress" is applied. Some workers, taking no cognizance of unconscious processes or of the intrapsychic meaning to the individual of current situations in the light of past experience, demand a visible, almost tangible, recent happening (presumably one that they themselves can understand as stressful) as acceptable stress. Just as one man's meat is said to be poison for another, so what is stressful to one, on the basis of his or her personality configuration and past life experiences, may to another be entirely innocuous.

Cormia[8] and Greenberg[19] report comparable findings in psychologic studies of 8 and 44 patients respectively, and these in turn reflect findings previously reported by Irwin.[14] In summary, these researchers found 80-90 percent of randomly selected patients with alopecia areata to have psychiatric problems that were in need of treatment. The majority of these patients were psychoneurotic with such symptoms as anxiety, depression, insomnia, or obsessive-compulsive symptoms; the majority also had experienced feelings of insecurity and inferiority for many years, and were shy and passive, unable to express strong feelings verbally or in action; in many cases, it was possible to trace these characteristics to childhood developmental difficulties; Lyketsos et al., in a 1985 study, confirmed these same personality characteristics.[24] Long-standing emotional problems were considered by these researchers to be of greater etiologic significance than were recent traumata, although a precipitating traumatic event could be identified in many cases.

In more recent years attention has been turned once again to the emotional sphere. In 1979 Toback and Rajkimur detected mild to moderate psychological disturbance in all of 10 alopecia areata children.[43] They based this diagnosis on the results of psychologic testing without benefit of psychiatric evaluation in depth, and further, since they fail to make clear the distinction between alopecia areata and trichotillomania, their findings are difficult to evaluate. More significant is the paper by Mehlman and Griesemer,[26] who observed the onset of symptoms in young children two weeks after they had undergone a traumatic experience that could be interpreted by them in terms of a loss. This loss, which though it varied from patient to patient, was one that represented a major threat to the child, and one that had profound significance to the child, in terms of his or her own early life experience. Interestingly, Wolf and Wolf report a similar situation, with the coincidental onset of alopecia areata in two siblings, within days of their mother leaving for an overseas vacation.[45] DeWeert et al. found an incidence of chronic emotional stress in 70 percent of 41 adult patients, and behavioral problems in 7 of 9 children, but they do not elaborate on these statistical findings.[10] Perini et al., in an attempt to better clarify and quantify emotional stress, subjected 48 alopecia areata patients to an extensive psychiatric evaluation that included a tabulation of recent life events comprising 64 possible situations, as well as an anamnestic history and a psychiatric interview in depth.[34]

Patients with alopecia areata in their study reported 123 events in the preceding 6 months, of which 63 were characterized as severe, as compared with figures of 22 and 10 in the controls; this breaks down into 2.56 events per patient and only 0.73 events per control. Events with objective negative impact such as those that were uncontrolled or undesirable, or that represented the loss of an important figure, were significantly more frequent in the patient group.

In summary, there seems to be little doubt from numerous studies over many years that a high percentage of patients with alopecia areata, because of early childhood difficulties, develop a type of personality configuration that confers on them a particular vulnerability to stress. When these patients are subjected to psychosocial stress above the average, whether that stress be from internal or from external sources, effective mechanisms for coping break down, and somatic symptoms develop. Because of "priming" of the scalp genetically or symbolically, alopecia areata is "chosen" for that symptom.

From a psychodynamic view-point, alopecia areata can be understood to represent a hysterical conversion reaction in some cases, as reported by Cormia,[8] and by Basset et al.,[3] while Mehlman and Griesemer,[26] and Cohen and Lichtenberg[7] found the genesis to be earlier in life, and rooted in ambivalent early mother-child relationships and separation difficulties.

Because alopecia areata is disfiguring, and often the cause of much personal distress, the argument is frequently advanced that hair loss has preceded any psychologic difficulties that are detected, and that this is very understandable; one is asked "wouldn't you be depressed, anxious, etc., if your hair fell out?" Whereas secondary symptoms of anxiety and depression certainly often arise and aggravate the current situation, it is clear from the studies cited above, that the majority of the patients reported had suffered from long-standing psychologic difficulties, difficulties that in many cases had been in need of treatment long before the hair-loss supervened.

Differential Diagnosis

The major considerations in the differential diagnosis of alopecia areata are trichotillomania, fungal infections, and traumatic alopecia secondary to traction from rollers or cosmetic hair processing such as hot-combing, permanent waving, or coloring. The clinical picture, with complete absence of hair centrally, peripheral exclamation point hairs, and fine vellus regrowth, is diagnostic. Fungal cultures are negative and the biopsy findings characteristic. In those cases where hair-loss starts diffusely, telogen effluvium and hereditary pattern hair loss may be considerations, until typical patches of alopecia develop and the condition declares itself.

Dermatologic Managment

The dermatologic treatments of alopecia areata are legion, and the reader is referred to standard texts in dermatology for a full discussion. They will only be listed here:

1. Reassurance and benign neglect. In many cases solitary lesions of short duration will resolve spontaneously.
2. Topical gucocorticoid lotions or gels.
3. Intralesional glucocorticoids.
4. Systemic glucocorticoids.
5. Production of irritant reactions by such agents as liquified phenol or topical anthralin.
6. Photochemotherapy with psoralcn and ultraviolet-A irradiation (PUVA)
7. Sensitization to the dibutyl ester of squaric acid, with subsequent maintainance of a low grade contact dermatitis on the involved scalp.

Psychiatric Management

An explanation of our understanding of the nature and the possible causes of alopecia areata is of paramount importance. Given the significance that our society places on beautiful hair, and the unconscious symbolic meanings that hair has for most patients, conscious and unconscious fantasies about their disease cause great distress for many. It is important to verbalize the unspoken fears by firmly asserting that the patients do not have cancer, an infection, or some serious underlying physical problem, and that they are in no way contagious. It is important also to reassure patients that the hair-follicles are not destroyed, that the potential for regrowth exists, and that in only a small percentage of cases is the condition rapidly or severely progressive.

Explain to the patient our current psychosociobiological view of disease and its particular relevance to alopecia areata. Institute topical treatment, with frequent short visits as indicated in the section on general principles of treatment. If it be-the adjustment to the condition of alopecia is particularly difficult, then psychotherapy is indicated. This includes several options: (1) supportive psychotherapy by the dermatologist; (2) referral to a local chapter of the Alopecia Areata Foundation, for group support; and (3) referral to a psychiatrist.

From the reported findings, the vast majority of patients suffer from a psychoneurosis, and will most benefit from psychoanalysis or psychoanalytic psychotherapy. There are many reports in the literature of successful treatment by this means, of which Pomey-Rey's is the largest series.[35] She treated 42 patients, 8 of whom had alopecia totalis, using psychotherapy, with or without antidepressants but with no other treatment. She achieved complete regrowth in all cases in anywhere from 6 months to 4 years. I myself have achieved full regrowth in the case of one adolescent patient with alopecia totalis, and good success in a number of patients with less extensive involvement, using psychoanalytic psychotherapy.

Since these patients have a tendency towards shyness, passivity, and inability to express feelings, those unwilling or unable to commit themselves to an insight-oriented approach might be expected to benefit from assertiveness training, and from therapeutic measures designed to build confidence.

If depression is overtly or covertly present, antidepressants should be prescribed.

Those patients for whom separation or "loss" (in its broadest sense) have proved traumatic, can be helped in developing coping skills for these eventualities, and manipulation of the environment to reduce stress can be suggested, if this is indicated.

Because children often demontrate more severe psychopathology, and because the long-term effects of childhood psychologic difficulties can have a devastating effect on the quality of adult life, special attention should be paid to one's psychiatric assessment of children, and psychiatric evaluation should be recommended early. Short-term treatment at an early stage may prevent more profound difficulties later, and may obviate the need for long-term treatment in the future.

Course and Prognosis

The prognosis is always uncertain and it is impossible to give a reliable opinion early in the course of the disease. Thirty percent of patients recover from the first attack within 6 months, and 50 percent within 1 year; the figure for 5 years is 70-80 percent, while 20-30 percent make no recovery. The immediate prognosis is more favorable for females than for males, and though 40-50 percent of cases will relapse within 5 years, apparent cure does occur in 30 percent of cases.[17] Rapid evolution, repeated episodes, ophiasis, associated atopy, loss of eye-brows and eye-lashes, and severe nail changes all adversely affect the prognosis.

Ikeda[21] subdivided alopecia areata into four types. Type I, which constituted 10 percent of cases, were patients who were atopic; in these cases the onset was early and the course prolonged; 75 percent developed alopecia totalis.

Type II, constituting 5 percent, had an onset after age 40 years, and a prolonged course with alopecia totalis developing in 10 percent. This group was associated with autoimmune desease.

Type III were prehypertensive young adults in whom one or both parents were hypertensive. These patients, who constituted 4 percent of the total, sustained a rapid course and in 39 percent of cases developed alopecia totalis.

Type IV were the remaining 83 percent who formed the "common" group, with an onset in later childhood or early adult life; these patients ran a course of under 3 years, individual patches regrew within 6 months, and only 6 percent developed alopecia totalis. Ebling and Rook find some merit in this classification.[12]

TELOGEN EFFLUVIUM

Clinical Picture

The shedding of large numbers of scalp hairs following a severe febrile episode, or childbirth, has been accepted medical lore since ages past, but telogen effluvium did not achieve its position as an entity until Kligman elegantly presented his findings outlining the clinical picture and the pathodynamics in 1961.[22]

When the human organism is stressed significantly, the scalp mounts a nonspecific response that leads to the premature precipitation of anagen hairs into the telogen phase; after a latent period of 2 to 4 months, there is a diffuse shedding of these telogen hairs in daily numbers of anywhere from 100 to 1000. Shedding depends on the number of follicles that are affected, and this number in turn is determined by the nature of the precipitating cause, its duration, and its severity; it may continue for as long as 6 or 8 months before regrowth is established. Though in some cases there may be recurrences, for the vast majority the condition is temporary and the potential of the follicles for regrowth is not lost; very severe cases, or cases with frequent recurrences may never achieve complete restitution.

Under normal circumstances less than 20 percent of scalp hairs are in the telogen phase, while in telogen effluvium that percentage is increased to as much as 50 percent or even higher. For most patients less than 25 percent of the total scalp hair is shed, and though subjectively it may assume the proportions of total disaster, objectively it may barely be perceptible. In very severe cases, when 50-60 percent of the total pelage is lost, the diffuse partial nonscarring alopecia is descernible to all; in some instances, a latent hereditary androgenic alopecia may be unmasked by such an episode.

Etiology

The stresses that are recognized to precipitate this transition from anagen to telogen include high fevers, parturition, hemorrhage, even including blood-donation,[38] iron deficiency, chronic systemic illness, certain drugs, and emotional stress, perhaps including the stress of jet-lag;[12] also, the physiologic neonatal effluvium of the infant should not be forgotten.

There is some variability in the extent and rate of shedding due to these different causes; for example, during pregnancy the transition from anagen through catagen to telogen is delayed and after parturition the restitution of hormone levels results in a quite rapid hair loss as the delayed hairs "catch up." High fevers also produce a rapid and short-lived effluvium, while the course following emotional stress is variable.

Psychogenic Telogen Effluvium

Two patterns of telogen effluvium associated with emotional stress are described; following a sudden and severe stress there may be a rather dramatic, rapid and extreme shedding;[22] in psychoneurotics, on the other hand, who suffer from chronic and overwhelming anxiety due to intrapsychic rather than external causes, slower and more insidious hair loss has been observed. This appears to be more prolonged and of lesser intensity than the hair loss attributable to the other causes mentioned.

Pathodynamics and Histopathology

It has been determined that catagen, the transition between anagen and telogen, lasts for a period of 2 weeks, while the remainder of the 3 of 4 month latent period between insult and time of shedding is required for the full development of the telogen hair, and the concurrent initiation of new anagen growth. This development involves loss of the epithelial sheath, shrinking away of the base of the follicle from the papilla, and a thrusting of the new anagen hair upwards through the base of the follicle.[22]

The histologic findings in telogen effluvium then show no abnormality other than an increase in the proportion of telogen follicles.

Management of Psychogenic Telogen Effluvium

No topical or systemic measures are of any benefit. In all cases, the somatopsychic aspect must be addressed. The distress caused to the patient by a hair-loss that to the causal observer is barely perceptible, may be extreme. Anxiety based on unspoken conscious fears and unconscious fears and fantasies may be paralyzing; the patient should be helped to verbalize these, and accept reassurance.

The extreme and rapid loss following a sudden and severe stress requires only the measures as described above. More prolonged and insidious loss due to chronic or overwhelming anxiety requires that the causes of the anxiety be addressed.

Psychotherapy should be undertaken, or psychiatric referral be recommended in the following instances: (1) if neurotic symptoms are interfering in other aspects of the patient's life; (2) if concern over the hair loss is obsessive and incapacitating; or (3) if depression is a feature. In this case antidepressants may be prescribed.

Hirsutism

Because of the relative infrequency of hirsutism as a complaint, and because of the recent elucidation of possible causes in many idiopathic cases, it is not my purpose to discuss hirsutism in any detail here; a number of points should be mentioned, however: (1) the very high incidence of hirsutism in schizophrenic females;[25] (2) the reportedly relatively common onset of hirsutism after a stressful episode, and most particularly a depressive episode;[27] (3) a reported association of stress with the onset of hirsutism of adrenocortical origin;[6] and (4) the possible role of prolactin in stress-induced and depression-induced hirsutism.

In hyperprolactinemic states there is an increase in adrenal androgen production, in face of a normal urinary 17 oxosteroid:17 oxogenic steroid ratio;[40] hirsutism is found in 50 percent of these patients. The secretion of prolactin is increased in depression, and after severe stress, and a role for the endorphins in controlling this has been suggested.[38]

Psychogenic factors therefore must be considered in the evaluation of any case of female hirsutism. The somatopsychic aspect also must not be ignored, for increased facial and body hair in itself serves as a stress for many fastidious women.

REFERENCES

1. Allen HB, Moschella SL: Ulcerative colitis associated with skin and hair changes. Cutis 14:85-88, 1974
2. Arnold H: Alopecia areata: prevalence in Japanese and prognosis after reassurance. Arch Dermatol Syph 66:191-196, 1952
3. Basset F, Israel L, Jadin A, et al.: Quelques considerations concernant l'étude psychosomatique des alopécies. Am Med Psychol 2:283, 1969
4. Brown AC: Autoimmune gonadal disease, in Brown AC, Crouse RG (eds): Hair, Trace Elements, and Human Illness. New York, Praeger, 1980, pp 313-333

5. Brown WH: The etiology of alopecia areata in relationship to vitiligo and possible scleroderma. Br J Dermatol Syph 41:299-321, 1929
6. Bush IE, Mahesh VB: Adrenocortical hyperfunction with sudden onset of hirsutism. J Endocrin 18:1-25, 1959
7. Cohen IH, Lichtenberg JO: Alopecia areata. Arch Gen Psychiat 17:608-614, 1967
8. Cormia FE: Basic concepts in the production and management of the psychosomatic dermatoses II. Br J Dermatol 63: 129-151, 1951
9. Cunliffe WJ, Hall R, Stevenson CJ, Weightman D: Alopecia areata, thyroid disease and autoimmunity. Br J Dermatol 81:877-881, 1969
10. DeWeert J, Temmerman L, Kint A: Alopecia areata: A clinical study. Dermatologica 168:224-229, 1984
11. DuVivier A, Munro DD: Alopecia areata, autoimmunity and Down's Syndrome. Br Med J I:191-192, 1975
12. Ebling FJ, Rook A: Hair, in Rook A, Wilkinson DS, Ebling FJG (eds): Text Book of Dermatology, 3rd ed. Oxford, Blackwell Scientific Publications, 1979, p 1777
13. Faergemann T: Lichen sclerosus et atrophicus generalisata, alopecia areata, and polymyalgia rheumatica found in the same patient. Cutis 23:757-758, 1979
14. Friedman P: Decreased lymphocyte reactivitiy and autoimmunity in alopecia areata. Br J Dermatol 105:145-151, 1981
15. Galbraith G, Thiers BH, Pandey JP: Gm allotype associated resistance and susceptibility to alopecia areata. Clin Exp Immunol 56:149-152, 1984
16. Galbraith GMP, Theirs BH, Vasily DB, Fudenberg HH: Immunological profiles in alopecia areata. Br J Dermatol 110:163-170, 1984
17. Gip L, Loden A, Molin L: Alopecia areata: a follow-up investigation of outpatient material. Acta Derm Venereol Stockholm 49:180-188, 1969
18. Goust JM, Fudenberg HH: T cell binding to B lymphoid cell lines in humans: A marker for T-B cell interaction? J Immunol Methods 59:29-38, 1983
19. Greenberg SI: Alopecia areata: a psychiatric survey. Arch Dermatol 72:454-457, 1955
20. Igarashi R, Takeuchi S, Sato Y: Immunofluorescent studies of complement C3 in the hair follicles of normal scalp and of scalp affected by alopecia areata. Acta Dermatovener (Stockholm) 60:33-37, 1980
21. Ikeda T: A new classification of alopecia areata. Dermatologica 131:421-445, 1965
22. Kligman AM: Pathologic dynamics of human hair loss 1. Telogen effluvium. Arch Dermatol 83:175-198, 1961
23. Lerchin E, Schwimmer B: Alopecia areata associated with discoid lupus erythematosus. Cutis 15:87-88, 1975
24. Lyketsos GC, Stratigos J, Tawil G, et al.: Hostile personality characteristics,

dysthymic states and neurotic symptoms in urticaria, psoriasis, and alopecia. Psychother Pschosom 44:122-131, 1985

25. Lohse E, Bjarnhjedinsson G: Frequency of hypertrichosis in schizophrenic women as compared to normal. Acta Psychiat Scand 20:185-211, 1945
26. Mehlman RD, Griesemer RD: Alopecia areata in the very young. Am J Psychiat 125:605-614, 1968
27. Meyer AE: Korperstorungen und sexualitat dargesteet am Beispiel des genuinen Hirsutismus. Praxis der Psychotherapie 8:262, 1963
28. Monjan AA: Stress and immunologic competence: studies in animals, in Ader R (ed): Psychoneuroimmunology. New York, Academic Press, 1981, pp 185-228
29. Muller S, Winkelmann R: Alopecia areata: an evaluation of 736 patients. Arch Dermatol 88:290-297, 1963
30. Obermayer ME: Alopecia Areata in Psychocutaneous Medicine. Springfield, IL., Charles C. Thomas, 1955, pp 294-304
31. Palmblad J: Stress and immunologic competence: studies in man, in Ader R (ed): Psychoneuroimmunology. New York, Academic Press, 1981, pp 229-257
32. Panconesi E: Psychosomatic dermatology in Panconesi E (ed): Clinics in Dermatology, Stress and Skin Disease, Psychosomatic Dermatology, Vol 2. Philadelphia, LB Lippincott, No 4, pp 143-148
33. Penders AJM: Alopecia areata and atopy. Dermatologica 136:395-399, 1968
34. Perini GI, Fornasa CV, Cipriani R, et al.: Life events and alopecia areata. Psychother Psychosom 41:48-52, 1984
35. Pomey-Rey D: About 80 cases of baldness and diffuse alopecias treated by a psychoanalytically inspired psychotherapy in association with psychotropes. Abstracts 16th, Congressus Int Derm, No 465:335, 1982
36. Price VH: Alopecia Areata. Publication of the National Alopecia Areata Foundation, P.O. Box 5027, Mill Valley, CA
37. Rook A: Common baldness and alopecia areata, in Rook A (ed): Recent Advances in Dermatology (ed. 4). Edinburgh, Churchill Livingstone, 1977, p 223
38. Rook A, Dawber R: Diseases of the Hair and Scalp. Oxford, Blackwell Scientific Publications, 1982
39. Sauder DN, Bergfeld WF, Krakauer RS: Alopecia Areata: An inherited autoimmune disease, in Brown AC, Crounse RG (eds): Hair, Trace Elements and Human Illness. New York, Praeger, 1980, pp 343-347
40. Seppala M, Hirvonen E: Raised serum prolactin levels associated with hirsutism and amenorrhoea. Br Med J iv:144, 1975
41. Solomon GF: Emotional and personality factors in the onset and course of autoimmune disease, particularly rheumatoid arthritis in Ader R (ed): Psychoneuroimmunology. New York, Academic Press, 1981, pp 159-182

42. Thiers BH, Galbraith GMP: Alopecia areata in Thiers BH, Dobson RL (eds): Pathogenesis of Skin Disease. New York, Churchill Livingstone, 1986, pp 57-64
43. Toback C, Rajkumar S: The emotional disturbance underlying alopecia areata, alopecia totalis and trichotillomania. Child Psychiatry Hum Dev 10(2):114-117, 1979
44. Todes-Taylor N, Turner R, Wood GS, et al.: T cell subpopulations in alopecia areata. J Am Acad Dermatol 11:216-223, 1984
45. Wolf D, Wolf R: Simultaneous alopecia areata in two siblings. J Am Acad Dermatol 11(5):897-898, 1984

Part 3: Conditions Probably Dependent on Genetic or Environmental Factors Whose Course is Often Affected by Emotional Stress

The conditions that will make up the substance of this section are those that though primarily dependent on genetic and environmental factors for their onset, have a course that is significantly affected by the emotional state, and by stress.

The conditions about which most has been written from the emotional perspective are psoriasis, atopic dermatitis, and acne vulgaris. But if we accept the concept of a constant psychosociobiologic interaction, it becomes clear that we could quite appropriately encompass the entire remaining field of dermatology under the same rubric. In health, the psychologic, social, or environmental and biologic forces are in a state of balance; a stress in any one of those spheres has the potential to tip the balance and permit illness to become manifest; these concepts have been discussed more fully in Chapter 3. It is the task of this section to address the possible contribution of psychologic factors in the precipitation or perpetuation of the dermatologic disorders under consideration, and to try to elucidate their genesis, and their results.

It is clearly not within the scope of this volume to discuss each of the conditions adequately from a dermatologic point of view; the reader is referred to the standard texts in dermatology for that information; only material pertinent to the psychologic aspects will be treated fully in the pages that follow.

Chapter 16

Psoriasis

Psoriasis, perhaps more than other demotoses, serves to illustrate the subtle interactions between genetic predisposition, environmental influences, and psychosocial factors that must take place before the disease can become manifest.

Long recognized as having a multifactorial etiology, population and twin studies have confirmed the clinical impression that one of those etiologic factors, and indeed a prerequisite for the development of psoriasis, is genetic predisposition. Evidence from specific genetic studies points to a polygenic transmission,[63] and a greater tendency towards the development of manifest disease, the greater the number of predisposing genes that are received in the genetic package.[9] Interaction with the environment is the next step, and certain environmental factors are known to have the potential to precipitate psoriasis in those who are predisposed. The greater the number of predisposing genes, the less will be the contribution from the environment that will be needed to generate clinical manifestation, and vice versa.[6]

AGENTS WITH THE POTENTIAL TO PRECIPITATE PSORIASIS

Trauma of any type to the skin may result in the development of a lesion; irritation from xerosis or from sweating must be considered in this light, as well as cuts, burns, friction, surgical incisions, or even the site of some previous rash, as for example a contact dermatitis or a drug eruption; this phenomenon is known as the Koebner reaction. *Infection* is a second possible "triggering" agent. Post-streptococcal guttate psoriasis is the situation most readily recognized,[66] but it is likely that viral infections too may be followed by exacerbation.[40] A third possible agent is *sunlight*. A small percentage of patients with psoriasis are photosensitive and get worse in the summer, though for the majority that is the best time. *Endocrine factors* are evidenced by the peaks of psorisis activity at puberty and at menopause that are reported,[30] while improvement during pregnancy is not uncommon. Certain *drugs* may exacerbate psoriasis;[5] these include lithium salts,[55] drugs that block β-adrenergic receptors,[56] and antimalarials.[5] *Psychogenic factors* will be discussed at length in a later section.

PATHOPHYSIOLOGY

The Koebner reaction, which is present in 33-50 percent of psoriatic patients,[3] suggests a psoriasis "readiness" inherently present in the entire integument; it suggests also that seemingly normal interlesional skin is not in fact normal.[23] This indeed is the case, for the number of dividing cells in seemingly uninvolved skin is twice normal,[26] and a number of the ultrastructure features characteristic of lesional skin can be detected in interlesional skin, though to a lesser degree than in the lesions themselves. For example, abnormalities in dermal capillaries that will be described later extend for some distance beyond the clinical lesions,[33] and though the blood flow in uninvolved skin is less than in lesional skin, it is still greater than normal (Fig. 16-1); arachidonic acid metabolites, which apparently play a part in the inflammatory component of psoriasis, likewise are elevated above control levels, in interlesional skin, though to a lesser extent than in psoriatic lesions.[27]

Though not yet fully elucidated, many pieces of the pathophysiologic puzzle have been assembled; these demonstrate pathological changes in a number of complex systems involving epidermal and dermal structures; they begin to explain some of the characteristic microscopic finding, and may allow us to begin to understand the possible pathways of some of the triggering mechanisms.

Vascular changes precede the epidermal changes, and consist of transformation of papillary capillaries from arterial to venous structures;[12] increased permeability allows exudation of serum and lymphocytes; papillary edema and spongiosis follow, and focal keratinocyte necrosis[11] has been attributed to a possible cell-mediated immune response.[17]

Ultrastructure studies of keratinocytes demonstrate the plasma membrane to be defective, and to have inadequate surface receptor binding sites; internal structural abnormalities are noted, and keratinization is defective.[17]

Cell proliferation kinetics suggest loss of normal homeostatic restraint.[3]

Further evidence of the abnormalities in the plasma membrane comes from studies of cyclic AMP (cAMP) metabolism in psoriatic epidermis. The intracellular levels of cAMP depend upon the balance between synthetic activity by adenylate cyclase, and degradation by cAMP phosphodiesterase; in psoriasis, this intracellular level is lower than normal, and increases only by 25 percent of normal after stimulation by epinephrine; stimulation by prostaglandin E raises the level by 50 percent of normal.[1,2] This is explained on the basis of a decreased synthesis due to the deficient receptors, together with increased degradation.[29] Increased intracellular levels of cAMP inhibit epidermal growth, and it is postulated that reduced levels may therefore result in hyperproliferative states.[61] The significance of the above findings in terms of the pathogenesis of psoriasis is supported by the fact that lithium salts, which inhibit adenylate cyclase, and hence cAMP

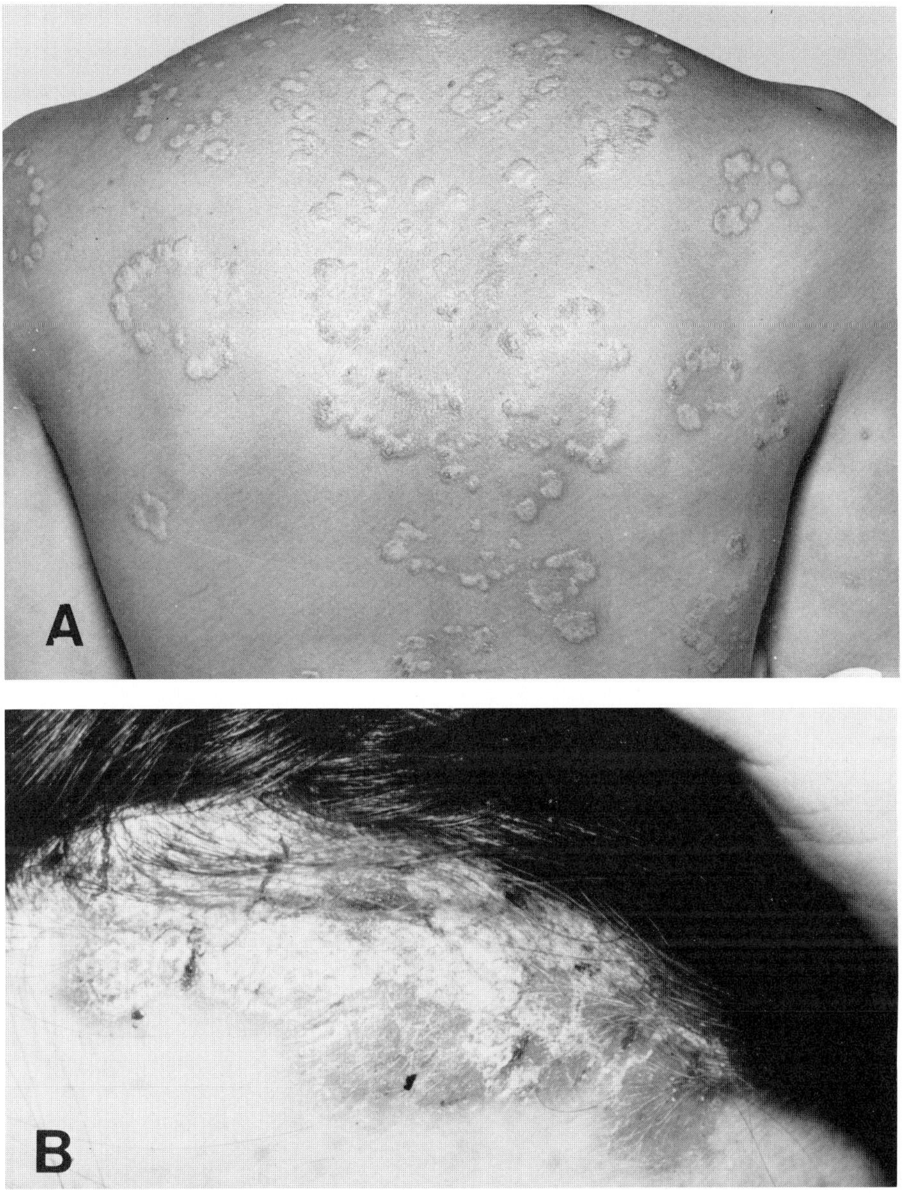

Figure 16-1. This patient demonstrates aggregates of scaly pink papules (A). The close-up (B) shows a well-demarcated plaque in a typical location, the scalp. The lesion is red and covered with a dense micaceous scale; bleeding fissures are evident.

synthesis,[24] and β-blockers, which block epinephrine stimulation of the cAMP cascade, both are known to precipitate or exacerbate psoriasis.[56]

Many of the ultramicroscopic findings described above can be explained on the basis of defective cAMP generation, and while levels of cAMP are decreased, cyclic GMP (cGMP) levels are consistently elevated in psoriatic epidermis, perhaps as a result of stimulation of the arachidonic acid cascade.[15]

Another possible effect of cAMP deficiency is in the production of ornithine decarboxylase, which is the rate-limiting enzyme for polyamine formation. These low molecular weight amines, putrescine, spermidine and spermine, are associated with cell-proliferation, and are found to be elevated in psoriasis.[38]

Levels of arachidonic acid are significantly higher in involved and uninvolved psoriatic skin than in controls, and the activity of phospholipase A2, the enzyme responsible for its liberation, is increased. Arachidonic acid and its metabolites are probably involved in psoriatic inflammatory changes; the cycloxygenase pathway for arachidonic acid metabolism results in the production of prostaglandins, and the lipoxygenase pathway in the production of leukotrienes.[62] Pospholipase A2 may be activated by a variety of noxious stimuli to set these metabolic cascades in motion. The end products of each of these cause vasodilatation, increased permeability of the post capillary venules, and leukocyte chemotaxis; included here is the chemoattraction of neutrophils, which may be the pathway for Muno microabsess production. Interestingly, phospholipase A2, is yet another agent that may be regulated by cAMP.[34]

The proteinases such as plasminogen activator have greatly increased activity in psoriatic epidermis, and conceivably too may be regulated by cAMP;[67] these proteinases may contribute to inflammation by the proteolytic activation of complement.[37]

Immunologic findings in the pathophysiology of psoriasis include: (1) Antibodies to basal cell nuclei and stratum corneum have been demonstrated;[18] (2) Immune complexes have been demonstrated in the circulation and in psoriatic scales; (3) Psoriatic serum suppresses blast transformation of T lymphocytes.[35] (4) Cellular immune mechanisms in psoriasis are decreased; although the absolute numbers of helper and supressor T cells are normal,[44] suppressor T cell function is decreased,[48] while macrophage chemotaxis and phagocytosis is enhanced.[36] It has been suggested that this increased macrophage activity may be a reflection of the defective β-andrenergic receptor function; and (5) Psoriatic patients have increased numbers of circulating polymorphonuclear leukocytes, with enhanced levels of activity; the beneficial effects of methotrexate and of leukapheresis and the exacerbating effect of lithium may perhaps all in part be attributed to their action on neutrophils.[3]

While it is not too difficult from the above simplified presentation of current information to surmise how environmental factors or damage to the skin from internal causes such as infections may set in motion some of these diverse, but interconnected trains of events, and precipitate psoriatic lesions, psychogenic mechanisms are more difficult to explain. That they in fact even do set pathogenic mechanisms in process has been a matter of controversy over the years, and evidence pertinent to that issue will be discussed in the next section before an attempt is made to try to arrive at some kind of integrated psychopathophysiologic understanding.

PSYCHOGENIC INFLUENCES

Clinical experience seems to indicate that for some patients psychosocial stress is a factor in the precipitation or exacerbation of psoriatic episodes, and in some cases indeed the major factor; clinical experience indicates also that many patients believe this to be irrefutable, regardless of the opinion of their physicians. The history of medical opinion on the impact of stress on psoriasis reflects the history of opinion on psychosomatic medicine in general, swinging back and forth between uncritical acceptance of soft evidence and hypercritical skepticism. Many observers have tended towards vagueness and lack of specificity in their assertions, presenting only impressions and generalizations that are difficult to evaluate, while others evaluate findings on the basis of external factors only; these observers ignore the importance of the contextual significance of events as a determinant of stressful potential, and demand stringent controls that in fact may have little relevance to the type of information being sought.

Thus Becker and Obermeyer note without further clarification that patients with psoriasis often exhibit "features of emotional instability" that they believe to be part of the "psoriatic constitutional diathesis"[41] and Obermeyer quotes a number of other authors of a similar opinion.[10,46] Of 72 adult patients studied by Wittkower and Russell,[68] 60 percent were described as "emotionally maladjusted" in a variety of different ways, but Whitlock, who reviews many of these early papers, ignores unconscious factors and the possible contextual significance of emotional events to these patients, and chooses rather to consider their emotional difficulties as the effect of the psoriasis and not a contributory cause;[65] this position is taken also by Shuster.[54] Symptoms of depression and anxiety crop up in many reports, but frequently the psychiatric findings are presented in descriptive terms only, with no attempt to elucidate their developmental or psychodynamic features.[20,49,53]

Susskind and McGuire,[59] in an attempt to clarify some of these allegations, studied 20 patients and found that a stressful event was associated with the onset of psoriasis in 8 patients, with relapse in 14, and with both onset and relapse in 4. These findings cannot be lightly dismissed because affective disturbances developed concomitantly with the somatic symptoms, following the stressful event. The patients experienced anxiety and unexpressed resentment, and exhibited features of depression; these symptoms were triggered by the stress.

Engel and Daneman,[19] and Goldsmith et al.[25] both confirmed a high incidence of psychiatric disease amongst psoriasis patients. In Engel and Daneman's group of 20 patients, 65 percent warranted one or more psychiatric diagnosis before treatment was started and in those 7 who completed the study, improvement or worsening of the emotional status parallelled that of the cutaneous lesions. Goldsmith et al.'s patients scored higher than did controls for symptoms of hysteria and depression; 30 percent of these were thought to be in need of psychiatric treatment on the basis of psychometric tests. Baughman and Sobel showed the severity of psoriasis to vary with stress in a study in 1971;[7] in 1976[8] these same workers, using different experimental parameters, were able to declare not only that their psoriasis patients were better emotionally adjusted than were their controls, but also that they were little disturbed in their social, occupational, and family roles by their disease. Unconscious factors were not explored in these studies, nor was the possibility of defensive denial acknowledged; this latter feature, defensive denial, has been suggested by Goldsmith et al. as one reason for treatment noncompliance.[25]

And so the pendulum has continued to swing back and forth in the intervening years, with the great preponderance of workers supporting a significant role for stress,[20,50,51] but with an occasional report presenting the opposing view.[42] All of these papers have relied on questionnaires, personality profiles, and subjective assessment of stress with only occasionally psychiatric in-depth interviews; the difference between the findings in Baughman and Sobel's first and second studies, quoted above, demonstrates clearly the conflicting information that may be obtained when only limited psychologic parameters are relied on.

More recently, objective physiologic measurements of endocrinologic and metabolic responses to stress have been made, in persons subjected to controlled experimental stressors.[4] All the findings in this study demonstrated that under the conditions of the test both psoriasis patients and controls experienced a selective increase in sympatho-adrenomedullary activity, as opposed to pituitary adrenocortical activity; the increase in the psoriatic patients was statistically greater than in the controls, and was reflected in proportionately higher levels of serum adrenalin; dopamine and norepinephrine remained unaffected, while serum cortisol was significantly lower in the psoriatics. Adrenalin is the neurotransmitter most responsible for the feelings of tension and discomfort that develop during stress; the patients reflected the physiologic effects of their relatively higher adrenalin levels in their greater complaints of tension and discomfort during the test conditions. Elevation of blood glucose, another measure of stress, was also significantly higher in the patient group.

From this study it is clear that psoriatic patients behave biochemically and metabolically differently, under conditions of controlled stress; they demonstrate a greater than normal degree of sympatho-adrenomedullary activation, characterized by significantly higher adrenalin levels and significantly lower cortisol levels.

TOWARDS A PSYCHOPATHOPHYSIOLOGIC UNDERSTANDING

The effect of stress on immune mechanisms is well known and has been documented in Chapter 3; this effect can certainly be invoked as one possible way in which stress may be anticipated to affect psoriasis adversely, as it does in many other immunologically mediated disease processes.

Given the pronounced rebound effect of glucocorticoid withdrawal in psoriasis patients, with which we are all familiar, the markedly reduced serum corisol levels of psoriatics under stress may provide a contributory pathway.

Farber et al., stressing the remarkable symmetry of psoriatic lesions, suggest a role for neurohumoral mediators, and more specifically the neuropeptide, substance-P. That substance-P is released as a part of the hypothalamic-hypophyseal stress reaction is well-known, and its role in mediation of flush reactions and itching has been discussed in previous chapters. Farber et al. lay out an elegant hypothesis that implicates substance-P in every phase of psoriatic pathology.[21]

The ubiquitous involvement of cAMP provides another avenue for further study. That intracellular levels of cAMP are lower in psoriasis, and associated with various of the aberrant phenomena as described above, that they are less reponsive to β-adrenergic stimulation than are those in controls, and that psoriatic patients are more sensitive to stressors in terms of sympathetic adrenomedullary responses, with higher levels of adrenalin than controls, all speak to complex interactions in many systems that involve cyclic nucleotides and that are intimately related to the stress reaction.

Perhaps more questions are raised by our current knowledge than answers given, but acceptable scientific explanations for observed clinical events seem at this time at lease to be within the realm of possibility.

MANAGEMENT

Dermatologic management will be along conventional lines. The general principles of *psychological* management are discussed in Chapter 5. In this context, the doctor-patient relationship is particularly important. In a study of 94 dermatology out-patients in a hospital setting, 38 of whom had psoriasis, Jowett[31] found that 60 percent had negative feelings about their appointments, and clearly felt that they were treated neither with interest nor respect by doctors whom they had no opportunity to get to know; 50 percent were dissatisfied also with the information and explanation that they received from these doctors.

Given the chronicity of psoriasis, the need frequently for complicated and sometimes unpleasant treatments, and the extent to which the disease may impair the quality of life for the individual, an encouraging, supportive, and positive doctor-patient relationship would seem to be mandatory for effective treatment, and we must pay attention to avoiding the kind of insensitivity that Jowett's patients encountered.

The relatively high percentage of psoriasis patients found to have concomitant or preceding psychiatric disease,[19,25] also makes it imperative that the physician be sensitive to the psychiatric needs of the patient, and that the physician work to create a positive therapeutic relationship. Many patients are found to be anxious and worried,[20,21] but perhaps more importantly, depressed. Matussek reports that, unlike more characteristic depressive patients, the psoriasis patients that he studied expressed their high levels of aggression outwards onto others, rather than inwards onto themselves;[39] this ready expression of aggression makes for an uneasy relationship unless the physician is aware of the possibility and able to address it directly, instead of permitting him or herself to feel defensive and angered. To be able to say calmly and evenly to an angry, hostile, and abusive patient, "I seem to have made you very angry" is usually disarming; it focuses the patient's attention back onto his or her own behavior, rather than focussing on the patient's complaints about others, and helps therefore to open up the patient's feelings for a discussion that may prove revealing and helpful to both.

Suicidal ideation, and even successful suicide, in patients with stress-related dermatoses is reported by Sanborn, et al.[47] In each case, the suicide was precipitated by a further psychosocial stress added to a life situation that was already difficult; in many cases the physician was totally taken by surprise by the event, another evidence that we are not always listening to our patients in a meaningful way; nor are we always in tune with what is going on behind the superficial resignation, or defensive denial of the seemingly adjusted patient.

Because of the nature of psoriasis, its treatment, and its effects, continuity of care in order to permit development of a positive therapeutic relationship is perhaps a goal that should be sought more assiduously, although within the context of a training program there are numerous obstacles to this ideal. Jowett[31] notes that enough attention is not paid to fostering communication skills in trainees, and with this I would concur, adding that attention to empathic understanding is often neglected also.

Special Treatments

Psychotherapy. There is a place for psychoanalysis, psychoanalytic psychotherapy, and supportive psychotherapy in the treatment of psoriasis, when the criteria for these modalities are met.

Hypnosis. Frankel and Misch[22] report successful treatment of a case of psoriasis recalcitrant to treatment for 20 years using a combination of hypnosis and psychoanalytic psychotherapy. This patient, who usually improved during the summer, was taught, by self-hypnosis, to induce a trance in which he imagined himself to be basking in the sun. His skin essentially cleared within 7 months, and more importantly, he began to recognize that his situation was not completely without hope.

Behavior therapy. Waxman[64] reports an equally prolonged and recalcitrant case that responded to combined hypnosis and dynamic psychotherapy, to which was added the behavioral technique of counter-conditioning. This patient too experienced both relief of skin lesions and a general improvement in personality functioning.

Gaining of insight. Both psychotherapy and hypnosis above illustrate the positive therapeutic effect of insight in cases of psoriasis associated with psychosocial stress. This is a point that Seville has also made,[52] and with which I can concur. A patient of mine, a 38-year-old married woman who has been in once-weekly psychoanalytic psychotherapy for the past 3 years has experienced severe flares of her psoriasis explosively, as new conflictual material has come into consciousness during the course of her treatment, only to clear equally dramatically as insight has been gained into the nature and genesis of the conflict. The fact that suggestion is found not to be beneficial,[57] would be in line with this finding.

This is an avenue of research that has been ignored for too long, and that may provide us with interesting information, as well as beneficial results.

Group therapy. Group therapy for psoriatic patients has been studied at a number of centers in the Netherlands since 1968. These studies have focused on improving the quality of life for patients with chronic illnesses, by decreasing illness behavior, anxiety, stress, and isolation, and increasing patient skills in self-care and in developing relaxation capabilities.[13] These workers have devised a successful group model in which the therapeutic team consists of a physician and a psoriasis fellow-sufferer, working together.[14]

Support groups. Psoriasis Associations give invaluable help to individual sufferers by decreasing their sense of isolation and alienation, by sharing coping skills, by fostering public education about the disease, and working towards greater social acceptance of persons with psoriasis in public, professional and recreational situations.[60]

Lessening psychosocial stress. The adopting of stress management techniques and improving coping mechanisms can be taught, but a better fundamental level of functioning, which will include the above, is best achieved by the personality changes that can be effected through psychoanalytic psychotherapy. Manipulation of the environment or hospitalization may be helpful in reducing stress also; one of the benefits of treatment at a facility such as that which has been established at the Dead Sea[43] must, I think, be the possibility of abdicating responsibility, and regressing to a level at which the patient can permit him or herself to be taken care of.

Psychotropic drugs. Short courses of anxiolytic drugs may be indicated in situations of external stress. Given the relatively high incidence of depression in patients with psoriasis it seems likely that the benefits of tricyclic antidepressants have not to date been adequately explored. Lithium should be avoided because of its adverse side-effects as should the use of propranolol, for example, for panic attacks.

Effects of Psoriasis on the Patient—The Somatopsychic Effect

Inevitably, a chronic and disfiguring disease that requires assiduous, long-term, often unpleasant treatment that may be painful or pruritic, and that produces unsightly and troublesome scaling, has the potential to affect adversely the quality of life of the sufferer.

Jowett and Ryan[32] report 38 patients with psoriasis of a mean duration of 13 years who were interviewed at length; these patients spoke poignantly about the impact of psoriasis on their lives. Eighty-seven percent complained of pruritus and other writers have associated pruritus with emotional difficulties in patients with psoriasis. The scales made patients feel unacceptable and "like the plague," and there was a tendency among them to project onto others their self-disgust, causing them to anticipate a negative reaction from others. They complained that there was a general level of ignorance about psoriasis in the community and they found little empathy with their discomfort; many felt (rightly or wrongly) that certain professional opportunities were closed to them, and they attributed interpersonal difficulties on the job and in the family to the disease. This tendency to project apparently resulted from lowered self-esteem, defensiveness, and sensitivity. For many there was anxiety about what they could expect from their disease, and from the prescribed treatments; 30 percent were depressed, and many felt that social, family, and sexual relationships had been adversely affected; many encountered difficulties in finding comfortable or esthetically acceptable clothing, or in finding leisure time activites that were comfortable for them.

These are aspects of the disease that in a busy clinic or practice situation are often not addressed, although clearly for the individual they are devastating; surely if we are interested in total health and well-being of our patients we cannot afford to ignore them, as Coles and Ryan remind us.[16]

Stankler[58] and Roenigk and Roenigk[45] have also addressed these issues, with similar findings; Roenigk and Roenigk found, not unexpectedly, that women tend to be more disturbed generally than men, and they provide us with some thoughts as to why this might be, on the basis of psychological developmental differences between the two sexes. Hill-Beuf and Porter[28]discuss the special needs of the child whose appearance is impaired, and point out that those who develop their disease earlier, experience less difficulty with self-esteem than do those whose impairment develops later. The early adolescent years are the most traumatic, and children who develop areas of competence that help to build self-esteem are able to achieve the best levels of adjustment.

Finally, the entire topic of improving the quality of life for the psoriasis sufferer has been beautifully and comprehensively summarized by Swanbeck and Jobling.[60]

REFERENCES

1. Adachi K, Halprin KM, Takeda J, et al.: Epidermal surface receptors which link pharmacological mediators to the adenylate cyclase system. Br J Dermatol 107(23):111-118, 1982
2. Adachi K, Yoshikawa K, Halprin KM, Levine V: Prostaglandins and cyclic AMP in epidermis. Br J Dermatol 92:381-388 1975
3. Anderson TF, Voorhees JJ: Psoriasis, in Theirs BH, Dobson RI (eds): Pathogenesis of Skin Disease. New York, Churchill Livingstone, 1986, pp 67-84
4. Arnetz BB, Fjellner B, Eneroth P, Kallner A: Stress and psoriasis. Psychoendocrine and metabolic reactions in psoriatic patients during standardized stressor exposure. Psychosom Med 47(6):528-541, 1985
5. Baker H: The influence of chloraquine and related drugs on psoriasis, and keratoderma blenorrhagicum. Br J Dermatol 78:161-166, 1966
6. Baker H, Wilkinson DS: Psoriasis, in Rook A, Wilkinson DS, Ebling FJG (eds): Textbook of Dermatology (ed. 3). Oxford, Blackwell Scientific Publications, 1979, p 1317
7. Baughman R, Sobel R: Psoriasis, stress and strain. Arch Dermatol 103:599-605, 1971
8. Baughman R, Sobel R: Emotional factors in psoriasis: recent findings in Farber EM, Cox AJ (eds): Psoriasis. New York, Yorke Medical Books, 1976, p 180-188
9. Beckman L, Bergdahl K, Sedergren B: Genetic markers in psoriasis. Acta Dermatol Vener (Stockh) 57:247-251, 1977
10. Borda JM: On the pathogenesis of psoriasis. Exc Med XIII 2, 104: Abst 380, 1948
11. Braun-Falco O, Christopher E: Structural aspects of initial psoriatic lesions. Arch Dermatol Forsch 251:95-110,1974
12. Braverman IM, Yen A: Ultrastructure of the capillary loops in the dermal papillae of psoriasis. J Invest Dermatol 68:53-60, 1977
13. Bremer-Schulte M: Medical education in relation to self activity of patients, in Kickbusch I, Hatch S (eds): Selfhelp in Europe. London, Croom Helm Ltd, 1983
14. Bremer-Schulte M, Cormane RH, van Dijk E, Write J: Group therapy of psoriasis. J Am Acad Dermatol 12 (1:1):61-66, 1985

15. Cantieri JS, Graff G, Goldberg ND: Cyclic GMP metabolism in psoriasis. Activation of Soluble Epidermal Guauylate Cyclase by Arachidonic Acid and 12-Hydroxy-5;8,10,14 Eicosatetraenoic Acid. J Invest Dermatol 74:234-237, 1980
16. Coles RB, Ryan TJ: The psoriasis sufferer in the community. Comment. Br J Dermatol 93:111-113, 1975
17. Cormane R, Hunyadi J, Hamerlinck F, et al.: The role of lymphoid cells and polymorphonuclear-leukocytes in the pathogenesis of psoriasis, in Farber EM, Cox AJ (eds): Proceedings of 2nd International Symposium on Psoriasis. New York, Yorke Medical Books, pp 47-54, 1977
18. Cormane RH: Immunopathology of psoriasis. Arch Dermatol Res 270:201-215, 1981
19. Engel MF, Daneman EA: Psoriasis: Joint dermatologic and psychiatric study. Dermatol Digest August:63-67, 1967
20. Farber EM, Bright RD, Nall ML: Psoriasis. A questionnaire survey of 2,144 patients. Arch Dermatol 98:248-259, 1968
21. Farber EM, Nickoloff BJ, Recht B, Fraki JE: Stress, symmetry and psoriasis: Possible role of neuropeptides. J Am Acad Dermatol 14(2):305-311, 1986
22. Frankel FH, Misch RC: Hypnosis in a case of long-standing psoriasis in a person with character problems. Int J Clin Exp Hypn 21: 121-130, 1973
23. Fraki JE, Briggaman RA, Lazarus GS: Uninvolved skin from psoriatic patients develops signs of involved psoriatic skin, after being grafted onto nude mice. Science 215:685-686, 1982
24. DiGiovanna JJ, Aoyagi T, Adachi K, Taylor JR: Inhibition of epidermal adenylate cyclase by lithium carbonate. J Invest Dermatol 74:246-247, 1980
25. Goldsmith LA, Fisher M, Wacks J: Psychological characteristics of psoriatics: implications for management. Arch Dermatol 100:674-676, 1969
26. Goodwin P, Hamilton S, Fry L: A comparison between DNA synthesis and mitosis in uninvolved and involved psoriatic epidermis, and normal epidermis. Br J Dermatol 89:613-618, 1973
27. Hammerstrom S, Lindgren JA, Marcel C, et al.: Arachidonic acid transformations in normal and psoriatic skin. J Invest Dermatol 73:180-183, 1979
28. Hill-Beuf A, Porter JDR: Children coping with impaired appearance: Social and psychologic influences. Gen Hosp Psych 6: 294-301, 1984
29. Iizuka H, Adachi K, Halprin KM, et al.: Cyclic nucleotide-phosphodiesterase in the uninvolved and involved skin of psoriatics. J Invest Dermatol 70:246-249, 1978
30. Ingram JT: The significance and managment of psoriasis. Br Med J(ii):823-828, 1954
31. Jowett S: Career, interpersonal trouble in acne, psoriasis, eczema patients. Skin and Allergy News 16:3, 1985
32. Jowett S, Ryan T: Skin disease and handicap: An analysis of the impact of

skin conditions. Soc Sci Med 20:425-429, 1985

33. Kerkhof van de PCM, Van Rennes H, De Grood R, et al.: Metabolic changes and the margin of the spreading psoriatic lesion. Br J Dermatol 108:647-652, 1983
34. Kragballe K, Voorhees JJ: Arachidonic acid and its metabolites in the pathogenesis and treatment of psoriasis, in Roenigk HH Jr, Maibach HI (eds): Psoriasis. New York, Dedder, 1984
35. Krueger GG, Hill HR, Jederberg WW: Inflammatory and immune cell function in psoriasis—a subtle disorder, I, In vivo and in vitro survey. J Invest Dermatol 71:189-194, 1978
36. Krueger GG: Psoriasis. Current concepts of its etiology and pathogenesis, in Dobson RL, Thiers BH (eds): Yearbook of Dermatology. Chicago, Yearbook Medical Publishers, 1981, pp 13-70
37. Lazarus GS, Frachi J, Briggaman R, et al.: The role of proteinases in the pathophysiology of psoriasis, in Roenig HH Jr, Maibach HI (eds): Psoriasis. New York, Marcel Dekker, 1985, pp 265-270
38. Lowe NJ, Breeding J, Russell O: Cutaneous polyamines in psoriasis. Br J Dermatol 107:21-25, 1982
39. Matussek P, Agerer D, Seibt G: Aggression in depressives and psoriasis. Psychother Psychosom 43:120-125, 1985
40. Nyfors A, Lemholt K: Psoriasis in children. A short review and a survey of 245 cases. Br J Dermatol 92:437-442, 1975
41. Obermeyer ME: Psychocutaneous Medicine. Springfield, IL, Charles C. Thomas, pp 325-339
42. Payne RA, Payne CMER, Marks R, et al.: Stress does not worsen psoriasis; a controlled study of 32 patients. Clin Exper Dermatol 10:239-245, 1985
43. Perry WJ: Sun, emollients therapy for psoriasis at Dead Sea Clinic. Skin & Allergy News 16:4:26, 1985
44. DePietro WP, Berger C, Harber LC, Edelson RL: Normal numbers of phenotypic helper, suppressor, and total T cell populations in psoriasis vulgaris: a quantitation by monoclonal antibodies. J Am Acad Dermatol 5:304-307, 1981
45. Roenigk RK, Roenigk HH: Sex differences in the psychological effects of psoriasis. Cutis 21(4):529-533, 1978
46. Russell B: Psoriasis. Practitioner 164:197-204, 1950
47. Sanborn PE, Sanborn CJ, Cimbolic P, Niswander GP: Suicide and stress-related dermatoses. Dis Nerv Syst 33:391-394, 1972
48. Sauder DN, Bailin PL, Sundeen J, Krakauer RS: Suppressor cell function in psoriasis. Arch Dermatol 116:51-55, 1980
49. Schaar van der WW: Psychometric investigation in 48 Dutch patients suffering from psoriasis. Psychother Psychsom 27:159-162, 1976-77
50. Seville RH: Psoriasis and stress. Br J Dermatol 97:297-302, 1977

51. Seville RH: Psoriasis and stress II. Br Med J 98:151-153, 1978
52. Seville RH: Psoriasis, stress, insight, and prognosis. Semin Dermatol 2(3):213-216, 1983
53. Shanon J: Psoriasis: psychosomatic aspects. Psychother Psychosom 31:218-222, 1979
54. Shuster S, Fisher EH, Binnell O: The effects of skin disease on self image. Br J Dermatol 99(16):18-19, 1978
55. Skoven J, Thormann J: Lithium compound treatment and psoriasis. Arch Dermatol 115:1185-1187, 1979
56. Sondergaard J, Wadskov S, Aerenlund Jensen H: Aggravation of psoriasis and occurrence of psoriasiform cutaneous eruptions induced by practolol (Eraldin). Acta Dermatol Venereol 56:239-243, 1976
57. Stankler L, Main RA: The effect of occlusion, suggestion, and hospitalization on psoriasis. Dermatol Digest 15:19, 1977
58. Stankler L: The effect of psoriasis on the sufferer. Clin Exper Dermatol 6:303-306, 1981
59. Susskind W, McGuire RJ: The emotional factor in psoriasis. Scot Med J 4:503-507, 1959
60. Swanbeck G, Jobling R: Organization of psoriasis treatment and psychosocial aspects. Acta Dermatol Venereol 112:61-63, 1984
61. Voorhees JJ, Ovell EA, Kelsey WH: Dibutyl cyclic AMP inhibition of epidermal cell division. Arch Dermatol 105:384-386, 1972
62. Voorhees JJ: Leukotrienes and other lipoxygenase products in the pathogenesis and therapy of psoriasis, and other dermtoses. Arch Dermatol 119:541-547, 1983
63. Watson W, Cann HM, Farber EM, Hall ML: The genetics of psoriasis. Arch Dermatol 105:197-207, 1972
64. Waxman D: Behavior therapy of psoriasis—a hypnoanalytic and counter-conditioning technique. Postgraduate Med J 49:591-595, 1973
65. Whitlock FA: Psychophysiologic aspects of skin disease. London, WB Saunders Co., Ltd, 1976, pp 197-201
66. Whyte HJ, Baughman RD: Acute guttate psoriasis and streptococcal infection. Arch Dermatol 89:350-356, 1964
67. Wilson EL, Reich E: Modulation of plasminogen activator synthesis in chick embryo fibroblasts by cyclic nucleotides and phorobol myristate acetate. Cancer Res 39:1579, 1979
68. Wittkower E, Russell B: Emotional Factors in Skin Disease. New York, Paul B. Boeber Inc, 1953, pp 109-120

Chapter 17

Atopic Dermatitis

The concept of multifactorial etiology has a long history in the case of atopic dermatitis. The relative significance of genetic, constitutional, and environmental factors has been debated in the literature at least since the latter part of the last century, though different valence has been accorded the multivariate elements by different writers.[61,68,73] The recognition that influences from the psychologic sphere were among these elements was reflected in the name "neurodermatitis disseminata," by which atopic dermatitis was formerly known.[12]

Any physical condition, and particularly one that is chronic and recurrent, and that has its onset in early infancy, inevitably must demonstrate a close interaction between soma and psyche in the ebb and flow of its course. This interaction has its genesis in the earliest interplay between these two agencies, an interplay that is crucial to the development of the internal body-image and that takes place within the dynamic context of the mother-child relationship.[31] Particularly is this the case for cutaneous symptoms, because the skin is of such central importance as an organ of perception in those very early months of life. This facet of psychosomatic disease was discussed in Chapter 1, and the early developmental issues that were explored then will be considered again later in this chapter, in the section devoted to psychopathology and psychodynamic formulations in atopic dermatitis.

A discussion of the clinical aspects of atopic dermatitis is beyond the scope of this volume, and is not central to my thesis. The reader is referred to the standard texts in dermatology for this information.

Whereas the relevance of the experimental information that follows and the need to include it in a text such as this may be questioned, it has seemed to me to be important. Past claims of causal relationships based on anecdotal evidence and nebulous information have sometimes donned a cloak of magic. We do now have available to us fragments of verifiable information from a multiplicity of sources, each subtly linked to the other and each connected, however distantly, to psychic activity; it has seemed to me to be important to trace each of those individual links in order better to understand the whole.

ETIOLOGY

There seems to be general agreement in the literature that genetic factors establish the tendency towards atopic dermatitis,[75] while factors in the environment determine the severity of the disease and the areas of involvement.[9,61]

Genetic Factors

The evidence for genetic predisposition comes from many sources, and a polygenic mode of transmission is suggested by the heterogeneity of the clinical and pathophysiologic manifestations.[20] Some of the evidence to support this hypothesis follows: (1) 79 percent of children develop atopic symptoms if both parents have allergic disease, while the figure is 58 percent, when only one parent is involved.[50] In only 21 percent of cases can neither a personal nor a family history of atopy be identified. (2) Concordance is ten times greater in monozygotic than in dizygotic twins.[9,11] (3) An elevated IgE level is a feature of atopic dermatitis; IgE production appears to be governed by two separate autosomal genes.[20] (4) A number of other genetically linked conditions may be associated with atopic dermatitis. These include autosomal dominant ichthyosis vulgaris,[75] reactive airway disease,[62] reduced sebum production,[75] the Wiskott-Aldrich Syndrome,[4] anhidrotic ectodermal dysplasia,[75] and alopecia areata.[73]

Environmental Factors

The skin of the atopic individual is inherently "itchy."[97] This "itchiness" is apparently due in part to an itch threshold that is lower, and a duration of itch that is longer following a stimulus than occurs in normal subjects;[37] it is due in part also to above average tissue levels of histamine.[44]

It is common clinical experience that factors in the environment that increase the tendency to itch can trigger an outbreak of dermatitis by stimulating the scratch response. The factors of which I speak include changes and extremes of temperature, sweating, xerosis, friction, draughts, contact with harsh or whiskery fabrics, dust, alkalies, detergents, bacterial infections, and hot or spicy foods.[73]

The question of specific allergic reactions in the etiology of atopic dermatitis is a matter of controversy, but is strongly supported by Tuft and other allergists.[55,70,75] Ingestion of specific food stuffs such as chocolate, milk, eggs, nuts, and citrus fruits have been inculpated, particularly in early childhood; inhalant allergens are also thought in some cases to be responsible for exacerbations. There is much to suggest, however, that the mechanism by which these exacerbations occur is not via a specific allergic reaction.[34]

Evidence will be adduced later in this chapter to support the significant part played by emotional stress in tipping the homeostatic balance, and triggering an attack of eczema.

INCIDENCE

The incidence of atopic dermatitis in children under 5 years is variously quoted as from 2.5-3.1 percent,[43,98] with a figure of 0.7 percent in adults.[45] In 60 percent of patients the onset is during the first year of life and in 85 percent during the first 5 years.[75] The female to male ratio for individuals of all ages is 1.2:1.0, although children with atopic dermatitis are more often male (Fig. 17-1).[75]

PATHOPHYSIOLOGY

A complex assortment of physiologic abnormalities have been demonstrated in patients with atopic dermatitis; these abnormalities allow of speculative hypotheses and point to areas for continuing research, but do not fully elucidate the pathophysiologic mechanisms involved in the disease process. Itching[68,75] and erythema[20] are variously quoted as the first event in the course of an outbreak, but it is generally agreed that the characteristic dermatitic lesions frequently do not appear until the skin has been scratched. This finding is of particular interest in light of the fact that the onset in infancy is usually deferred until after the second month, when the capacity for co-ordinated scratching has developed.

The Role of IgE

The frequently observed elevation of IgE levels appears to represent a non-specific feature of atopic dermatitis, and may be reflective of a basic defect in immune regulation.[20] Though present in 43-80 percent of patients, often paralleling the severity of the disease, and highest when dermatitis is associated with others of the atopic disorders, this elevation is not specific for atopic dermatitis and is seen in other dermatoses.[71] In a similar vein, atopic dermatitis may be seen in patients with no IgE, in those who have agammaglobulinemia.[74]

Further support for the nonspecific nature of this IgE elevation comes from failure of the majority of radio allergosorbent text (RAST) tests to correlate with the clinical symptoms,[42] and by similar inconsistency in the ability of suspected food allergens to trigger exacerbation[8] In some instances ingestion of specific foods can, however, be demonstrated to precipitate an outbreak, if for example a reactive erythema or urticaria is subsequently scratched.[8]

That circulating immune complexes containing IgE have been demonstrated following food challenge in patients with eczema is also interesting, and raises the possibility that deposition of these complexes in the tissues could generate the characteristic skin lesions.[13]

IgE binds avidly to mast cell membrane receptors, and provides one mechanism for mast cell degranulation and histamine release. There are many nonIgE dependent mechanisms also, whereby mast-cell degranulation can be accomplished.[100]

Defects in the regulation of IgE production that may help to explain the above findings will be discussed in the following section.

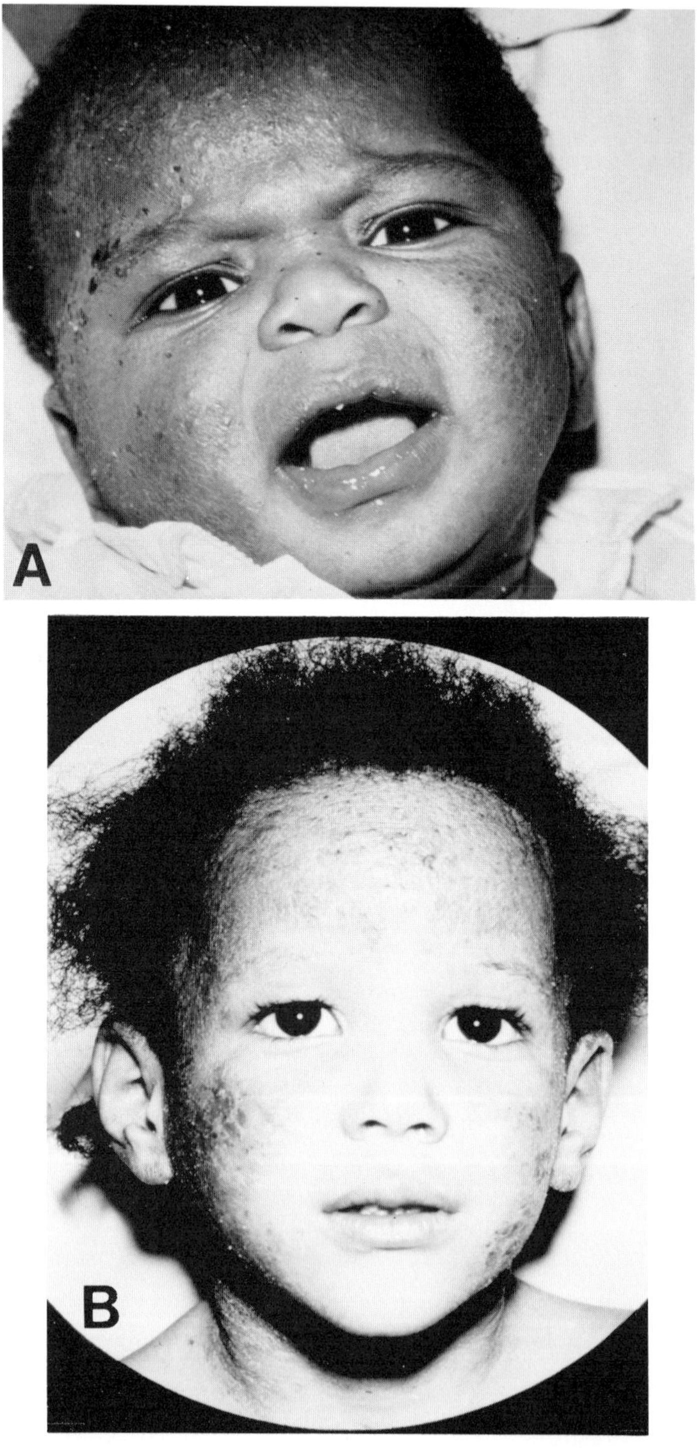
A
B

Defects in Cell-mediated Immunity

Extensive studies have been undertaken to elucidate the defective cell-mediated immunity observed in clinical practice; these defects are expressed in enhanced susceptibility to cutaneous bacterial, viral, and dermatophyte infections,[36] and decreased susceptibility to contact sensitisation.[72] A decreased delayed response to candidal, streptococcal, and trichophyton antigens is also noted.[21] That this defect is partial only, is demonstrated by the absence of an enhanced susceptibility to systemic infections, or to internal malignancy.

Studies using monoclonal antibodies against individual T-cell subsets reveals a decrease in the total T-cell population[18] and a decrease in suppressor/cytotoxic T cells.[54] The basic defect appears to be in a specific subset of helper T-cells whose function it is to induce suppressor-cell differentiation.[56] That this deficit is one of maturation rather than a more fundamental aberration is supported by the finding that T-cell responses are normal after incubation of the defective cells with thymic hormone extract.[19] T-cell responses may also be normal in patients during remission, and in those who have outgrown their disease.

While synthesis of IgE from unstimulated atopic peripheral lymphocytes has been reported in vitro, in vivo, current information suggests that B-cell activation and IgE synthesis in atopic patients is modulated by helper factors from T-cells, which are active in the presence of IgE and specific antigen.[83] This abnormal IgE synthesis is suppressed, when atopic T-cells are incubated with those from normal peripheral blood.

The Role of Histamine

That histamine plays a fundamental role in the atopic process has long been known, but the specifics of that role continue to unfold. Mast cell concentrations

---

Figure 17-1. Infantile and juvenile atopic eczema. The 9-month-old (A) shows all the characteristics of chronic disease. The diagnostic lichenoid skin-colored or pink papules that are the primary lesion are perceptible only at the margin of the large exudative, crusted red plaques on cheeks and forehead. An extra fold is visible on the lower eyelids (Dennie's sign). The eyes are bright and the look is anxious. In the 4-year-old (B) these same lesions are beginning to look lichenified. The crusting is often a sign of infection with staphylococcus aurus. The deliberate underexposure highlights the sparing of the perinasal and perioral areas. (The lantern sign—an area of lightness in a halo of pink.) Again note the bright eyes and anxious look.

are increased in the dermatitic skin of the atopic,[65] tissue histamine levels are raised,[44] and histamine is released in response to levels of IgE that are lower than are required by normal mast cells.[17] These increased histamine levels together with the characteristically lowered itch threshold, in large part account for the intractable pruritus that is the hallmark of atopic dermatitis; scratching, by releasing leukotrienes, proteases, and other chemical mediators, then serves to enhance the histamine-provoked itch.[88]

It has been suggested that histamine may determine the characteristic location of atopic lesions. Intramuscular injection of histamine in atopic subjects results in a disproportionate increase in the skin temperature of the face, neck, and flexures, the sites most commonly involved in atopic dermatitis.[103] This finding may reflect rather, however, simply an increase in the transudation of histamine as a result of the inflammatory changes.

Finally, it has been suggested that it may be histamine that causes the impaired neutrophil and monocyte chemotaxis that is characteristic of active atopic dermatitis.[40] While this impairment may explain the susceptibility of the atopic to infection with Staphyloccus aureus, the acute exacerbations so often associated with bacterial colonisation may well have an immunologic basis. This possibility is suggested by the increased levels of IgE antibodies specific for Staphylococcus aureus that can be detected in the serum of atopic patients.[1]

Vascular Responses

A number of vascular responses historically were considered to be idiosyncratic to and diagnostic of atopic dermatitis; these reactions included white dermographism[101,102] and a paradoxical blanch to topically applied nicotinic acid,[93] and to methacholine chloride.[55] These same reactions subsequently have been observed in a number of other inflammatory dermatoses and are now thought merely to reflect the inflammatory process in a nonspecific way.[55]

Neurotransmitters and the Cyclic Nucleotides

A theory of partial blockade of β-adrenergic receptors has been invoked as a possible basis for many of the reactions observed in atopic dermatitis.[91a] Such a blockade, it is suggested, would result in relatively increased cholinergic and α-adrenergic responses, and in a mild generalized disorder of autonomic functioning.[20]

Hyperreactivity to cholinergic agonists is expressed in: (1) the blanch response to methacholine;[101] (2) the hyperresponsive sweat reaction that is part of the atopic picture;[48] and (3) the increased histamine release in response to methacholine.[55]

Increased sensitivity to α-adrenergic agonists is reflected in: (1) the increased piloerection that is part of the atopic picture;[75] (2) the cutaneous vasoconstriction, and pupillary dilatation that follows phenylephrine application;[38] and (3) the abnormal cold-pressor test, and acral vasoconstriction that are reported in atopics.[75]

In order to understand the effect of a partial blockade of β-adrenergic receptors, consideration must be given to the function served by those receptors in the epidermis.[91a] Adrenergic receptors are sites on cell membranes that interact with catecholamines and structurally related compounds. α- and β-rcccptors have been identified, according to their relative sensitivity to epinephrine, norepinephrine, and isoproterenol.[3] The response of these receptors to stimulation by adrenergic agonists is mediated through adenylate cyclase, and results primarily in increased levels of intracellular cyclic AMP (cAMP) and/or cyclic GMP (cGMP).[55] Beta-receptors are stimulated in this fashion, not only by calecholamines, but also by histamine and by prostaglandin E.

An inverse relationship exists between adenylate cyclase activation and intracellular cAMP levels on the one hand, and cell reactivity on the other. The adenylate cyclase response to prostaglandin E and to isoproterenol is found to be impaired in atopic lymphocytes. A similar partial blockade in atopic mast cells and basophils has been invoked to explain the increased histamine release observed in atopics through a relative failure in cAMP controlled inhibition of histamine synthesis and release. The effect of this failure in control is further enhanced by the increased sensitivity of atopic cells to acetyl-choline noted above; this also contributes to histamine release through its effect on intracellular levels of cGMP.[49]

While there is evidence to suggest that the lowered cAMP levels result from partial blockade of β-adrenergic receptors and reduced adenylate cyclase activity as described above, increased phosphodiesterase activity has also been identified,[33] and plays its part in maintaining lowered levels of cAMP through increased cAMP breakdown.

It is now recognized that chemical mediators other than histamine are also involved in the atopic process. As has been noted above, erythemia and/or pruritus or in some cases urticarial wheals frequently are the first lesions, and precipitate the scratch response that triggers the characteristic eruption of atopic dermatitis.[55]

The role of humoral mediators in the genesis of these three elements, erythema, pruritus, and urticaria, has been discussed in previous chapters under the appropriate rubric. The mediators in question in addition to histamine include the bradykinins, prostaglandins, substance-P, vasoactive intestinal peptide, and the opioid peptide, met-enkephalin. Once scratching has taken place, the way is then open for proteases and the other mediators of inflammation to do their work.[88]

PSYCHOPATHOLOGY

It has been noted previously that the etiology of atopic dermatitis is multifactorial and that the inherent diathesis may long remain undetected, revealing itself only when the delicate balance is upset between those factors that promote health on the one hand, and constitutional and environmental factors that render the patient susceptible to atopic expression on the other.

That emotional factors may be involved in the constitutional as well as in the environmental predisposing forces is made abundantly clear in the literature. As has been described previously for psoriasis, so in atopic dermatitis, a higher percentage of patients than controls carry a psychiatric diagnosis, and psychiatric symptoms are often present before the eczema becomes manifest. Early observers speak rather broadly of "emotional instability,"[29,70,79] without developing more specific diagnostic formulations. But Hall-Smith and Norton,[35] in a random sampling of patients who attended the Dermatology Clinic of a community general hospital, found that out of 150 patients sampled 98 (60 percent) suffered psychiatric symptoms in need of treatment. Of these 150 patients, 50 appear to have had some form of atopic dermatitis, 40 percent of whom were diagnosed as obsessional neurotics with symptoms of anxiety. Kidd and Watt in a comparable study quote similar findings,[51] and Kuypers,[53] Greenhill and Finesinger,[32] and Musaph[68] also stress the association of obsessive-compulsive features with atopic dermatitis; Levy[57] on the other hand, in a study of 50 atopic patients found a high incidence of hysterical neurosis.

In contrast to the obsessional and hysterical psychoneuroses, the literature does not support an association between atopic dermatitis and the severe personality disorders, or psychosis. My own experience parallels this; I too find that there is no consistent psychological pattern, but there seems to be a more frequent association with obsessive-compulsive neurosis than with hysterical neurosis, and generally speaking, a negative association with personality disorder or psychosis.

Alexithymia is mentioned by a number of authors.[92] This condition, in which the patient has an impoverished phantasy life and no access to the language with which to express emotion, is sometimes a part of somatisation syndromes,[69] and may be seen in atopic dermatitis. A symptom rather than a diagnosis, alexithymia may exist side by side with features of neurosis as well as with more profound psychiatric disturbances. In line with this concept and in support of the above observations is the fact that the inner life of the severe obsessional is often restricted. In contrast, and as Panconesi has observed, the rich phantasy life and ready access to emotional experience seen in hysterical neurosis is less likely to be observed in atopic dermatitis[73] unless hysterical conversion mechanisms are operative. Anxiety particularly, but also depression, either as symptoms of neurosis, or as "somatopsychic" responses to the dermatosis itself, are common findings.

PSYCHODYNAMIC FORMULATIONS AND THE GENESIS OF ATOPIC DERMATITIS

Because the onset of dermatosis often is almost at the onset of life, the observation of patients with atopic dermatitis from infancy onwards provides a living laboratory for the study of the psychodynamic factors operative in precipitating or perpetuating the dermatosis.

The reader is referred to Chapter 1 for a discussion of the way in which the skin functions as an organ of perception very early in life, and its crucial significance in this capacity for healthy growth and development, and for the establishment of an intact body image and a solid self-esteem. I have described how early and adequate cutaneous tactile stimulation in a warm and loving environment is necessary for normal physical, emotional, and intellectual development both in animals and in man. Of the works previously cited, that of Spitz[89] is most clinically significant here. Two features appear repeatedly in the relevant literature: disturbances in the mother-child relationship, and difficulty in handling aggression: it will be seen in the material that follows that the latter is but one of the many profound consequences of the former.

The Mother-Child Relationship

In his observation of institutionalized infants from birth, Spitz found the difference to be in two areas only between the 28 who had atopic dermatitis, and the 165 who did not; a congenital predisposition and the characteristics of the interaction between mother and child.

Inherent Predisposition

At birth, those infants who subsequently developed atopic dermatitis demonstrated a cutaneous reflex excitability much greater than normal. This was demonstrated in scores for the cremasteric and rooting reflexes that were significantly higher than in the control infants.

Characteristics of the Mother-Child Relationship

On the surface, the eczema mothers appeared to be anxious and over-solicitous, regarding their infants as fragile and vulnerable and fearing irrationally to do them damage. Observation made it clear that this attitude was a defense against a profound unconscious hostility, which precluded a normal mode of relating. Not only did the mothers at times put their infants in reality situations that were dangerous, they also feared to handle them, touch them, or care for them, so that these children whose inherent need was greater than the average, were systematically deprived of essential cutaneous contact.

Because their own personalities were immature, these mothers had little capacity to control or compensate for their unconscious anxiety, and so transmitted to their offspring emotional signals that were inconsistent and often chaotic.

Effects of the Impaired Relationship

The effects on growth and development. The laying down of memory traces and the capacity to imitate are the learning tasks for the infant in the early months of life; the mastery of these tasks takes place through interaction with the mother and results in internalization and integration of her actions and attitudes, which become a part of the developing "self" of the infant. The continuing interaction and acquisition of skills through this "identification" with mother, together with the mastery of motility, permits the infant gradually to develop autonomy and an identity of his or her own, and so to separate emotionally from the mother. These tasks progress more smoothly, evenly, and with greater rapidity in a warm and loving environment, so it is not unexpected to find that Spitz observed delay in development of these skills for the eczema infants.[90]

Delayed also was growth and development in the area of social relationships. In only 15 percent, as compared with 85 percent of the control infants, did the normal stranger-anxiety develop at 8 months. This anxiety, which is generated in the presence of strangers and when mother is absent, demonstrates that a point in development has been reached where a visual image of the mother persists in the memory of the infant even in her absence, and so enables him to distinguish her from strangers. This persisting memory, or "object-constancy," is a necessary prerequisite for mature relationships to develop later, and occurs satisfactorily only in the context of a harmonious mother-child relationship.

Effects on the affects and drives. The ability to control such emotional responses as feelings, wishes, and drives is also developed within the context of the early mother-child relationship. It has been observed that it is not until an external stimulus is interpreted for the infant through the mother's own response to that stimulus that an emotional reaction is generated in small infants. As an example, during the Air Raids in war-time England, infants were only seen to experience anxiety once their mothers became anxious and transmitted that unrest to the child through emotional signals.[24]

Mothers with emotional conflict inevitably, if unwittingly, will transmit signals to their infants that though congruent with the two sides of their conflict, are inconsistent and confusing. Spitz observed that eczema mothers gave to their infants emotional signals that were ostensibly appropriate to the given situation, but as unconscious conflict surrounding her baby began to surface, the mother became anxious, and that anxiety caused those signals to be suppressed, and a new set generated. These new signals, derived as they were from a different internal attitude, and one that represented an over-compensation for the first, were neither consistent with her deeper feelings nor with her actions towards the child. Confusing signals such as these will inevitably generate anxiety within the child and may contribute to the high level of tension and activity so often observed in infantile eczema.[79]

As an example, a patient of mine, a 35-year-old woman and mother of four children, found herself pregnant once again. She had felt that financially and emotionally four children were the most she could handle, and it had been her intention to return to her profession to prepare for their college years, once the youngest was in school. She was distraught to be pregnant again, for she received little emotional support from her husband yet her principles would not permit her to seek an abortion.

When the new baby arrived, he was restless and demanding. A poor sleeper from the beginning, he had her up several times each night, and she was exhausted. Unconsciously, she bitterly resented this baby who had sabotaged all her plans, and who interfered with her sleep. In consequence, she handled the child roughly, and though warm and loving to her other children, her attitude to this new infant seemed rather cold. As she gradually became aware of these negative feelings at some level, anxiety supervened, the negative feelings were suppressed, and an over-solicitousness for the wakeful baby motivated her to take him into bed with her each night. Her anxiety was transmitted to him, he became more tense and demanding, and the atopic dermatitis that he developed at 2 months became intractable. His importunity was greatest at night, and now she resented his presence also in her bed, but because of ambivalence she could not permit herself to put him out. Whenever his wishes were threatened, he became angry and frustrated, his itching became intolerable, his scratching uncontrollable, and his mother in turn more solicitous; this vicious cycle was stoked cyclically by her ambivalent feelings and her anxiety (Fig. 17-2).

The handling of aggression. Inconsistency in the emotional climate creates a milieu in which it is difficult for emotional energy to be discharged.[87] It is the mother's ability to master her own aggression that enables the infant to test limits and gain mastery over his. With the receipt of confusing signals, it is difficult for the infant to risk expressing directly the rage and frustration that he experiences in face of a mother that is not in tune with his needs; his intense emotion must be suppressed.

Other Authors on the Mother-Child Relationship

Spitz's careful observation of atopic infants throughout the first year of life has provided a paradigm for the characteristic developmental pattern in this disorder.

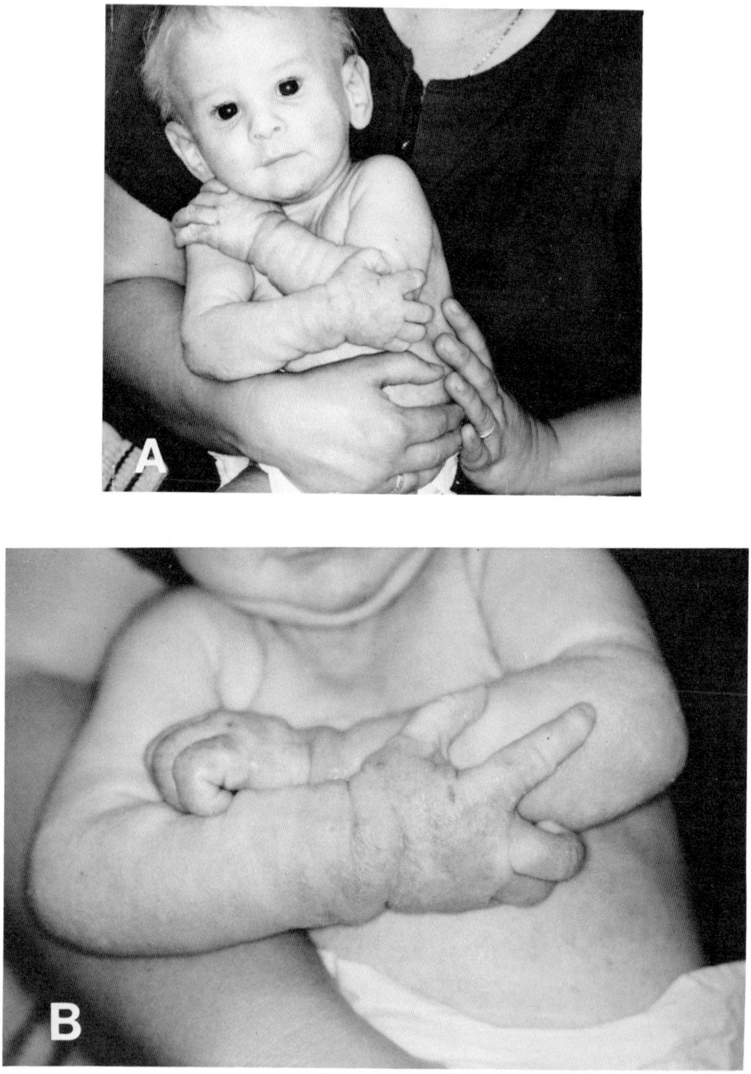

Figure 17-2. (A, B) Infantile atopic eczema. This 9-month-old was in a frenzy of scratching and rubbing throughout his visit to the office. He was scratching with both hands and also rubbing his legs together incessantly. The fury of his scratching can be seen in B. The bright eyes, anxious look, and general tension expressed by increased body tone were very evident.

Since these were institutionalised mothers that he described, it could be argued that the sample was biased, although his controls were well-matched. Confirmation of his findings with regard to the quality of the mother-child relationship typical of patients with atopic dermatitis, however, comes to us from a number of other sources.

Rosenthal[80,81] reported that in 26 infants with atopic eczema, the mother's overt avoidance of physical contact with her infant was an outstanding feature. Williams[104] observed the characteristic lack of "fit" between the cutaneous and emotional needs of the infant, and the mother's rejection. Marmor et al.[60] confirmed maternal emotional immaturity and repressed hostility, and observed maternal rejection in 13 of 22 cases. In one third of their cases, separation from the mother, though perhaps experienced by the infant as rejection, was for realistic reasons, rather than from unconscious maternal hostility. Miller and Baruch,[67] Miller,[66] Lynch et al.[59] and more recently Vaughan,[94] and Fritz[27] among many others, report a distorted or impaired mother-child relationship; they observe unconscious hostility and rejection on the part of the mother, as an almost constant finding.

My own experience suggests that not infrequently it is the other side of the unconscious maternal ambivalence that is expressed. Her negative feelings are repressed and replaced by an over-solicitousness and over-indulgence that permits no behavioral limits to be imposed on the child. The child's resultant demanding and uncontrolled behavior distorts the mother-child relationship.

Sequellae in the Patient as a Result of the Disturbed Relationship

Each one of the sequelae that follow is likely to be aggravated when an additional stress is added, and puts at risk the rather vulnerable homeostatic balance of the atopic. Each situation may lead to scratching, and so, to exacerbation.

High Levels of Anxiety

Certainly in childhood atopic dermatitis high levels of anxiety are a frequent clinical observation. Confirmation of this increased anxiety comes from psychological testing in adults. Atopic patients demonstrate both a greater tendency towards anxiety, and higher actual anxiety level than do controls.[22,28,52]

Suppression of Emotion

Aggression. Because of the factors relevant to aggression stated above, atopic patients are characterised by a tendency to suppress all emotion and an inability effectively to handle the aggressive drive.[14,52] These tendencies are common to many psychosomatic disorders. As a result, aggression may be turned against the self: nonneutralized aggressive energy is expressed in somatic terms as symptom,[39,87] or as self-destructive excoriation, and masochism is common.

Sensual and affectionate feelings. Attention has been paid in the literature also to the use of the skin for the expression and discharge of sensual feelings that cannot be expressed directly. At the level of cutaneous erotism, paroxysmal excoriation may represent unconscious erotic gratification;[66,91] it may alternatively be used to satisfy the residual longings for cutaneous contact from the earlier infantile period, when the mother failed to satisfy the needs for tactile stimulation. The other side of this wish for tactile gratification may be expressed in the disfigurement from scratching, as though to say, "if you will not love me, then I will make myself unlovable." At a less deeply unconscious level, scratching is commonly used manipulatively in a demand for attention. Perhaps because of early deprivation, these demands, focused through the skin, are sometimes insatiable.

Examples of the use of the skin for the expression of aggression in any clinical practice are legion; there is no one who cares for children who has not observed the atopic child scratch convulsively when upset or angry. Less commonly observed is the sensual use of the skin, but one patient of mine stands out.

The mother of this 40-year-old woman suffered a deep depression post-partum, and subsequently held herself very distant from her daughter; a disturbed and angry woman, her attitude alternated between cold indifference and frank hostility. My patient learned to derive great pleasure from stroking fabrics; more particularly she learned to bite her nails down to the quick, so that at times of depression and loneliness she could rub the sensitive bared fingertips over skin or clothing to comfort herself and to replace the fondling of which she had been deprived in infancy by her depressive mother. In therapy sessions, her loneliness, isolation, and sense of abandonment are almost palpable as she quietly rocks and rubs her dress with her bared fingertips.

Effect on Body-image and Self-esteem

In similar fashion, cutaneous contact by stroking, rubbing, or excoriating may be used by the patient to define boundaries and to confirm for the patient his or her body-image and sense of self,[6] when the inner sense of these structures is impaired. For the developmental reasons that have been described, self-esteem is frequently poor in atopic patients, and this is further diminished by the visible and disfiguring dermatosis.

We each assign a different value and ascribe a different inner meaning to different areas of the body; the head and face followed closely by the genitals, have for most people the greatest inner significance.[6] It has been suggested that patients who are more disturbed emotionally when stressed, will scratch most those areas most highly valued; this may evidence a greater self-destructive urge, or a more greatly diminished self-esteem; feeling oneself to be unlovable, the disfigurement makes one even more so.

Scratching as a Conditioned Response

Regardless of the basic psychopathology, and the underlying psychodynamic forces that motivate the drive to scratch, there is no question that scratching also frequently becomes a conditioned response, as has been demonstrated by Jordan and Whitlock.[47] Atopic patients appear to develop this conditioned response very readily, a fact in part attributable to their generally high levels of anxiety.[22,28,46]

TOWARDS A PSYCHOPATHOPHYSIOLOGIC UNDERSTANDING

Even the most skeptical observers accept the concept of a strong psychosomatic interaction in the precipitation and perpetuation of atopic dermatitis.[47] Brown has demonstrated experimentally what is common clinical experience: that potentially stressful events are significantly common in the period preceding the onset of eczema.[15] He reminds us again that in evaluating stress, it is not the event itself that is significant, but rather the meaning of that event to the individual in terms of the individual's intimate relationships, hopes, aspirations, and self-esteem in light of his or her current life-circumstances and past experience. Brown notes further that because of the defense mechanisms employed by many atopic patients, this kind of information is not always readily accessible.

It remains my task to try to arrive at some understanding of the possible mechanisms whereby stress can bring about the pathophysiologic changes that we see in atopic dermatitis. Given the multiplicity of pathophysiologic findings that I have described, it seems unlikely that any unitary theory will satisfy all of our requirements, but interactions in three major areas seem to be involved: sympathetic tone, histamine release, and the immune system. Each of these is mediated by the hypothalamus, as is graphically depicted in Table 3-1.

Increased Sympathetic Arousal

Faulstich et al. have demonstrated an increased sympathetic arousal in atopic patients; this is exemplified by increases in electromyographic activity, and heart rate in response to experimentally induced psychophysiologic stress that are significantly above those of the controls.[23] This finding is consonant with the increased levels of anxiety previously described.[22,28]

This disproportionately heightened sympathetic tone in face of a partial blockade of β-adrenergic receptors will, according to Szentivanyi's theory,[91a] result in relatively greater increases in α-adrenergic and cholinergic activity; each of these three factors, partial β-blockade, and enhanced α-adrenergic and cholinergic activity, can contribute to the increased histamine release that has been described.

Vascular Response

Enhanced vascular responses in atopic patients result in variations in blood flow in response to stress that are significantly greater than those in the controls.[30] These variations generate erythema and pruritus, and because of the inherently lowered itch threshold, stimulate the urge to scratch. A number of mechanisms may be involved; these include increased histamine release as described above, a direct cholinergic vascular response, and release of the other stress-related vasoactive neuropeptides that I have previously discussed.

Immune Regulation

The reader is referred to Chapter 3 for a more extensive review of the influence of emotional factors on immune regulation. Suffice it to say here that stress has been demonstrated to influence virtually every aspect of immunologic activity;[2] and thus may be expected to exacerbate all those elements of the atopic process that are mediated by the immune system.

It remains to be demonstrated experimentally in appropriately controlled studies, the specific pathways that link emotional experience with somatic expression in patients with atopic dermatitis, but given the inherent predisposition in terms of genetic endowment and early life-experience, it is evident that stress has the capacity to trigger pathophysiologic mechanisms in a number of ways. These include:

1. Enhanced histamine release via enhanced IgE production, via Type 1 immunologic responses, and via the effect of neurotransmitters on cyclic nucleotide metabolism.
2. Centrally or peripherally mediated pruritic and vascular reactions that lead to scratching.
3. An increased sweat response.
4. Increased susceptibility to bacterial, viral, and fungal infections, with a secondary release of the chemical mediators of inflammation that cause itching and lead to scratching.

COURSE AND PROGNOSIS

In 60 percent of patients the onset of dermatitis is in the first year of life, and 85 percent within the first 5 years:[75] of these children, 30-50 percent will subsequently develop asthma or hay fever.[82] Although the disease may appear, clear, or relapse at any time, there is a greater tendency for spontaneous resolution during infancy, at puberty, and after the second decade; while a figure of 30 percent is quoted for patients over 20 years of age,[82,90] continuation past 30 years is uncommon, and only 2 percent of patients are said to be over 45.[45] The course in many cases is continuous, though remissions of up to as long as 2 to 10 years may occur. Vickers, in a 20 year study of 2000 patients, found that onset after 6 months of age, a discoid pattern, parental discord, and social problems all had an adverse effect on prognosis. In contrast, early onset, a seborrhoeic pattern, and a treatment approach that reduced itching to a minimum were favorable to a good outcome.[95] Ninty-three percent of this series were recovered by age 15 years, but no figures are available either for relapse after puberty or for the later appearance of any of the adult manifestations of atopy.

Nummular eczema and chronic vesicular eruptions of the hands and feet (dyshidrotic eczema, pompholyx—see Figure 17-3) are reaction patterns that may follow a chronic and recurrent course and that in a percentage of cases are atopic in origin. Though a prior history of dermatitis may not be obtainable, other atopic manifestations are often in the background. Similarly up to 50 percent of patients with chronic ano-genital pruritis are thought to have atopic dermatitis.[82]

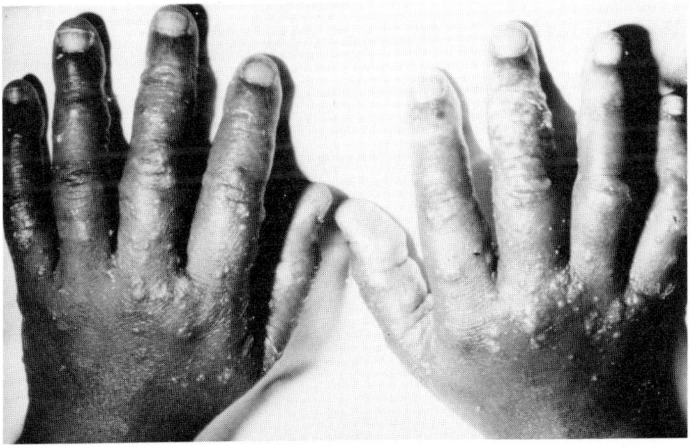

Figure 17-3. Dyshidrotic eczema. When palmar and plantar hyperhidrosis is associated with the atopic diathesis eczematous eruptions of the hands and feet may result. Because the hyperhidrosis has a psychogenic origin, lesions of this kind are often very recalcitrant. This 5-year-old also had large bullae on the palms and less severe dermatosis of the feet. Note the size of the primary lesions typical of the location.

MANAGEMENT

Dermatologic Management

The successful long-term management of severe atopic dermatitis is perhaps one of the most frustrating challenges in clinical dermatology, and one that will test the physician's ingenuity to the full. A full discussion of current and conventional specific treatment modalities can be found in the standard dermatology texts; space does not permit their inclusion here. Where relevant they will be alluded to in the next section, in general terms only.

Since the prognosis appears to be significantly and favorably affected by aggressive treatment at the onset,[95,96] and by the implementation of modalities that control the urge to scratch, it is towards this end that the various treatment approaches will be directed.

Psychological Management

The general principles of the psychological management of psychocutaneous disease are discussed in Chapter 5.

The importance of a positive therapeutic relationship between doctor and patient is addressed in Chapter 16, and that discussion is equally relevant to the treatment of atopic dermatitis.

Patient Education

Infantile and childhood atopic dermatitis. If the patient or parent is to work cooperatively in a positive therapeutic relationship, he or she must have a thorough understanding of the disease in all its aspects; patient education as a therapeutic tool cannot be over-emphasized.

The expectable course and prognosis must be made clear to the mother. She must understand that although there is much she can do to help her child, it is unlikely that she will be able to keep the child's skin always clear; she must learn to tolerate imperfections and criticism from family and friends without guilt or self-blame. The need for long-term and adequate hydration and use of emollients should be stressed.

The mother must understand the need to avoid repeated bacterial or viral infections. Routine prophylactic use of antibacterial cleansers such as 4 percent chlorhexidine gluconate (Hibiclens Antimicrobial Skin Cleanser, Stuart, Wilmington, DE) should be recommended, as should avoidance of contact with persons with herpes simplex.

The question of food allergies will be raised, and the physician must be prepared to make clear his or her own position in this regard. I personally do not find a cause and effect relationship between specific foods and atopic flares, and do not recommend dietary restrictions unless an urticarial response suggests a relevance.

The mother must understand the inherent "itchiness" of her child's skin, its susceptibility to irritants, and the crucial role of scratching in development of overt lesions. The role of frequent hot baths, alkaline soaps, harsh or whiskery fabrics, draughts, heat, or sweating in triggering the itch response must be explained. A description of this inherent "itchiness" has perhaps not been bettered since Erasmus Wilson wrote, in 1868:[105]

> The great, the urgent symptom of the whole, is the teasing, the intense, the violent itching; sometimes the itching is constant, with frequent exacerbations; sometimes there are intervals of repose which are apt to be disturbed by changes of temperature, and then a violent attack of pruritis recommences; but the crowning suffering of all occurs at night; the child is often frantic with itching; it scratches with all its force, digging its little nails into the flesh, while the blood and ichor run down in streams. At last, worn out with suffering and exhaustion the child sleeps, probably to be awakened again several times in the night, by a repetition of the same agony. This constant suffering naturally wears out the child's powers, and added to the mal-assimilation, brings about the state of atrophy previously described. But it is remarkable how little the strength and spirits of the child are affected by these separate paroxysms of suffering; in the morning, after a night of distress, the little thing is fresh and lively, eager for food, and ready for the battle of the day; while the nurse or mother is languid and powerless, from watching and anxiety.

Through an appropriate concern about the possible local and systemic complications of the long-term or excessive use of glucocorticoids, there has in recent years been a barrage of admonition in the lay and medical press that has amount to "overkill"; as a result, many mothers are terrified of the concept of "steroids," and resistant even to their appropriate or minimal application.

It is of paramount importance for these mothers to understand that the effects from itching are a far greater hazard than are those from topical glucocorticoids; for itching leads to scratching, and thereby to an exacerbation of the eruption that can leave the way open to physical and emotional distress, and to all of the complications of atopic dermatitis. It is far better to use effective short courses of potent preparations than prolonged but ineffective courses of less potent agents. One of the factors favorable to a good long-term prognosis is early control by the adequate use of antihistamines and topical glucocorticoids.[95]

Vickers was able to demonstrate remissions of up to 1 year following short courses of clobetasol cream in a tapered-down schedule, in children who had previously been unresponsive to coal tar derivatives and emollients.[96] Interestingly Vickers observed a growth spurt following control of the dermatitis, in some of these children who had previously been in the lower percentiles. This raises interesting questions about the short stature frequently seen in children with severe atopic disease: is it secondary to psychosocial factors?[84] Is it secondary to the uncontrolled disease itself? Or is it secondary to the injudicious use of glucocorticoids (Fig. 17-4)?

The mother must be educated about the ways her child will try to manipulate her, and be alert to the danger of the child's disrupting the entire family, through the use of his or her skin; he or she is likely to play on the mother's guilt and sympathy, monopolize her time, and drain her energy, at the expense of siblings and father. The mother must be encouraged not to over protect the child, and to help him or her live as normal a life as possible. The desired objective is to have a child who is independent, and who can acquire the skills to take charge of his or her own medication and skin care.

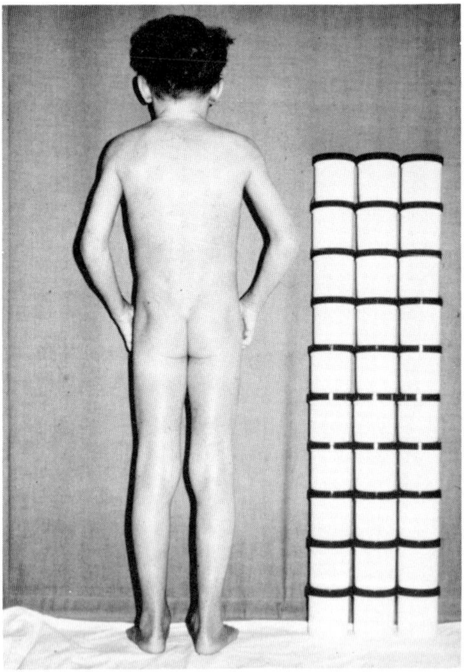

Figure 17-4. Chronic atopic dermatitis. This greatly undersized 12-year-old had had extensive atopic dermatitis for at least a decade. An inquiry from the State Welfare Department alerted us to the fact that in the course of 3 months this patient had consumed 30 lbs of 0.1 percent Triamcinolone cream. The patient spent hours each day rubbing himself with cream. Eucerin was used in similar quantities.

It is well known that some frustration of unfettered infantile demands is necessary, if satisfactory emotional growth and development is to take place.[89] While we understand that scratching will exacerbate the dermatitis, at the same time we must recognise that no mother can permit herself to succumb to the insatiable demands for love and attention that are expressed by her child in terms of misery and distress through anxiety, wakefulness, restlessness, itching, and paroxysmal excoriation.

It is the ambivalent mother who is most at risk here, because her unconscious guilt about feelings of hostility towards her child may motivate her to over-react, and to do everything within her power to prevent the child's aggressive excoriation. The more the child's demands are gratified, the more dependent does the child become on that gratification. The child's behavior regresses in the face of frustration and he or she becomes ever more tiresome, intrusive, clinging, and demanding. Inevitably this regressive behavior will arouse further hostility and frustration in the mother, and resentment in other family members, so that a vicious spiral develops.

In contrast, the mother without conflict will be able to tolerate displays of aggression in her child; she will empathise with the child's distress and feelings of frustration, but she will nevertheless permit scratching or crying until the child gradually comes to recognise that these weapons do not empower him or her to control the mother. Once this is clear, the child's insatiable demands are likely to be given up, and the two can work together to relieve his or her distress.

Williams, recognising the importance of directly or indirectly expressed maternal rejection, educated mothers in appropriate interaction with their atopic infants as part of the treatment; he hoped to relieve the children of the need to express angry feelings towards their mothers.[104] Forty-five percent of 33 patients whose mothers were educated in this way were symptom-free after 24 months, while the same was true for only 10 percent of the controls.

In my own practice a rather characteristic group of patients illustrates this point.[50] These were children, eight in all, in whom maternal ambivalence was such that the mother was unable to deny any call on her time whatever. In each case the entire family had been held hostage by the patient, and demands had been met even to share the parental bed, in order that one or other parent might in turn constantly stroke or rub the patient to soothe the itchy skin throughout the night. For the parents this intrusion on their privacy could not but be inhibiting and frustrating, and for the child, while it provided a gratification that was hard to give up, it perpetuated infantile dependency and heightened anxiety by generating intense emotional responses that were difficult for a small child to handle.

In each of these patients the eczema had remained wholly recalcitrant, despite very aggressive dermatologic treatment, until the parents had been educated as to the psychodynamics of the interaction, and supported in a gentle but firm denial of the child's unreasonable demands, particularly those with regard to the bedroom, and the parental bed.

What is it that determines which child will clear in infancy or at puberty, and which will continue with dermatitis into adult life, in a remitting or relentless and unremitting course?

When inherent predisposition, environmental factors, and emotional status are in equilibrium, there will be no disease, but an uneven weighting of any one of these three may trigger an exacerbation.

Clearly the child with the greater inherent predisposition will be at greater risk from relatively more minor changes in environment or emotions, and for the infant, the environment includes also the emotional milieu of the mother-child relationship. Scratching and chronic changes, whatever the circumstances, will perpetuate the disease.

If the physical milieu is not manipulated to reduce the drive to scratch, chronic disease will result; similarly if aberrations persist in the emotional milieu, in terms of unanswered emotional needs or continued generation of anxiety and aggression, scratching will persist and chronic disease ensue. Psychosocial stress strong enough to overwhelm the psychologic defenses and permit emotional regression at any time may permit reactivation of immature emotional responses. Generation of non-neutralised aggressive energy then results in a resurgence of the drive to scratch, and exacerbation may ensue.

Older children and adults. The same educational objectives pertain in older children and adults. The part played by anxiety or stress in triggering the itch response should be plainly stated in such a way that the patient does not feel judged, but rather can begin to look at him or herself from that perspective.

Adolescents should be educated about bathing habits and about overheating and sweating if they participate in athletics; occupational irritants should be discussed with adults, where relevant.

Specific Therapies

Although there is some impression in the literature that *psychotherapy* is not helpful in the management of atopic dermatitis, many authors report positive results from that modality.

Psychoanalysis and *psychoanalytic psychotherapy* are both helpful in cases where the criteria for these treatments are met, and the patient well-motivated.[52,85] *Short-term therapies* are reported successful, particularly those directed towards helping the patient to express directly their suppressed or repressed hostility.[78,86,99] Brown and Bettley found that while one third of atopic patients will complain spontaneously of psychiatric symptoms, one third will do so only when asked; the remaining "super-stable" one third, rather than being free of emotional difficulties, they felt, were merely highly defended, and emotionally restricted. Asa result, these authors took into brief psychotherapy (limited arbitrarily to 4 months) a half of a group of 72 adult patients who were randomly assigned.[16] They found that the rate of clearing was doubled in those patients who received psychotherapy in addition to standard dermatologic therapy, but only if those patients had overt emotional difficulties, and if they were well-motivated.

Hypnosis has been used to help control the itching response. Because of the heightened anxiety levels previously mentioned,[22,28] *stress-management techniques*, and *autogenic training* may be helpful for symptom relief in some cases; manipulation of the environment may also be indicated to reduce stress. *Behavior modification therapies* have also received attention,[10] because scratching can be viewed as a conditioned response.[46] Progressive relaxation[77] systematic desensitisation,[10] and a number of other techniques designed to make the patient ignore the itching and so permit the skin to heal, have been employed. Melni et al. describe a method designed to encourage behavior incompatible with scratching. They found a significant improvement in patients who received this approach in addition to corticosteroid creams over those who used creams alone.[64] In children, parents have been recruited to apply behavioral techniques to their children,[5] with some success. Needless to say, these methods eradicate only the symptom of scratching; they are not applicable to patients with more profound emotional problems.

The place of *support groups* has been discussed in detail in the previous chapter, and the same remarks apply here. The National Eczema Society provides appropriate services in Great Britain,[7] and a similar group is reported from Australia.[63]

Psychotropic drugs have a place in treatment also. *Tranquillizers* should be restricted to short-term administration at times of physical illness, or external stress; the long-term use of these drugs is not appropriate in the treatment of chronic disease.

Tricyclic antidepressants are extremely useful in the treatment of atopic dermatitis. Depression is a not uncommon concomitant, while the marked antihistamine effect provides superior antipruritic activity. These drugs are prescribed according to the schedule described in the section on psychotropic drugs in Chapter 5.

Monoamine oxidase inhibitors are discussed by Friedman et al. They report dramatic results in atopic dermatitis from the use of high doses of phenelzine; side effects were rather common. This drug should be reserved for very severe and recalcitrant cases.[25,26]

THE SOMATOPSYCHIC EFFECT

As is the case with psoriasis, so the emotional toll on the eczema sufferer and his or her family is a heavy one. The mothers of atopic infants frequently feel inadequate because of their inability to control the disease, and guilty because their child is in distress. The extra work in caring for the child, and lack of sleep from the child's restlessness conspire to make her short-tempered and resentful, and guilty on that account also. Siblings become demanding and difficult because they feel that they do not get enough attention, and the financial burden of medical care adds to the marital stress that is not uncommon.

Although Hill-Beuf and Porter found that in impaired children those whose impairment developed earlier, suffered less emotional disturbance than did those whose developed later,[41] many young children have significant difficulties. Emotional developmental arrest, or regression because of dependence on the mother, and the aberrant nature of the mother-child relationship, lead to a babyishness that is resented by siblings and peers, while the physical appearance may cause the child to avoid friendships, for fear of rejection. Loss of school-time through periods of illness contributes to the loneliness and the emotional immaturity.

In older children and young adults close relationships are often avoided, again for fear of rejection, and out-door activities shunned lest exposure bring ridicule. Many patients are "loners." As is the case with psoriasis, eczema sufferers fear that employment opportunities will be closed to them because of their appearance, and to this is added the realistic risk of exposure to irritants that will preclude certain occupations.

Physical appearance, cost, the need for time-consuming and often unpleasant treatments, the damaging effect of greasy preparations on clothing, and the resentment of healthy siblings, all serve to make the patient feel "different," inferior, and resentful and may contribute to the already considerable unconscious anger and hostility, and to feelings of depression.[57]

REFERENCES

1. Abramson S, Dahl MW, Walsh G, et al.: Antistaphylococcal IgE levels in patients with atopic dermatitis. J Am Acad Dermatol 7:105-110, 1982
2. Ader R (ed): Psychoneuromimmunology. New York, Academic Press, 1981
3. Ahlquist RP: Study of adrenergic receptors. Am J Physiol 153:586-600, 1948
4. Aldrich RA, Steinberg AG, Campbell DC: Pedigree demonstrating a sex-linked recessive condition characterized by draining ears, eczematoid dermatitis, and bloody diarrhoea. Pediatrics 13:133-139, 1954
5. Allen DE, Harris FR: Elimination of a child's excessive scratching by training the mother in re-inforcement procedures. Behav Res Ther 4:79-84, 1966
6. Anderson PC, Cross TN: Body cathexis and neurodematitis. Comprehens

Psychiat 4:40-46, 1963

7. Ardill L: The National Eczema Society. Practitioner 22:1059-1062, 1984
8. Atherton DJ, et al.: A double-blind cross-over trial of an antigen avoidance diet in atopic eczema. Lancet 1:401-403, 1978
9. Banna SL: Concordances in atopic twins. J Allergy Clin Immunol 71:100A, 1983
10. Bar LHJ, Kuypers BRM: Behavior therapy in dermatological practice. Br J Dermatol 88:591-598, 1973
11. Bonini S, Rasi G, Trillo ME, et al.: Atopy in twins. J Allergy Clin Immunol 71:100A, 1983
12. Brocq L, Jacquet L: Notes pour servir a l'historie des neurodermites: ou lichen circumscriptus des anciens auteurs, ou lichen simplex chronique de M. le Dr. E. Vidal. Ann Dermatol Syphie (Paris) 2:634, 1892
13. Brostoff J, Carini C, Wraith D, Johns P: Production of IgE complexes by allergen challenge in atopic patients, and the effect of sodium cromoglycate. Lancet 1:1268-1270, 1979
14. Brown DG: Emotional disturbance in eczema. A study of symptom reporting behavior. J Psychosom Res 11:27-40, 1967
15. Brown DG: Stress as a precipitant factor of eczema. J Psychosom Res 16:321-327, 1972
16. Brown DG, Bettley FR: Psychiatric treatment of eczema: A controlled trial. Br Med J 2:729-734, 1971
17. Butler JM, Chan SC, Stevens SR, et al.: Increased leukocyte histamin release with elevated cyclic AMP-phosphodiesterase activity in atopic dermatitis. J Allergy Clin Immunol 71:490-497, 1983
18. Byrom NA, Timlin DM: Immune status in atopic eczema: A survey. Br J Dermatol 100:491-498, 1979
19. Byrom NA, Staughton RCD, Campbell JA, et al.: Thymosin-inducible "null" cells in atopic eczema. Br J Dermatol 100:499-510, 1979
20. Cheng DS, Hanifin JM: Atopic dermatitis, in Theirs BH, Dobson Rl (eds): Pathogenesis of Skin Disease. New York, Churchill-Livingstone, 1986
21. Elliot ST, Hanifin JM: Delayed cutaneous hypersensitivity and lymphocyte transformation. Arch Dermatol 115:36-39, 1979
22. Faulstich ME, Williamson DA, Duchmann EG, et al.: Psychophysiological analysis of atopic dermatitis. J Psychosom Res 29:415-417, 1985
23. Faulstich ME, Williamson D: An overview of atopic dermatitis: towards a bio-behavioral integration. J Psychosom Res 29:6:647-654, 1985
24. Freud A: The Writings of Anna Freud, Vol III. New York, International University Press, 1973, pp 169-170
25. Friedman S, Kantor I, Sobel S, et al.: On the treatment of chemotherapy of neurodermatitis with a monoamine oxidase inhibitor. J Nerv Ment Dis 166:117-125, 1978

26. Friedman S, Kantor I, Sobel S, et al.: A follow-up study of the treatment of neurodermatitis with a monoamine oxidase inhibitor. J Nerv Ment Dis 166:349-357, 1978
27. Fritz GF: Psychological aspects of atopic dermatitis. A viewpoint. Clin Peds 18:360-364, 1979
28. Garrie EV, Garrie SA, Mok T: Anxiety and atopic dermatitis. J Consult Clin Psychol 42:742,1974
29. Goeckerman WH: Discussion of Brunsting LA, Atopic dermatits (disseminated neurodermatitis) in young adults. Arch Dermatol Syph 34:6, 935-957
30. Graham DT, Wolff S: The relation of eczema to attitude and to vascular reactions of the human skin. J Lab Clin Med 42:238-254, 1953
31. Greenacre P: Early physical determinants in the development of the sense of identity. J Am Psychoanal Assn 6:612-627, 1958
32. Greenhill MH, Finesinger JE: Neurotic symptoms and emotional factors in atopic dermatitis. Arch Dermatol Syph 46:187-200, 1942
33. Grewe SR, Chan SC, Hanifin JM: Elevated leukocyto cyclic AMP phosphodiesterase in atopic disease: A possible mechanism for cAMP-agonist hyporesponsiveness. J Allergy Clin Immunol 70:452-237, 1982
34. Hagerman G: The importance of food factors in atopic dermatitis. Acta Dermato Venereologica. S Hellerstrom 65 years, 1966, p 81
35. Hall-Smith SP, Norton A: Psychiatric survey of a random sample of skin out-patients. Br Med J 2:417-421, 1952
36. Hanifin JM: Atopic dermatitis. J Am Acad Dermatol 6:1-30, 1982
37. Haruack K: Experimental itch as a diagnostic method. Acta Dermatol Venereologica, suppl 92:40-41, 1980
38. Henderson WR, Shelhammer JH, Rheingold DB, et al.: Alpha-adrenergic hyperresponsiveness in asthma. New Eng J Med 300:642-647, 1979
39. Heseltine GF: The site of onset of eczema and personality trait differences: an exploratory study. J Psychosom Res 7:241-246, 1963
40. Hill HR, Quie PG: Raised serum IgE levels and defective neutrophil chemotaxis in three children with eczema and recurrent bacterial infections. Lancet 1:183-187, 1974
41. Hill-Beuf A, Porter JDR: Children coping with impaired appearance: Social and psychological influences. Gen Hosp Psychiat 6:294-301, 1984
42. Hoffmann DR, Yamamoto FY, Geller B, Haddad Z: specific IgE antibodies in atopic eczema. J Allergy Clin Immunol 55:256-67, 1975
43. Hurwitz S: Clinical Pediatric Dermatology. Philadelphia, WB Saunders, 1981, p 39
44. Johnson HH, de Oreo GA, Lascheid AP, et al.: Skin histamine levels in chronic atopic dermatitis. J Invest Dermatol 34:237-238, 1960

45. Johnson ML: Prevalence of Dermatologic Disease among Persons 1-74 years of age. United Staes, Advance Data from Vital and Health Statistics, No. 4, Jan 26, 1977
46. Jordan JM, Whitlock FA: Emotions and the skin: the conditioning of the scratch response in cases of atopic dermatitis. Br J Dermatol 86:574-585, 1972
47. Jordan JM, Whitlock FA: Atopic Dermatitis. Anxiety and conditioned scratch responses. J Psychosom Res 18:297-299, 1974
48. Kaliner M: The cholinergic nervous system and immediate hypersensitivity. J Allergy Clin Immunol 58:308-315, 1976
49. Kaliner MA, Orange RP, Koopman WJ, et al.: Pathopharmacologic enhancement of the IgE mediated release of histamine, and slow reacting substance of anaphylaxis in the rat, in Lepow IH, Ward PA (eds): Inflammation: Mechanisms and Control. New York, Academic Press, 1972
50. Kaufman HS, Frick OL: The development of allergy in infants of allergic parents: A prospective study concerning the role of heredity. Ann Allergy 37:410-415, 1976
51. Kidd CB, Watt, KIM: Neuroticcism and distribution of lesions in patients with skin disease. J Psychosom Res 11:253-261, 1967
52. Koblenzer CS, Koblenzer PJ: Infantile atopic dermatitis. (In preparation)
53. Kuypers, BRM: Atopic dermatitis: some observations from a psychological viewpoint. Dermatologica 136:387-394, 1968
54. Leung DYM, Rhodes AR, Geha RS: Enumeration of T cell subsets in atopic dermatitis using monoclonal antibodies. J Allergy Clin Immunol 67:450, 1981
55. Leung DYM, Rhodes AR, Geha RS: Atopic dermatitis in dermatology, in Fitzpatrick TB, Eisen AZ, Wolff K, et al. (eds): General Medicine (ed 3). New York, McGraw Hill, 1986
56. Leung DYM, Saryan JA, Frankel R, et al.: Impairment of the autologous mixed lymphocyte reaction in atopic dermatitis. J Clin Invest 72:1482-6, 1983
57. Levy RJ: The Rorschach pattern in neurodermatitis. Psychosom Med 14:41-49, 1952
58. Liddle GW, Hardman JG: Cyclic adenosine monophosphate as a mediator of hormone action. N Eng J Med 285:560-566, 1971
59. Lynch FW, Hinckley RG, Cowan DW: Psychosomatic studies in dermatology. Arch Dermatol Syph 51:251-260, 1945
60. Marmor J, Ashley M, Tabachnick N, et al.: The mother-child relationship in the genesis of neurodermatitis. Arch Dermatol 74:599-605, 1956
61. Marsh DC, Meyers DA, Bias WB: The epidemiology and genetics of atopic allergy. New Engl J Med 305:1551-1559, 1981

62. Masuda T, Naito A, Kinoshita M, et al.: Acetylcholine inhalation test in atopic dermatitis. J Allergy Clin Immunol 40:193-201, 1967
63. McSkimming J, Gleeson L, Sinclair M: A pilot study of a support group for parents of children with eczema. Aust J Dermatol 25:8-11, 1984
64. Melni L, Frederiksen T, Nore P, et al.: Behavioral treatment of scratching in patients with atopic dermatitis. Br J Dermatol 115:467-474, 1986
65. Mihm MC Jr, Soter NA, Dvorak HF, et al.: The structures of normal skin and the morphology of atopic eczema. J Invest Dermatol 67:305-312, 1976
66. Miller HL: Psychodynamic mechanisms in a case of neurodermatitis. Psychosom Med 10:309-316, 1948
67. Miller HL, Baruch DW: Psychosomatic studies of children with allergic manifestations. I. Maternal rejection. Psychosom Med 10:275-278, 1948
68. Musaph H: Itching and Scratching. Philadelphia, FA Davis Co, 1964
69. Nemiah TC, Freyberger H, Siffneos PE: Alexthymia: a view of the psychosomatic processes, in Hill OW (ed): Modern Trends in Psychosomatic Medicine, Vol 3. London, Butterworth, 1976, pp 430-439
70. Obermeyer ME: Psychocutaneous Medicine. Springfield, IL, Charles C. Thomas, 1955, pp 202-214
71. O'Laughlin S, Diaz-Perez J, Gleich G, Winkleman R: Serum Ig E in dermatitis and dermatosis. Arch Dermatol 113:309-315, 1977
72. Palacios J, Fuller EW, Blaylock WK: Immunological capabilities of patients with atopic dermatitis. J Invest Dermatol 47:484-490, 1966
73. Panconesi E: Stress and Skin Disease. Psychosomatic Dermatology, Clinics in Dermatology 2:4. Philadelphia, JB Lippincott, 1984
74. Peterson RDA, Page AR, Good RA: Wheal and erythema allergy in patients with Agammaglobulinemia. J Allergy Clin Immunol 33:406-411, 1962
75. Rajka G: Atopic Dermatitis. London, WB Saunders 1975
76. Rajka G: Atopic dermatitis, in Rook AJ, Maibach HE (eds): Recent Advances in Dermatology 6. New York, Churchill-Livingstone, 1983, p 109
77. Ratliff RG, Stein NH: Treatment of neurodermatitis by behavior therapy. Behav Res Ther 6:397-399, 1968
78. Rogerson CH: The role of psychotherapy in the treatment of the asthma-eczema-prurigo complex in children, Br J Dermatol 46:368-378, 1934
79. Rogerson CH: Psychological factors in skin disorders. Br J Dermatol 59:6-13, 1947
80. Rosenthal MJ: A psychosomatic study of infaantile eczema. 1. The mother-child relationship. Pediatrics 10:581-591, 1952
81. Rosenthal MJ: Neuropsychiatric aspects of infantile eczema. Arch Neurol Psychiat 70:428-451, 1953
82. Roth HL, Kierland RR: The natural history of atopic dermatitis. Arch Dermatol 89:209-214, 1964

83. Saryan JA, Leung DYM, Geha RS: Induction of human IgE synthesis by a factor derived from T-cells of patients with hyper IgE states. J Immunol 130:242-247, 1983
84. Schanburg SM, Kuhn C: Maternal deprivation: an animal model of psychosocial dwarfism, in Usdin E, Sourkes T, Moussa BH, Youdi M (eds): Enzymes and Neurotransmitters in Mental Disease. New York, Wiley, 1980, pp 373-393
85. Schecter M: Psychoanalysis of a latency boy with neurodermatitis, in Eissler RS (ed): Psychoanalytic Study of the Child, Vol 26. New York, Quadrangle Books, 1973, pp 529-564
86. Schoenberg B, Carr AC: An investigation of criteria for brief psychotherapy of neurodermatitis. Psychosom Med 25:253-263, 1963
87. Schur M: Comments on the metapsychology of somatization, in Eissler RS (ed): The Psychoanalytic Study of the Child. New York, University Press Inc, 1955, Vol 10, pp 119-164
88. Soter NA, Lewis RA, Corey EJ, Austen KF: Local effects of synthetic leukotrienes (LTC4, LTD4 and LTB4) in human skin. J Invest Dermatol 80:115-119, 1983
89. Spitz RA: The First Year of Life. New York, University Press, 1971
90. Stifler WC: A 21-year follow-up of infantile eczema. J Pediat 66:166, 1965
91. Stokes JH: The effect on the skin of emotional and nervous states; masochism and other sex complexes in the background of neurogenous dermatitis. Arch Dermatol Syph 22:803-810, 1930
91a. Sventivanyi A: The beta-adranergic theory of atopic abuosuiability in bronchial asthma. J Allergy 42:203-232, 1968
92. Tantam D, Kalucy R, Brown DG: Sleep, scratching, dreams in eczema. A new approach to alexithymia. Psychother Psychosom 37:26-35, 1982
93. Uhehara M, Ofuji S: Abnormal vascular reactions in atopic dermatitis. Arch Dermatol 113:627-629, 1977
94. Vaughan VC III: Emotional undertones in eczema in children. J Asthma Res 3:193-197, 1966
95. Vickers CFH: Factors influencing the prognosis of infantile eczema—another 10 years. Br J Dermatol 99(16):22, 1978
96. Vickers CFH: Juvenile atopic dermatitis. Skin and Allergy News, April 1986, p 40
97. Vidal E: Du Lichen (Lichen, prurigo, strophulus) Ann de Dermat et Syph 17:131-154, 1886
98. Walker RB, Warin RP: Incidence of eczema in early childhood. Br J Derm 68:182-183, 1956
99. Walsh MN, Kierland RR: Psychotherapy in the treatment of neurodermatitis. Staff meetings of the Mayo Clinic 22:578-584, 1947

100. Wasserman SI: The mast cell and its mediators, in Goldsmith LA (ed): Biochemistry and Physiology of the Skin. New York, Oxford University Press, 1983, p 880
101. West RJ, Johnson LA, Winkelman RK: Delayed Blanch phenomenon in atopic individuals without dermatitis. Arch Dermatol 85:227-228, 1962
102. Whitfield A: On the white reaction in dermatology. Br J Dermatol 50:71, 1938
103. Williams DH: Skin temperature reaction to histamine in atopic dermatitis. J Invest Dermatol 1:119-129, 1938
104. Williams DH: Management of atopic dermatitis in children. Control of the maternal rejection factor. Arch Dermatol Syph 63:545-560, 1951
105. Wilson E: A Practical and Theoretical treatise on the Diagnosis, Pathology and Treatment of Diseases of the Skin. London, Churchill, 1842, p 115

Chapter 18

Further Applications of Psychosomatic Principles to Dermatology

It is perhaps foolhardy for us to ignore the observations of wise and experienced clinicians, even when those observations (though repeated over and over again) are anecdotal at best and not subject to support from laboratory tests or reproducible and measurable findings; to do so serves only to close in certain directions, the pathways to advancing knowledge.

Psoriasis is a case in point; earlier dermatologists repeatedly observed situations where stress seemed to precipitate or aggravate the disorder,[20] but lack of controlled studies to support their clinical observations apparently dampened interest and blocked temporarily that particular avenue of research. Attention instead was focussed in other directions, tremendous strides were made in our understanding of the disease process, and stress gradually came to be left out of the equation as a factor to be considered seriously. As more and more pieces of the pathophysiologic puzzle begin to fall into place, in more and more instances do we find facets of the disease where, because of capabilities that are now subject to experimental scrutiny and confirmation, stress can be expected to influence pathophysiology. These facets, which are outlined in Chapter 16, seem to be providing a stimulus for confirmatory laboratory studies; examples would be the studies that demonstrate how psoriatic patients behave differently, biochemically and metabolically, than controls, under experimental conditions of stress.[4] Farber's hypothesis with regard to substance-P is interesting in a similar vein,[10] and provides another area where solid psychophysiologic research should prove fruitful.

But to date, studies that rigorously and scientifically confirm the psychosomatic interactions that clinical experience insistently avers must take place are few. Much information is speculative at best. The field for future psychoimmunologic, psychoendocrinologic, and psychometabolic research is fertile indeed, but in order to make advances, we must be emotionally able to tolerate unproven hypotheses.

If we accept the premise of a psychosociobiological view of illness, as presented throughout this text,[29] then thc principles that I have elaborated in the preceding two chapters can be applied to the entire spectrum of disease: for our purposes, this encompasses the entire spectrum of dermatologic disease.

The proportion contributed by each of the three compartments, inherent predisposition, environment, and psychosocial stress, will vary from disease to disease, and from patient to patient, but in each case, when the three are in equilibrium, there will be no disease; when the balance is tipped by an uneven weighting of any one of the three, disease will result.

LICHEN PLANUS

Lichen planus, for example, clearly fits the psychosociobiological view of disease. Familial cases are reported,[18] suggesting genetic factors, and an inherent predisposition is supported also by the readiness with which some persons develop a lichenoid reaction; a contribution from the environment is evident in those cases caused by photographic developers,[6] or where the eruption represents a reaction to certain drugs.[7] The situation with regard to emotional factors is less clear-cut; formerly believed to have strong psychogenic components,[20] recent texts and papers have tended to down-play[26] if not to out-right deny[2] this aspect. But once again clinical observation would seem to support the possibility of an emotional trigger, even if such a trigger has not been confirmed experimentally. An anecdote (unsupported) will serve to make my point:

A 60-year-old woman had no previous history of any kind of skin disease. Recently retired from a singularly successful professional career, where she had risen unusually high in her field for one of her sex and race, she was planning to pursue a rigorously intellectual avocation. Her elderly husband was involved in an accident. Within days of the accident this woman developed extensive lichen planus. Her husband made a rather slow and incomplete recovery from his injuries; he did not resume driving, remained dependent on my patient to get around, and to care for him, and became demanding and critical of her every move. This woman was unable to pursue her avocation because of his helplessness and his demands, and she no longer had her profession. She was in fact tied to the house more than at any time since her children were small. She became depressed and angry with her husband, but also guilty because anger was unacceptable to her. During the course of the following year her itching was intractable and her lesions so hypertrophic that they failed to respond to any modality; on several occasions hypertrophic tissue was removed from thighs, legs, and lower back by laser vaporization (Fig. 18-1). She finally obtained some relief only when antidepressant doses of a tricyclic agent were added to an intensive topical regimen, and when she was enabled to explore, even if only superficially, some of her feelings of anger and resentment.

And what of the psychopathophysiologic mechanism? It now seems likely that lichen planus results from an immunologic process, the reflection of a cell-mediated immune response;[3] increased numbers of Langerhans cells are seen in early lesions, the dense infiltrate in the area of the damaged dermo-epidermal junction is composed almost exclusively of helper-T-cells, and a lichen planus-specific antigen has been detected within the epidermis.[21] Once cell damage has occurred, humoral mediators can be expected to be released and inflammation initiated.

The effect of stress on immune mechanisms, on T-cell subsets, and on the release of the humoral mediators of inflammation has been discussed at length throughout this text.

ACNE VULGARIS

Acne vulgaris is another condition in which pathogenesis results from the complex interaction of a number of variables, and that accords well with the psychosociobiological view of disease.

A genetic predisposition that may involve differing elements of the disease process independently, sets the stage;[9] a variety of environmental factors that include local trauma and friction, certain cosmetics and petroleum byproducts,[23] medications,[13] sweating, and excessive sun-light exposure,[14] are known to aggravate it; androgenic hormones are crucial, and the place of stress will be discussed later.

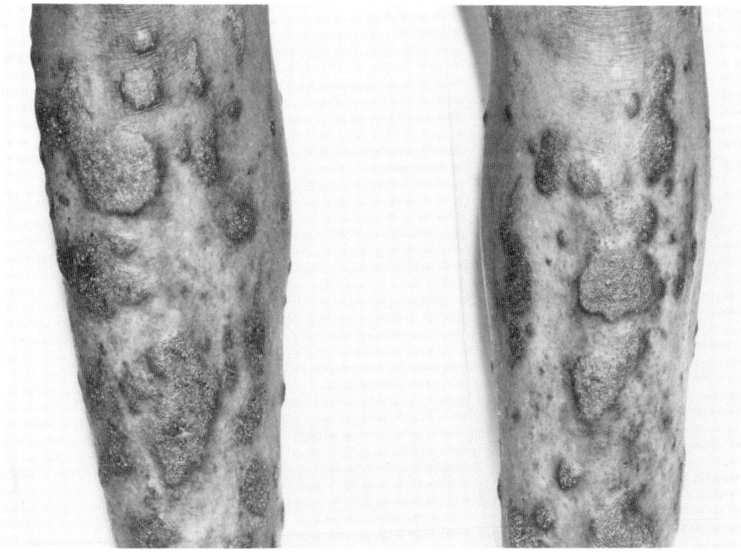

Figure 18-1. Hypertrophic lichen planus. Rubbing and scratching in a case of lichen planus may produce hypertrophic lesions of this type. Recovery even with aggressive therapy might take months or even years

The pubertal burst of circulating androgens promotes enlargement of the sebaceous glands and the increased secretion of sebum. This sebum secretion is a prerequisite for acne to develop, and may or may not be the only contribution of androgens to the disease.[9] While in males the gonads provide the source, in females in addition to ovarian androgens, particularly in the post-adolescent age-group, excessive adrenal androgen appears to play a significant part.[17]

Given this central importance of the sebaceous gland to the acne process, the control of sebaceous activity becomes relevant and the participation of a number of pituitary hormones, other than those directly related to androgen production, is not without interest; growth hormone, prolactin, melanocyte stimulating hormone (MSH), and possibly other neurohumoral agents are involved;[27] the question of a specific sebotropic hormone is currently controversial.

The inflammatory component is dependent on the presence of bacteria within pilosebaceous follicles; of these, proprionibacterium acnes are the most significant and their appearance in large numbers at puberty correlates well with the adolescent increase in sebum production.[27] Free fatty-acids, generated by lipolysis of sebum by bacterial lipases, contribute to the inflammatory response.[15,25]

Another possible source of inflammation, however, is from immunological activity and evidence is accumulating to suggest that this may indeed by the case. Immunoreactants have been identified in follicles and in perilesional skin,[8] circulating anti-P. acnes-antibody levels correlate well with the degree of inflammation that is clinically expressed,[24] and P. acnes has a demonstrated capacity to activate complement[28] by both pathways and so set in motion the inflammatory process (Fig. 18-2).

To summarize rather simplistically then: inborn abnormalities in the process of keratinization of the follicular epithelium of sebaceous follicles become evident at puberty, coincident with an age appropriate hormonally stimulated enlargement of sebaceous glands and increased sebum production. These two changes conspire to produce occlusion of those follicles by comedone formation. An inflammatory component is contributed by follicular bacteria through generation of free fatty acids, through immunologic mechanisms, or perhaps through both of them.

That any one of these steps, in addition to follicular keratinization, may be affected by genetically determined variations is clear and may help to account for the spectrum of clinical presentation.

A variation in the course of acne in response to stress conforms both to common lore and to clinical experience. Adolescents complain about flare-ups before the Prom, college students at exam-time, and adults before important social or professional engagements. A review of the literature confirms what our practice tells us, that no particular personality type characterizes the acne-sufferer,[22] that for many patients stress is the major trigger for exacerbations,[16] and particulary those exacerbations characterized by an inflammatory component,[11] and that acne may have a profound psychological effect on the sufferer.[22]

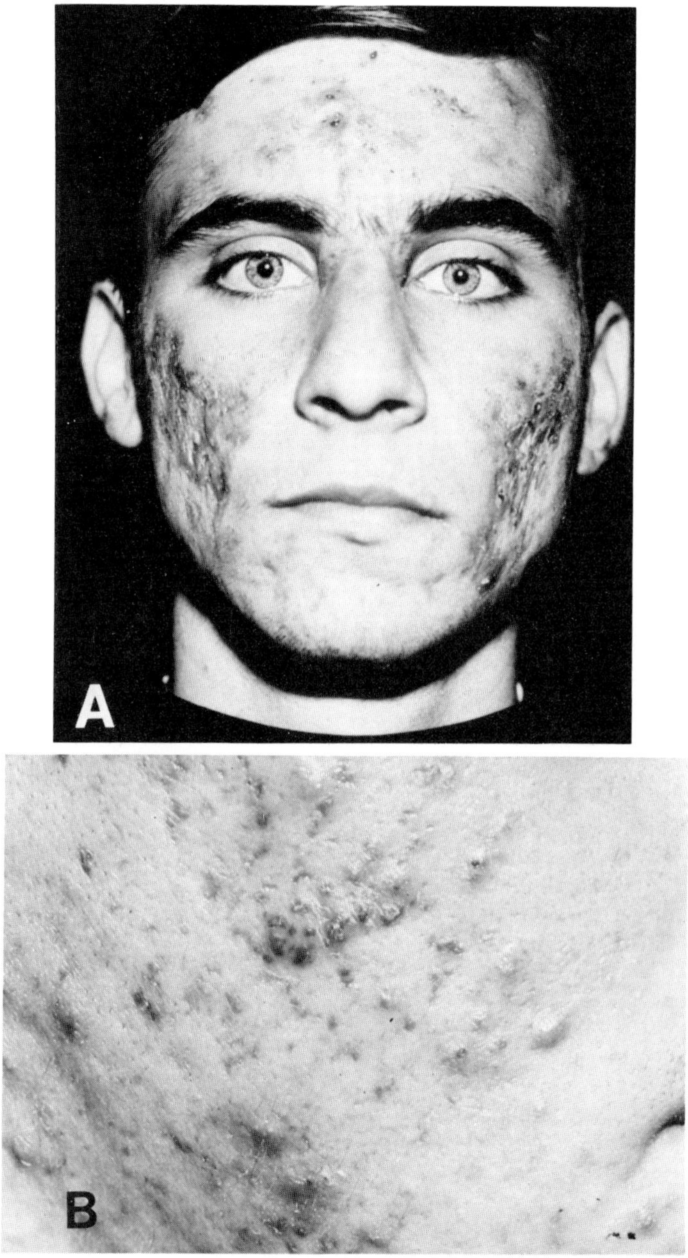

Figure 18-2. Acne Vulgaris. (A) The spectrum of lesions, comedones, inflammatory papules, pustules, and scars (icepick scars) in a moderately severe case. (B) The devastating scars caused by severe cystic acne is hopefully a thing of the past, since the availability of Accutane Capsules (Roche Laboratories, Nutley, NJ). The somatopsychic effect of the acute lesions and the deforming scars can readily be imagined.

From a theoretical stand-point, it is clear that psychosocial stress may effect the pathophysiologic process of acne at a number of separate points, though many of these effects await experimental confirmation. These points include the hypothalamic-pituitary-adrenal axes, through which androgen, growth hormone, and prolactin activity are regulated, and sebum secretion increased, the release of the stress-related vaso-active neuropeptides, and the humoral mediators of inflammation; the humoral and cellular components of the immune system, both of which are susceptible to psychoneuroendocrine modulation; and modification of the host response to bacteria[1] are some of these.

Just as there is no characteristic personality profile for the acne patient, so there is no universal somatopsychic effect; this effect will vary from patient to patient, and will depend largely on the preexisting psychological substrate. Panconesi, and I believe with validity, regards the feelings of inferiority, the emotional immaturity and instability, and the fears of sexual inadequacy so often seen in young acne patients as being simply a part of the adolescent condition.[22] Understandably, if these feelings are already present for other reasons, they can only be made worse if acne supervenes.

In cases in which early childhood experience has failed to establish a solid body-image and a positive self-esteem, acne during the psychologically vulnerable period of adolescence can be an especially severe blow. Studies have shown that children who are physically impaired are most vulnerable to adverse psychological effects if those impairments are sustained during adolescence.[12]

The consequences are the consequences of a diminished self-esteem and in severe cases also a distortion of the body image. They include a depressive affect, social withdrawal, difficulties in peer relationships, and poor school performance. In more severely affected youngsters, depressive symptoms may lead to disciplinary problems and severe family conflict; substance abuse may become a problem. Not infrequently treatment compliance becomes a weapon in bitter struggles between adolescent and parent, and for this reason I have made it a practice to hold adolescent acne patients responsible for their own skin care, and insist on seeing them in the office without a parent present. Some adolescents whose stability is already fragile may use the acne as an excuse for complete isolation, refusing to attend school or engage in any activities. Some may experience their body image as distorted and display obsessional concerns or dysmorphic delusions. Acne excoriee, as a compulsion, and symptomatic of emotional difficulty, has already been discussed. These are already vulnerable youngsters, however, and the acne is an aggravating factor at most; it is at the same time a vehicle for expression of the underlying emotional difficulty.

Medansky illustrated this same point from the opposite side, when he noted that for some adolescents even quite severe acne did not interfere with popularity, school work, or prowess in sports.[19] Panconesi suggests that such youngsters have "charisma" or leadership qualities,[23] and of course qualities of leadership are dependent for their existence on a solid self-esteem.

In studies to evaluate personality, or the degree of psychological difficulty experienced by acne sufferers, psychometric testing is of little benefit unless such testing includes projective tests, or is supplemented by in-depth psychiatric interviews. The reason is that in general these tests take at face-value information given by the patient; that information is only what the patient wishes the physician to know, for unconscious as well as for conscious reasons. It has already been edited, as a result of the psychological defense mechanisms. That 17 percent of patients have less anxiety than do controls argues for strong defenses of the type that have been described in the "super-stable" patient with atopy, as described by Brown and Bettley.[5]

FURTHER APPLICATIONS

All of the material presented to this point, by interpreting health and disease in terms of the relative state of equilibrium or dysequilibrium in the balance between individuals, in all of their aspects, on the one hand, and the environment, in the broadest sense, on the other, permits of a unified concept.

With such a unified view, there need be neither confusion nor mystery when we try to understand from a psychosomatic perspective, diseases that the constraints of space and time have not permitted me to include here.

For example, there are few physical conditions that do not involve in some way the immune system, vascular responses, the mediators of inflammation, or some element that is subject to neurohumoral modulation in the genesis of their symptomatology; each of these mechanisms, we know, is subject to modification in circumstances that by their overt or inner meaning are stressful to the individual. From this perspective, certainly the autoimmune diseases, bullous dermatoses, cutaneous infections, and even cutaneous malignancies are subject to modification in their course and outlook, under such circumstances.

It is our job then, in the evaluation of any patient, whatever the diagnosis, to try to determine what part, if any, stress may be playing in tipping the balance to permit disease. We must be prepared to address this issue and take action where indicated. We must be prepared also to determine what purpose the disease serves in the patient's inner life and what effect it has on his or her functioning.

REFERENCES

1. Ader R (ed): Psychoneuroimmunology. Academic Press, New York, 1981
2. Allen CA, Beck FM, Rossie KM, et al.: Relation of stress and anxiety to oral lichen planus. Oral Surg, Oral Med, Oral Path 61:44-46, 1986

3. Arndt KA: Lichen planus, in Fitzpatrick TA, Eisen AZ, Wolff K, et al. (eds): Dermatology in General Medicine (ed 3). New York, McGraw-Hill, 1986, p 968
4. Arnetz BB, Fjellner B, Eneroth P, et al.: Stress and Psoriasis. Psychoneuroendocrine and metabolic reactions in psoriatic patients during standardized stressor exposure. Psychosom Med 47(6):528-541, 1985
5. Brown DG, Bettley FR: Psychiatric treatment of eczema: A controlled trial. Br Med J 2:729-734, 1971
6. Buckley WR: Lichenoid eruptions following contact dermatitis. Arch Dermatol 78: 454-457, 1958
7. Cutler TP: Lichen planus caused by pyrimethamine. Clin Exp Dermatol 5:253-256, 1980
8. Dahl MG, McGibbon GH: Complement and immunoglobulin in inflammatory acne vulgaris. Br J Dermatol 101:633-640, 1979
9. Dobson RL: Acne, in Theirs BH, Dobson RL (eds): Pathogenesis of Skin Disease. New York, Churchill Livingstone, 1986, p 35
10. Farber EM, Nickoloh BJ, Recht B, Fraki JE: Stress, symmetry and psoriasis: possible role of neuropeptides. J Am Acad Dermatol 14(2):305-311, 1986
11. Griesemer RD, Nadelson T: Emotional aspects of cutaneous disease, in Fitzpatrick TM, Eisen AZ, Wolff K, et al. (eds): Dermatology in General Medicine (ed 2). New York, McGraw Hill, pp 1353-1363
12. Hill-Beuf A, Porter JDR: Children coping with impaired appearance: social and psychological influences. Gen Hosp Psychiat 6:294-301, 1984
13. Hitch JM: Acneform eruptions induced by drugs and chemicals. JAMA 200:879-880,1967
14. Hjorth N, Sjolin KE, Sylvest B, et al.: Acne aestivalis: Mallorca acne. Acta Dermatol Venereol 52:61-63, 1972
15. Kellum RE: Acne vulgaris. Studies in pathogenesis: Relative irritancy of free fatty acids from C2 and C16. Arch Dermatol 97:722-726, 1968
16. Kenyon FE: Psychosomatic aspects of acne. Br J Dermatol 78:344-351, 1966
17. Lucky AW, McGuire J, Rosenfield RL, et al.: Plasma androgens in women with acne vulgaris. J Invest Dermatol 81:70-74, 1983
18. Mahood JM: Familial lichen planus. A report of nine cases from four families, with a brief review of the literature. Arch Dermatol 119:292-294, 1983
19. Medansky RS, Handler MR, Lynn D: Self-evaluation of acne and emotion: a pilot study. Psychosomatics 22:379-383, 1981
20. Obermeyer ME. Psychocutaneous Medicine. Springfield, IL, Charles C. Thomas, 1955
21. Olsen RG: Lichen planus dermopathy: Demonstration of a lichen planus specific epidermal antigen, in affected patients. J Clin Lab Immunol 10:103-106, 1983

22. Panconesi E: Psychosomatic dermatology, in Clinics in Dermatology (Vol. 4; No. 2) Stress and Skin Diseases: Psychosomatic Dermatology. Philadelphia, JB Lippincott, 1984, pp 135-138
23. Plewig G, Fulton JE, Kligman AM: Pomade acne. Arch Dermatol 101:580-584, 1970
24. Puhvel SM, Hoffman IK, Sternberg TH: Corynebacterium acnes. Presence of complement fixing antibodies to C acnes in patients with acne vulgaris. Arch Dermatol 93: 364-366, 1966
25. Puhvel SM, Sakamoto M: A re-evaluation of fatty acids as inflammatory agents in acne. J Invest Dermatol 68:93-97, 1977
26. Samman P: Lichen planus and lichenoid eruptions, in Rook A, Ebling JG, Wilkinson DS (eds): Textbook of Dermatology (ed 3). London, Blackwell, 1979, p 1483
27. Strauss JS, Downing DT, Ebling FJ: Sebaceous glands, in Goldsmith LA (ed): Biochemistry and Physiology of the Skin. New York, Oxford University Press, 1983, pp 587-588
28. Webster GF, Leyden JJ, Normal ME, et al.: Complement activation in acne vulgaris: In vitro studies with P. acnes and P. granulosum. Infect Immunol 25:523-529, 1978
29. Weiner H: Psychobiology and Human Disease. New York, Elsevier, 1977, pp 3-13

Index